AROMATHERAPY
AN A–Z

ALSO BY PATRICIA DAVIS

SUBTLE AROMATHERAPY
A CHANGE FOR THE BETTER
ASTROLOGICAL AROMATHERAPY

WARNING

Make sure that the essential oils you buy
are as pure as possible. Be suspicious of cheap oils.
All the essential oil supplies in this book are recommended by
the publisher and author although the quality of oils can vary
from batch to batch. Buy essential oils as you would fine
wines. Fine wines, that is, without the colour,
but with twice the nose.

AROMATHERAPY
AN A–Z

The most comprehensive guide to
aromatherapy ever published

Patricia Davis

ILLUSTRATED BY SARAH BUDD

Vermilion
LONDON

*This book is dedicated to
my sister, Barbara, who provided
the initial impetus for its creation*

5 7 9 10 8 6 4

First published in the United Kingdom in 1988 by
The C. W. Daniel Company Ltd

Revised and enlarged edition published in 1999 by
The C. W. Daniel Company Ltd

This edition published in 2005 by Vermilion
an imprint of Ebury Publishing
Random House UK Ltd
Random House
20 Vauxhall Bridge Road
London SW1V 2SA

Random House Australia (Pty) Limited
20 Alfred Street, Milsons Point, Sydney
New South Wales 2061, Australia

Random House New Zealand Limited
18 Poland Road, Glenfield
Auckland 10, New Zealand

Random House (Pty) Limited
Isle of Houghton, Corner of Boundary Road & Carse O'Gowrie,
Houghton 2198, South Africa

Random House UK Limited Reg. No. 954009
www.randomhouse.co.uk

Papers used by Vermilion are natural, recyclable products made
from wood grown in sustainable forests

A CIP catalogue record is available for this book
from the British Library

ISBN: 9780091906610
ISBN: 009190661X

Designed by The Bridgewater Book Company Ltd
Printed and bound in Great Britain by William Clowes Ltd, Beccles, Suffolk

CONTENTS

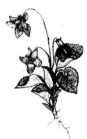

ACKNOWLEDGEMENTS

I offer my sincere thanks to the following people who have helped to make this book possible:

To Carola Beresford-Cooke, Yves de Maneville, Germaine Rich, Frances Treuhertz and Dr. Michael Weztler of Bristol Cancer Help Centre for so generously sharing their knowledge. To Robert Tisserand for permission to use material from the 'Essential Oil Safety Data Manual' and to reproduce the list of hazardous oils prepared for the International Federation of Aromatherapists, who I also thank. To Gordon Burns for the enthusiasm and sensitivity he brought to the task of decorating the book, and an especially big thank you to Anne Chance who read and corrected the manuscript and made very many valuable suggestions.

Finally, to my family, colleagues and students who have nagged, cajoled and encouraged me to complete the book, and to Ian Miller of C.W. Daniel for his patience and support during the long time it took me to do so.

HAUGHLEY, SUFFOLK
30 June 1987

ACKNOWLEDGEMENTS
ENLARGED EDITION

I would like to offer my sincere thanks to these people, who contributed valuable information to the Enlarged Edition:

Gill Farrer-Halls, for talking to me about her work with people with AIDS, Jan and Linda Kusmirek for technical information, Richard Offutt for sharing his experience of using Rosemary for people with epilepsy and Sheila Tozer for insights into acupuncture.

ACKNOWLEDGEMENTS
NEW ILLUSTRATED EDITION

I would like to offer a huge vote of thanks to Sarah Budd for her illustrations, which have added so much to the information in this book, as well as to its appearance.

Thanks also to Carolyn Swain for winkling out a few faux pas in the last edition, thereby enabling me to correct them.

AUTHOR'S PREFACE
TO THE ENLARGED EDITION

Seven years have passed since this book was first published (eight since I finished writing it) and a great deal has changed in that time so I am very glad to have had the opportunity to revise the book where it no longer reflected the current situation and to respond to feedback from readers.

In particular, a far greater variety of oils is available to therapists now than then, and it is easier to get organically-produced oils. Conversely, a lot of poor quality oils are widely available and falsification of all kinds is rife, in some cases very sophisticated, so we need to be aware of the pitfalls that implies.

Far more people are now aware of aromatherapy and make use of it to maintain their own health and well-being. New patterns of disease have emerged, and new approaches to healing. Aromatherapy is being used increasingly alongside conventional medicine. This spread and popularisation of aromatherapy has many obvious benefits, but also some dangers, as more untrained people experiment with essential oils. One of my primary concerns has always been with safety and I hope that this revised and enlarged edition will contribute to the safe use of essential oils by professional and lay readers alike.

TOTNES, DEVON
February 1995

AUTHOR'S PREFACE
TO THE NEW ILLUSTRATED EDITION

It amazes me that a whole decade has passed since the first edition of this book appeared – it must be true that time passes quickly when you are happy!

A great deal has changed, though, in that time, and I am delighted once again to have had the occasion to make a few additions and adjustments to the book. Major changes were made when preparing the Enlarged Edition, published in 1995, but I have welcomed the opportunity to add one or two more oils, correct some errors that had crept in (mea culpa!) and make certain other adjustments.

It has also been very exciting to watch the book metamorphose into this handsome new format, and to have been able to include the new illustrations which add so much to the information contained in it.

TOTNES, DEVON
September 1998

AROMATHERAPY
An introduction

❧

The art – and science – of using plant oils in treatment.
Aromatherapy is a truly holistic therapy, taking account of the mind, body and spirit of the person seeking help, as well as their lifestyle, eating patterns, relationships, etc.

Although the word aromatherapy was first used in the present century (maybe we ought to spell it 'aromathérapie' in this context as the originator was a Frenchman) to describe the use of essential oils from plants as a form of treatment, the principles on which it is based are very, very old.

Aromatherapy has its roots in the most ancient healing practices of humankind, for the plants from which we now derive essential oils had been used for thousands of years before the technique of distilling oils was discovered. Archaeologists have found traces of many plants of known medicinal value in the burial places and living sites of early humans (the plants can be identified by analysis of the fossilised pollen), and it is very unlikely that their users knew nothing of their healing properties, even if these were stumbled across by accident in the first place.

The earliest people probably discovered by chance that some of the leaves, berries and roots they gathered for food made sick people feel better, or that their juices helped wounds to heal. They probably also observed the plants that sick animals chose to eat. Such knowledge would have been very precious to people who depended entirely on the resources in their immediate environment and, once discovered, would be handed down within the tribe as part of their shared wisdom.

When the twigs of certain bushes or trees were thrown on the fire as fuel, the smoke and aromas they gave off may have made people drowsy, or happy, or excited, or maybe even given rise to

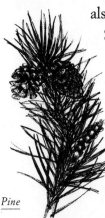

Pine

'mystical' experiences. If the same sensation was felt by all the people around that fire, and if the same thing happened next time that some twigs from the same bush were burnt, then that bush would be recognised as producing that effect, and possibly regarded as 'magic'. The 'smoking' of patients was one of the earliest forms of medicine, and as religion and medicine were closely bound up with each other, the use of special smokes also formed part of primitive religions. When early people made offerings to their gods of aromatic plants, they were making a very real sacrifice, for they were giving away to the gods something that was very precious to them.

The use of holy or magic smoke, in the form of incense, has survived in almost all major religions in both East and West, and the use of fumigation with aromatic plants remained standard medical practice right up to the present century. For example, until relatively recently, French hospitals burnt Thyme and Rosemary in the wards as a disinfectant.

Thyme

Ironically, the practice was discontinued at about the same time that research proved how effective both these plants are as bactericides! In some less advanced (?) parts of the world, fumigation is still standard practice.

The Egyptians were using aromatics 3,000 years before Christ for medicinal and cosmetic purposes, and to embalm their dead. They set great store by perfume for both public and private use. On important state occasions incense was burnt and slave girls danced with perfumed cones on their heads, which would melt and gradually disperse in the air as they performed. We know from various papyrus documents (the earliest dating from about 2,890 B.C.) some of the plants they used medicinally and the methods of use. They made pills, powders, suppositories, medicinal cakes and purées, ointments and pastes for external use, etc., from a wide variety of trees and plants, as well as animal and mineral substances. They also used plant ashes and smokes. Plants used included aniseed, castor oil, cedar, coriander, cumin, garlic, grapes and water melon among many others.

Whether or not the earlier Egyptians knew how to distil essential oils is open to debate. No mention of distilled oils is found in the earliest documents, and none of the containers found in tombs would have been suitable for storing essential oils. Large numbers of ointment and cosmetic jars and oil bottles have been found in pyramids, with traces of the original contents still intact. These were mostly fatty ointments or gummy pastes, and the aromas of Frankincense, Styrax, etc., were still perceptible. There are records on clay tablets of oils of Cedar and Cypress being imported, which tells us that an international trade in oils already existed, but these appear to have been infused oils. However, the evidence of wall-paintings shows that, at least by the 3rd century B.C. the Egyptians had a primitive form of distillation.

A little further east, in the Mesopotamian basin between the Tigris and the Euphrates, the Babylonian doctors recorded their formulae and prescriptions on clay tablets, the earliest of which are in the cuneiform script of the Sumerians. Unlike the Egyptians, they did not record the quantities to be used (which were presumably common knowledge), but gave careful details of when the remedy must be prepared and taken – usually at dawn, before eating. A Babylonian king ordered the planting of a garden of medicinal plants, and we learn that it contained apple and quince trees, cucumbers, pumpkins, garlic, onions, fennel, saffron, thyme, mustard, caraway, coriander, roses, juniper and myrrh – in other words, many of the plants which we use today in herbal medicine and aromatherapy.

The ancient Greeks acquired much of their medical knowledge from the Egyptians, as well as making further discoveries of their own, such as the fact that the odour of certain flowers was stimulating and refreshing while that of others was relaxing and soporific. They used olive oil (an abundant commodity in Greece, then as now) to absorb the odour from flower petals or from herbs, and used the perfumed oil for both medicinal and cosmetic purposes. Greek soldiers carried with them into battle an ointment made

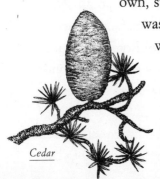

Cedar

from Myrrh for the treatment of wounds. Hippocrates, still revered as the 'father of medicine', mentions a vast number of medicinal plants in his writings, including a large number of narcotics – opium, belladonna and mandrake among them – as well as food plants such as rhubarb, quince, etc. He wrote 'Let your medicine be your food and your food be your medicine', but he placed even more importance on the moral qualities needed to be a physician, such as discernment, self-effacement and devotion. The 'Hippocratic Oath' is still taught to medical students: perhaps if they were taught some of Hippocrates' methods the world of medicine would be in less of a mess!

Rosemary

Many Greek doctors were employed by Rome as military surgeons, personal physicians to Roman emperors, etc. Galen, who was physician to Marcus Aurelius, started out as surgeon to a school of gladiators, and it is recorded that no gladiator died of his wounds during Galen's term of office. Perhaps this is not surprising, as he knew a fantastic number of 'simples' from which he prepared his remedies. He wrote a great deal on the theory of plant medicine and divided plants into various medicinal categories, which are still known as 'Galenic'. He invented the original 'cold cream' which was the prototype of virtually all ointments in current use. Another Greek, Dioscorides, was a doctor in the Roman army in the reign of Nero. He collected medicinal plants in many countries around the Mediterranean and by 78 A.D. he had collected the information about these plants and their uses into the five huge volumes of his 'Materia Medica'.

The works of Hippocrates, Galen, Dioscorides and others were translated into Arabic languages and after the fall of Rome, surviving Roman physicians who fled to Constantinople took their books and knowledge with them. Via Constantinople, from the translations of Graeco-Roman medical works and the famous medical library of Alexandria, knowledge built up in antiquity passed to the Arab world. The first great Arab physician of whom we have detailed

11

knowledge was Abu Bahr Muhammed ibn Zakaria al-Razi (865–925 A.D.) who wrote over two dozen books on medicine, many of them consisting of collections of herbal formulae.

But the greatest of the Arab physicians was undoubtedly Abu Ali al-Husayn ibn Abd Allah ibn Sina (980–1037 A.D.) known to us as Avicenna. He studied logic, geometry, metaphysics, philosophy, astronomy and all the other natural sciences known in his day, as well as medicine – in fact he was a perfect example of what we would now call a 'Renaissance Man'. He was a child prodigy, already famous as a doctor at the age of 18. He, too, left valuable written records describing over 800 plants and their effects on the human body. Not all of these have been identified as he sometimes used their local, vernacular names, but among those that can be reliably identified we find camomile, lavender, rose and others used in modern aromatherapy. He described the all-fruit diet, spinal manipulation and various forms of massage in great detail.

However, his greatest importance in the history of aromatherapy is that he is credited with inventing the technique of distilling essential oils. It now seems more likely that he did not invent the technique but perfected it, as archaeologists have found primitive stills pre-dating his lifetime, but he probably refined the method by adding cooling coils.

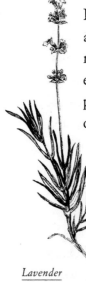

What was happening in Europe between the fall of the Roman Empire and about the 10th century (the epoch known as the Dark Ages due to the lack of coherent records) we don't really know, but it is almost certain that there was an established tradition of using herbs, much of which survives in present day folk medicine. We do know that by the 12th century the 'Perfumes of Arabia', i.e. essential oils, were famous throughout Europe. Crusading knights brought back with them not only the actual perfumes, but the knowledge of how to distil them. Lacking the aromatic, gum-yielding trees of the Orient, the Europeans used Lavender, Rosemary, Thyme and all the aromatic shrubs that are native to the Mediterranean, and were soon cultivating them much further north.

Lavender

Rose

Mediaeval manuscripts contain references to Lavender water and many methods of making infused oils. The invention of printing soon led to these formulae being published in books known as 'Herbals', and by the 16th century anybody who could read could have access to recipes for infused oils, aromatic waters, decoctions, infusions and other methods of treatment with plants. The women of a household would have made all these remedies for home use, as well as pomanders, lavender bags and other herbal sachets to perfume the home and protect linen from moth. More complex remedies were bought from apothecaries, who also sold the precious essential oils, known then as 'chymical oils', though great houses had their own still rooms. Floors were strewn with herbs that gave off their volatile oils when walked on, and pomanders or little bouquets of aromatic herbs, known as 'tussy-mussies' were carried in public places to ward off infection, especially the Plague. These practices have often been dismissed by historians as superstition, but in fact most of the herbs used are now known to be powerful disinfectants, bactericides and even antiviral agents. Others are known insecticides or insect repellents, and were valuable against the fleas, lice and flies that carried disease.

Some of the most celebrated herbals were those compiled by Gerard, Banckes and Culpeper in England, Brunfels, Fuchs and Bock in Germany, Nicolas Monardes in Spain – who included plants from the newly-discovered Americas, Charles de l'Ecluse in France and Pietro Mattioli in Italy. Mattioli's herbal, which was closely based on the work of Dioscorides, was translated into many European languages and sold 32,000 copies, making it one of the 16th century's best sellers!

Throughout the Middle Ages and the Tudor era, all forms of plant medicine were used by doctors, apothecaries and lay people alike, but by the 17th century the growing new science of experimental chemistry gave rise to new uses of chemical substances in medicine. Nicolas Culpeper wrote passionate denunciations of doctors who used poisonous substances, such as mercury, but was dismissed by many as being either old fashioned, clinging to his quaint old herbs, or just jealous of the doctors' financial success and position in society. Our current concerns about the side-effects of dangerous drugs is nothing new. Fortunately, though, attitudes towards 'alternative' practitioners are now somewhat more enlightened! The spate of witch burning in the 17th century coincided with the rise of early chemotherapy, and was as much inspired by the medical establishment's wish to suppress the knowledge of the village 'wise-women' as by the religious establishment's wish to stamp out heresy.

Of course, not all the new experimentation was harmful and some important minerals were discovered as a result, some of which – selenium for example – are only now being fully understood in their relationship to health and well-being. The chemist Friedrich Hoffman (1660–1742) did much research into the nature of essential oils, as well as investigating natural mineral waters at various spas. But the damaging aspect of this growing specialisation was the way it took medicine out of the hands of ordinary people.

Chemists continued to research the active ingredients of medicinal plants throughout the 18th and 19th centuries, and identified many substances such as caffeine, quinine, morphine, atropine, etc., which have valid uses, though this search for isolated active principles in plants was already leading away from the use of whole substances in a natural way. Essential oils continued to be used, though, many remaining in the pharmacopoeia until well into the present century. A smaller number are still in general pharmaceutical use (Lavender, Myrrh and Peppermint, for example). Gradually, though, they began to be supplanted by synthetic drugs, mostly derived from coal-tar products, especially in the second half of this century, with the disastrous results that we all know.

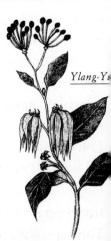

Ylang-Y

I would like to break off here to consider the use of plants for healing in the Far East, especially in India and China, where they are part of an unbroken tradition, thousands of years old – in

Garlic

contrast to the situation in Europe where we are only now re-discovering our 'lost' heritage of knowledge.

In India the use of plants reflects the religious and philosophical view of man as part of the continually changing process of nature. The most ancient religious texts, such as the Rigveda from 2,000 years B.C., contain formulae, as well as invocations to the plants themselves: 'Simples, you who have existed for so long, even before the Gods were born, I want to understand your seven hundred secrets!... Come, you wise plants, heal this patient for me.' Indian medicine was exclusively plant-based, reflecting the vegetarian principles of the main religions. The Buddhist King, Ashoka (3rd century B.C.) organised and regulated the cultivation of medicinal plants. Great attention was paid to the conditions in which the plants grew, and the people who handled them: 'They must be gathered by a pure and holy man . . . who has previously fasted. They must be harvested only in places that are not easily accessible to men, with fertile soil and good drainage, and not near any temple or holy place, or near any burial ground . . . .' The medicinal plants of India became famous throughout Asia and eventually found their way into Western medicinal formulae, as well as forming the basis of present-day traditional Indian medicine (Ayurvedic medicine). They include benzoin, caraway, cardamon, clove, ginger, pepper and sandalwood; cannabis, castor oil, sesame oil, aloes and sugar cane. The essential oils of the first seven of these plants are all used currently in aromatherapy.

China also has an ancient and unbroken tradition of herbal medicine, which is used alongside, and complementing, acu-puncture. Again, many of the plants have been known and used for many thousands of years, the earliest records being in the Yellow Emperor's Book of Internal Medicine, dating from more than 2,000 years B.C. The great classic of Chinese medicine, known as Pen ts'ao kang-mou, lists no less than 8,160 different formulae, compounded from nearly two thousand different substances, most of them plants. This represents a greater range of plants than in any other tradition

15

of medicine. Many of the plants used in China are known in the West, too: daisy, gentian, liquorice, walnut, peach, plantain, rhubarb, etc. China tea is a remedy for chills, headaches and diarrhoea. Opium was used as a treatment for dysentery as early as 1,000 B.C. but was not smoked until the 16th century A.D. when, under the Ming dynasty, alcohol was forbidden.

Camomile

Returning to Europe and the present day, we find not only an intensification of research into synthetic drugs, backed by big industry (it was Barbara Griggs who pointed out that you can't patent a plant, so there is little profit in plant medicine), but also renewed interest in the use of plants in a more whole and natural form.

Interest in essential oils and their properties has formed part of this trend since the 1920s, when René-Maurice Gattefossé, a chemist in his family's perfume company, became interested in the medicinal aspects of the oils. He discovered that many of the essential oils used in the company's products were better antiseptics than the chemical antiseptics being added to the same products. He burnt his hand badly in a laboratory explosion, and used Lavender oil to help heal the burn. The effectiveness of Lavender turned his attention to the use of this and other oils in dermatology and he did a great deal of research into their medicinal use. He first coined the word 'aromathérapie' in a scientific paper in 1928, and published a book of the same name in 1937.

Other French doctors, scientists and writers have continued this work, most notably Dr. Jean Valnet, a former army surgeon who used essential oils to treat severe burns and battle injuries. Later, he treated patients in a psychiatric hospital with the oils and with other plant products, with great success, despite the scepticism of the hospital staff. His book 'Aromathérapie' (translated as 'The Practice of Aromatherapy') is the 'bible' of serious aromatherapy practice. Marguerite Maury, Fabrice Bardeau and Marcel Bernadet have all added to our knowledge through their practices and their books.

In England, although awareness of aromatherapy as a serious discipline is more recent, it has become a widespread and valued form of holistic therapy. Standards of training and practice are very high, and aromatherapy is increasingly practised in hospitals. The majority of therapists, though, work within the wider spectrum of holistic medicine.

A properly trained aromatherapist will look far beyond the mere application of essential oils, and will seek to help the whole person in maintaining a balance of mental, physical and spiritual health. Essential oils lend themselves readily to a sensitive and subtle approach, for every one of them has many properties, unlike synthetic drugs or even active principles isolated from a plant, which are 'tailored' to treat a specific symptom. Essential oils are often balancing in their effects, helping the body to return from an imbalanced state which leads to illness, to the ideal balance representing health and well-being. Many aromatherapists embrace the Oriental idea of Yin and Yang – opposing energies which exist in a state of dynamic balance. When all the energies in the body and mind are in a state of balance, the person is in a state of health.

Some concrete examples of a lack of balance might be extremes of heat – fever or hypothermia, high blood pressure or low blood pressure, over or under production of various hormones . . . I'm sure you can think of many more.

The same principle applies to the mental and emotional planes, too. Depression, hysteria, wild swings of mood (which at the most extreme might be classified as manic depression) are all states of imbalance. Essential oils exert a subtle influence on the mind and, combined with the loving care of a sensitive therapist, offer a truly holistic, gentle and natural alternative to psychotropic drugs.

Melissa

Another important quality of essential oils is the wide variety of ways in which they can be used. Massage with essential oils is the most important method of treatment, for it combines the effects of the oils themselves, with the important element of human contact between the aromatherapist and the person seeking help.

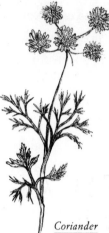

Coriander

The second most important use of essential oils is probably in aromatic baths. Water itself has many therapeutic properties, as anyone who has ever sunk into a hot bath after a tough day will know, and when these are combined with essential oils, each enhances the potent effect of the other. Baths are the simplest method of use, and can be a valuable way of continuing the benefit of aromatherapy treatment between visits to a practitioner.

The oils can be used in hot or cold compresses for various physical conditions, and mixed in creams, lotions and aromatic waters to help with the health of the skin, whether it is in treating such conditions as eczema and acne or in promoting a healthy, and therefore beautiful, complexion.

Essential oils are readily absorbed through the skin, and whenever they are used in massage, baths, skin preparations or compresses a certain amount of the volatile essence is inhaled. The aroma alone can have a subtle but real effect on the mind, and via the mind, on the body. Inhaling the oils also has a direct effect on the body, as some part of the oil will be absorbed via the lungs and will enter the bloodstream in that way.

Do not embark too lightly upon self-treatment with essential oils. Properly used, they are very safe indeed, but some oils present hazards that anyone using them should be aware of. Even small amounts of oil can build up to a toxic level in the body over a period of time, and some of the oils are very poisonous indeed. Deaths from essential oil poisoning have been reported in the medical press, and two cases of accidental poisoning (fortunately not fatal) have come to my personal attention in recent years. My major intention in writing this book has been to encourage the safe use of essential oils so that as many people as possible can enjoy the health benefits and sheer enjoyment they offer without risk.

ALPHABETICAL
ENTRIES

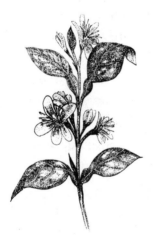

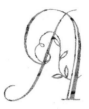

Abscesses

An abscess is usually treated in aromatherapy by means of hot compresses placed over the swelling, to reduce pain and inflammation and 'draw out' toxic matter. For a dental abscess, hot compresses should be applied to the face until a dentist can be consulted.

The most effective oils for treating an abscess are Camomile (especially for a dental abscess), Lavender and Ti-tree (singly or in combination).

The person's general health should also be considered. Advice on a non-toxic diet and maybe vitamin/mineral supplementation may be needed, especially if the condition is recurrent.

Absolute

This is the term used to describe materials which are obtained from the plant by means of enfleurage or solvent extraction. Enfleurage yields a material known as a pomade – a mixture of fat and essential oil – and solvent extraction produces a concrete consisting of fats, waxes, essential oils and other plant materials. The pomade or concrete is treated with alcohol to extract the absolute. These methods are used to extract the essence from flower petals where distillation would distort the delicate perfume, and the three with which we are mainly concerned in aromatherapy are the absolutes of Rose, Jasmine and Orange Blossom (Neroli). Other floral absolutes, such as Carnation, Gardenia, Mimosa, Hyacinth etc., are employed in high quality perfumery but are used only very rarely for therapeutic purposes.

Absolutes differ from essential oils (i.e., those obtained by distillation) in that they have an extremely high perfuming and therapeutic power, and need to be used in low concentrations. They are normally coloured, and are usually thicker and more viscous than essential oils. Rose absolute may solidify in the bottle at room temperature, but quickly becomes liquid again when held in the hand.

The purist view is that absolutes should not be used in aromatherapy because they may contain traces of the solvents such as acetone, ethanol or hexane, used to extract the absolute from the pomade or concrete. An exception is where natural ethanol has been used. In practice, many aromatherapists do use absolutes in small amounts without problems.

Kazanlik Rose

see also **CONCRETE, ENFLEURAGE, EXTRACTION.**

Acids

Acids (in this context) are a category of organic plant molecules which occasionally occur in essential oils. Many of them are water-soluble, so you will find them in the hydrolat (q.v.) rather than the corresponding oil. They are very good anti-inflammatory agents, and generally calming. Some of them are analgesic. Examples: benzoic acid, in Benzoin (large amounts), Ylang-Ylang, etc.; geranic acid, in Geranium, Rose, etc., and salicylic acid, in Birch.

Acne

One of the joys of being an aromatherapist is knowing that acne can be successfully treated, without potentially dangerous drugs or chemicals.

The condition – commonest in adolescents, but sometimes persisting well into the twenties – is due to over activity of the sebaceous glands in the skin (q.v.) combined with bacterial infection. Too much of the oily substance, sebum, is poured onto the surface of the skin. Dirt from the environment, particles from clothing, and dead cells which continually flake off from the surface of the skin, stick to the sebum and form a 'breeding ground' for bacteria. Pores become blocked, forming blackheads, and become infected, causing the familiar 'spots'. Liquid seeps from these and infects the surrounding tissues.

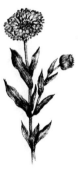

Aromatherapists can tackle acne in several ways. Essential oils are used to treat the skin externally to help clear infection and reduce the amount of sebum produced. Massage may be used to stimulate the circulation and help the body to eliminate toxins. The aromatherapist will advise on a non-toxic diet – probably the most important part of the treatment – and make sure that the sufferer is taught a proper skin hygiene routine. The collaboration of the acne sufferer in his/her own treatment is vital, and can help to alleviate some of the feelings of helplessness and hopelessness that are common with acne.

A variety of essential oils may be used to help this condition, and the therapist may need to try a number of different oils until the best one for the individual is found, and may also vary the oils from time to time during the course of treatment. The most helpful oils include Lavender and Ti-tree which are both bactericidal. Lavender is soothing and healing and promotes the growth of healthy new skin. Bergamot also has many properties that help acne, but should be restricted to winter because it is a photosensitiser. Bergamot is astringent, as well as anti-depressant (useful, because many young people become depressed about their acne, and the depression may even make the condition worse). Oil of Geranium can be used to balance the secretion of sebum. These oils can be used in facial massage (diluted in a carrier oil) and mixed into creams and cleansing and toning lotions for use between treatments.

Rosemary and Geranium, among other oils, are used for body massage to stimulate the lymphatic system, and so help clear the body of toxins. As the condition improves, wheatgerm oil can be blended in a carrier with Lavender and Neroli and used to reduce any scarring.

21

Treatment may need to be continued for many weeks, or even months, and it is even possible that the condition may appear to get worse initially, so careful counselling is needed to avoid discouragement.

If acne is seen in a person past their mid-twenties, it is possible that it is due to an allergy, and a different approach will be needed (see **ALLERGY**). (See also entries under **SEBUM, SKIN,** etc.)

Acupressure

see **SHIATSU.**

Acupuncture

Acupuncture is one of the therapies which combine extremely well with aromatherapy. A few people are trained in both disciplines, but more often an aromatherapist will work in collaboration with an acupuncturist.

Acupuncture is a very ancient system, having originated in China over 5,000 years ago. It is deeply rooted in the Taoist philosophy which recognises two opposite and complementary energies, YIN and YANG, flowing through nature. Human beings are seen as a part of this whole, and Yin and Yang energies flow through the body in a network of pathways called meridians, Yang energy passing down the back of the body and Yin energy up the front of the body. The two are maintained in a subtle and constantly changing balance. While this balance exists, and energy flows freely, health is experienced, but if a meridian is blocked at any point, an excess or deficiency of energy will be created and illness may arise. By inserting very fine needles at appropriate points on the meridians, the acupuncturist can remove the blockage and restore health.

The skilled reading of pulse points enables the acupuncturist to detect imbalances of energy before disease manifests on the physical level, and acupuncture has been used in China for thousands of years as a system of preventative medicine.

Traditional acupuncture takes into account the fact that five Elements (Fire, Earth, Metal, Water and Wood) and five Seasons (Spring, Summer, late Summer, Autumn and Winter) also affect the energy in the body. The time of day may also be significant, as each meridian is most active at different times throughout each 24 hours.

Acupuncture is only one part of traditional Chinese medicine, and some acupuncturists in the West are trained in, and practise, it as a whole. Others use needles on the meridian points but place less emphasis on the underlying philosophy, and some G.P.s and hospital doctors take very short courses (3 weekends in some instances) enabling them to use acupuncture points symptomatically, mainly for pain relief.

Some of the plants which have long formed part of the traditional oriental system also yield essential oils which can be incorporated into the treatment on this basis. Some writers have classified a number of essential oils as Yin or Yang, but in my experience many of the classifications are dubious, and it is more helpful to look at the properties of the oil and which organs or body systems it affects when using aromatherapy in conjunction with acupuncture.

For a fuller description of **YIN** and **YANG** see the entry under that heading.

Addition

The problem of addiction to such drugs as heroin and cocaine is an immense one, and some would question whether aromatherapy has any part to play in solving it. What is certain is that some therapists have been working with former addicts successfully, using sedative and antidepressant oils to combat situations in which the client is under pressures that could lead to a relapse into the old drug habit.

It is interesting that when given a choice of oils for massage, former addicts have time and again chosen Clary Sage – an oil which is described as 'euphoric'. Perhaps it gives some of the relief from immediate pressures that they previously sought in drugs? This suggests to me that aromatherapy could be just as valuable in the treatment and prevention of addiction as in helping former addicts. The tragic fact is that although addicts may be found in all strata of society, so many are underprivileged – lacking money, employment, education and housing – and would be totally unable to afford treatment from any alternative therapist, even if they were aware of the possibilities. I do know of some aromatherapists with a social conscience who are offering treatment through voluntary agencies but they are few in number and can help only the tiniest minority of drug users. There is a great need for more work in this field.

Hard drugs are not, of course, the only substances to which people may become addicted. Many people are addicted to nicotine, alcohol, tranquillisers, coffee and various foods. Support and help from a sympathetic aromatherapist combined with dietary advice and skilled counselling has helped many people free themselves from such addictions. All the antidepressant essential oils are valuable. Bergamot seems to be particularly helpful in food addiction, but the final choice must always depend on the client's personal preference. Bergamot, Camomile, Clary, Lavender, Rose, Jasmine and Ylang-Ylang spring first to mind but are far from the only possibilities. Changing the oils used at regular intervals is recommended: it is virtually impossible to become physically addicted to an essential oil, but some people may come to regard a particular oil as a 'prop' if it is used continually.

see also entries under **ALCOHOLISM** *and* **TRANQUILLISERS.**

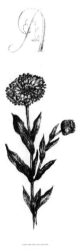

23

Adulteration

Because essential oils are relatively expensive to produce there is always a temptation to adulterate them to increase profits. This is particularly true where the demand for a particular oil outstrips the supply, and in the case of costly oils such as Melissa and the flower absolutes. Adulteration takes many forms: it may consist of adding a little of a cheaper oil to 'stretch' an expensive one, isolating various chemicals from cheap and plentiful oils and adding them to dearer ones, or adding totally synthetic substances to an essential oil.

Aromatherapists are not the only users of essential oils, and for some industrial uses adulterated oils may be quite acceptable. For example, manufacturers of household cleaners, cheap perfumes, cosmetics and toiletries are not concerned about the authenticity of an aromatic ingredient as long as it smells alright and the price falls within their budget. There is nothing wrong in this, provided we do not expect any therapeutic benefit from using the end product.

In aromatherapy, though, we need to be sure that our basic materials are exactly what they purport to be: pure, natural products extracted from specific plants with nothing added. Nothing else will give the therapeutic results we – and our clients – expect. We owe it to our clients to be certain of the origin and purity of everything we use in our daily practice.

The best safeguard is to buy from importers who specialise in supplying aromatherapists, who understand that our needs are not the same as those of industrial clients, and can guarantee the origin and purity of the oils they sell.

Aerosol Generators

Aerosol generators release essential oils into the air in the form of micro-droplets. This is done by means of an electrically-operated air pump, and should not be confused with aerosol sprays, which use harmful gases to turn their contents into a fine, mist spray.

Melissa

The amount of essential oil released into the air can be regulated, partly by choosing different sized generators, and partly by the controls on the machine. The oils are neither heated nor chemically changed in any way, which represents some advantages over more traditional ways of vaporising oils. Aerosol generators are also sometimes called diffusers.

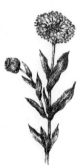

Ageing Skin

The skin may deteriorate in a number of ways with age. Apart from wrinkles, which are discussed in a separate entry, there may be discolouration, dryness, a crepey appearance and sagging and possibly thread veins in the cheeks. Aromatherapy treatments, and creams made with essential oils, can help to minimise all of these problems.

A good supply of oxygen to the growing layer of the skin is important for the health and appearance of the skin, and massage helps because it stimulates the local circulation. Massage directly on the face must always be very gentle, but a vigorous massage of the scalp will increase the blood circulation to the whole head, including the face. This is something that anybody can do for themselves daily, although the facial massage is best left to a trained person, and should form the basis of treatment for all the problems mentioned above.

The outermost, visible layer of the skin (the epidermis) is composed entirely of dead cells, and the health and appearance of the skin depends to a large degree on the layer of new cells constantly growing beneath it. The rate of renewal may slow with age, so cytophylactic essential oils (those which stimulate healthy new cell growth) are important to counteract this. Neroli and Lavender are the most important of these oils, and both are suitable for older skins.

Most skins become less oily as they grow older. You have probably noticed that people whose skin was oily in youth preserve a young looking skin much longer. The production of sebum, a natural oil which lubricates the skin, is at its peak in adolescence, and slowly declines thereafter. Massage with such oils as Geranium, Jasmine, Neroli or Rose will help to restore the natural balance to some degree, but it will probably also be helpful to add to the amount of oil on the skin surface by using richer carrier oils, such as avocado, jojoba, peach kernel or a little wheatgerm. These can be used in the form of creams as well as massage oils.

Frankincense, Sandalwood and Carrot-seed are all good oils for the treatment of older skins, also Patchouli for anybody who likes its rather individual smell. Any of these will help to counteract the dullness and crepey texture, especially when combined with regular massage. If, in spite of such treatment the skin still looks muddy in colour, face-packs with yoghurt help to give a fresher appearance. Simple facepacks made from fresh avocado pulp, or ground almonds mixed with a little honey are also very good when used for older skins.

Thread veins (broken capillaries) are sometimes a problem for older women. Oils of Camomile, Celery, Parsley or Rose can help to diminish them, though it may be several months before improvement is seen. Use them in massage oils, and in creams or lotions to be applied to the skin daily, as they really must be used regularly to have any effect. As the treatment needs to be continued for quite a long time, it is best to alternate the oils rather than use them together. Extremes of heat should be avoided, also very hot drinks, smoking and alcohol.

The skin reflects the general health of the body, and everything that contributes to that will delay and minimise the ravages that time makes on the skin: exercise, excellent nutrition, adequate sleep and avoidance of unnecessary pollutants.

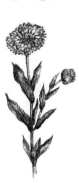

see also entries for **REJUVENATION** *and* **WRINKLES.**

25

A.I.D.S.

In considering A.I.D.S. (Acquired Immune Deficiency Syndrome), I think we should start from the same basic premises as with cancer: that we are not 'treating', still less offering a cure, and that no aromatherapist should take sole responsibility for any A.I.D.S. patient, but must work in collaboration with the doctor in charge. Within that framework, there is scope for a great deal of valuable work, ranging from emotional support and relaxing therapies for patients, through treating opportunistic infections to the very important area of strengthening the compromised immune system itself, and in fact the enormous value of all these things has already been shown by aromatherapists working in hospitals, through various A.I.D.S. charities and support groups, and in their own practices.

The possibility of strengthening the immune system is an area which has largely been overlooked by orthodox medicine, with so much emphasis being placed on the search for a vaccine. Aromatherapists, medical herbalists, acupuncturists and nutritionists, among others, use techniques which are designed to support and strengthen the body's own immune response, and this is very important when we realise that many people who are diagnosed as H.I.V. positive never develop A.I.D.S.

Strengthening the immune system is important because the H.I.V. virus attacks the body's immune system (how it does so is discussed in greater detail in a separate entry headed H.I.V.) and people who are known to be carrying the H.I.V. virus, but who do not develop A.I.D.S. almost certainly have a more efficiently functioning immune system than those who do become ill.

All the oils mentioned elsewhere in this book as being beneficial to the immune system are very helpful, especially those that strengthen the action of the spleen, adrenal glands and lymphatic system. It is also important to support the liver, as this organ plays a vital role in detoxifying the body. This is doubly important if the person with A.I.D.S. is taking prescribed drugs. Wherever possible, the aromatherapist should try to work in collaboration with a medical herbalist, and/or acupuncturist, as these therapies support and enhance each other.

Some people have the full A.I.D.S. syndrome before they come into contact with any alternative therapist, but we can still do much to help. The H.I.V. virus itself does not give rise to symptoms: the patient succumbs to opportunistic infections when the body's natural defences no longer work properly. These may at first be relatively minor and may include oral thrush (caused by candida albicans yeast), skin, lung and bowel infections. Enlarged lymph nodes may persist over a lengthy period – say three months. (This is by no means always so, since they may be associated with severe 'flu, glandular fever, etc.) This is an area where essential oils can be a great help in combating infection, which often includes a particularly virulent form of pneumonia, and this becomes even more important, since it may be life-threatening to somebody in this weakened state. Much of the work of medical staff in hospitals caring for A.I.D.S. patients is concentrated on combating such infections, and they are generally supportive of patients who wish to try other therapies. Some essential oils which have proved effective in this situation are Niaouli, Ti-tree, Eucalyptus radiata (having the same properties as Eucalyptus globulus but more easily assimilated) and Thyme, in the form of the chemotype, Thuyanol IV, which is particularly antiviral. One objection to these particular oils, though, is that people with A.I.D.S. have often had more than enough of 'medical' smells, and don't want to have that sort of aroma around them when they have their aromatherapy treatment. It may be better to look at immunostimulant or anti-viral/antibacterial oils that smell pleasant, such as Manuka, Ravensara or Rosewood.

Far more important, though, is helping to improve the quality of life, by offering relaxing massage, baths, mood-enhancing oils and emotional support. Massage is important, because of the element of touch. Everyone needs to be touched, but for people who are sometimes treated as 'untouchable' it is vital. For some people with A.I.D.S. just knowing that the aromatherapist is happy to touch them is the most important part of the therapy. Effleurage and long, slow massage strokes seem to give the most comfort. If somebody is weak or in pain, it will only be possible to use the lightest strokes. Sometimes is is only possible to massage a small area of the body, but whatever is possible is valuable.

The choice of essential oils can be almost infinite, and depends entirely on the physical and emotional needs of the individual. Oils which have been found particularly valuable by aromatherapists working with people with A.I.D.S. include Bergamot, Camomile, Clary Sage, Frankincense, Geranium, Grapefruit, Jasmine, Marjoram, Neroli, Rose, Rosewood, Sandalwood and Violet Leaf.

A possible contra-indication to the use of essential oils is chemotherapy. This may often be given to treat Karposi's Sarcoma, a rare form of cancer which affects many

A.I.D.S. patients. The whole question of essential oils and chemotherapy is discussed in the entry for **CANCER**, so I will not repeat it here, but do please read that section in conjunction with this.

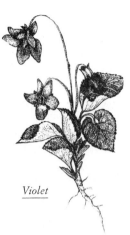

If you are an aromatherapist thinking about doing such work you need to be free from any prejudice about sexuality or lifestyle as many of your clients will be gay or bisexual men and intravenous drug users, though the number of women with A.I.D.S. is increasing. You will also need to interact with the families, friends and lovers of people with A.I.D.S. Be aware that some of the people you work with are going to die, and ask yourself whether you can cope emotionally with this.

Violet

You should also be aware that you may encounter prejudice yourself from people who fear you may pass the H.I.V. virus to them. Such fears are completely irrational, as the virus can only be transmitted via body fluids such as blood and semen, but the fear is real all the same. Giving aromatherapy to a person with A.I.D.S. presents no danger as long as neither therapist nor client have any broken skin (it is perfectly safe to cover minor cuts, etc. with a plaster).

Where therapists really do need to take care of themselves is in ensuring that they get support in the form of people who are prepared to listen to them whenever needed. Do whatever you need to maintain your own health and try not to get over-tired. Don't try to do too much – the emotional pressure of working with people who are very ill, from whatever cause, plus all the taboos that attach to A.I.D.S. can quickly lead to burn-out. Having said that, I must add that everybody I know who has worked in this area has found deep satisfaction in doing so.

SPECIAL NOTE: It is illegal for any non-medically trained person to give treatment for any sexually-transmitted disease, as a first referral, but they may do so in collaboration with, or with the consent of, the doctor in charge of treatment.

Please read the entries on **CANCER, H.I.V.** and on the **IMMUNE SYSTEM** in conjunction with this section.

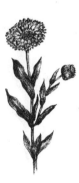

27

Airsprays

One of the simplest ways to introduce essential oils into the air is to mix them in water and use them as a spray. They mix better if dissolved in alcohol or some other dispersant before adding to the water, but a simple mixture of essential oil and water will work well enough for a short time if it is vigorously shaken. The oil will not completely dissolve in water, but enough of it will remain suspended in the water to form a good spray. A simple plant spray will do this job quite well, but if it is made of plastic or metal do not leave any essential oil mixture in it after using, as both plastics and metals interact with the oils and change them. Some plant shops sell small decorative ceramic plant sprays, and I recycle glass spray bottles.

Air sprays can be used for a wide variety of purposes, from simply perfuming a room to combating infection. Insect repellent oils in an airspray are effective at keeping a room, or the entire home, free from flies in summer, and deodorising oils, such as Bergamot, will clear unwanted smells from the air. But the most important use of such sprays is in treating infectious illnesses, and preventing the spread of infection. During epidemics of 'flu or childhood illnesses such as measles, chickenpox, etc., antiviral or bactericidal oils such as Ti-tree, Bergamot, Eucalyptus and Lavender sprayed repeatedly in the sickroom and around the house will speed the patient's recovery and help to protect other members of the household from infection.

Use 20 drops of essential oil to 200 mls of water for perfuming, air freshening or deterring insects, and twice this amount as a spray during illness or epidemics.

Lavend

Alcohol

Essential oils dissolve very readily in alcohol, and various forms of alcohol are used when making perfumes and other preparations from essential oils and various combinations of the oils.

Isopropyl alcohol (or isopropanol) is sometimes used in making rubs, deodorants and aftershaves, although it is rather 'savage' to the skin, and needs to be used in very small amounts, along with floral waters or distilled water. Some large retail chemists sell it, though they may limit the amount you can buy at any time.

Ethyl alcohol, or perfume grade alcohol (ethanol) is subject to a Customs and Excise duty, and can only be bought with a special licence.

For home making of smallish amounts of aftershaves, skin toners and deodorants, vodka (the highest proof you can find) is a good substitute, and if you visit the continent and can bring back some eau de vie, that would be even better. Brandy makes a good basis for a mouthwash.

Alcoholism

While it would be very wrong to suggest that aromatherapy can 'cure' or 'treat' alcoholism, there are ways in which a sympathetic therapist can support a person who is trying to overcome a problem with drink.

Massage may help to reduce the underlying stresses which have led to a dependence on alcohol, and here virtually any of the relaxing and antidepressant oils may be used. The choice will depend very much on individual preference and circumstances.

Detoxifying oils, such as Fennel and Juniper, are valuable in helping to clear the body of poisons that accumulate over long periods of excessive drinking, and the feeling of increased well-being that detoxification can give may be a boost to the morale. It is important to remember, though, that there may be a short-term reaction to the detoxifying process during which the individual will actually feel worse, as toxins which have been stored in the liver and other body tissues are released into the bloodstream.

Skilled counselling, support groups and other therapies are all very necessary, and the aromatherapist should not attempt to work in isolation.

see also the entry for **ADDICTION.**

Alcohols

❧

One of the categories of organic molecules found in essential oils. They can be subdivided into different groups according to which type of Terpene was involved in their production within the plant (see **TERPENES**) and the therapeutic action differs from group to group. Monoterpenic alcohols are the most common: they are generally non-toxic and gentle to the skin.

Monoterpenic alcohols are anti-infectious (antibacterial, antifungal and antiviral) and good immunostimulants, with a generally tonic action. Examples include borneol, in Lavender, Nutmeg, Pine, etc.; citronellol, in Citronella, Geranium, Palmarosa, etc.; geraniol, in Geranium, Palmarosa, Rose, Neroli, Petitgrain, etc.; lavandulol, in Lavender, etc.; linalol, in Lavender, Neroli, Nutmeg, Ylang-Ylang, etc.

Sesquiterpenic alcohols are not so prevalent and often found only in a specific plant. They have a weaker anti-infectious action, but are good immunostimulants, tonic and stimulant. Examples include cedrol, in Cedar; farnesol, in Palmarosa, Rose, Ylang-Ylang; nerolidol, in Neroli; santalol, in Sandalwood, etc.

Di-terpenic alcohols occur only in very small amounts in essential oils but even in tiny amounts they are very active. They often have an oestrogenic action. Examples: sclareol, in Clary Sage and salviol, in Sage.

You will realise that all the alcohols have names ending in 'ol' which makes it fairly easy to identify them when looking at the chemistry of any oil. However, the Phenols – which are highly irritant to the skin and mucous membrane, also have names ending in 'ol', so be careful not to confuse them.

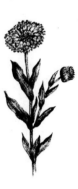

Aldehydes

❧

Another of the categories of organic molecules in essential oils. Aldehydes are highly anti-inflammatory and calming to the central nervous system. Some lower blood pressure, others help reduce temperature in a fever. Examples include citral, in Lemon, Lemongrass, Citronella, Geranium, etc.; citronellal, in Citronella, Eucalyptus, Lemon, Melissa, etc.; phellandral, in many of the oils extracted from trees; anisic aldehyde, in Aniseed, Vanilla, etc., and cinnamic aldehyde, in Cinnamon Bark (large amounts) and Cinnamon Leaf (small amounts). As you can see, the aldehydes either have names ending in 'al' or the word aldehyde included in their name so they are easily identified in lists of constituents.

NOTE: Despite the generally anti-inflammatory action of this group, cinnamic aldehyde is a severe skin irritant. If it is present in significant amounts in any oil, do not use that oil on the skin.

Allergy

The term allergy was originally coined in the early years of this century to describe an abnormal reaction of the body to foreign proteins, for example, the pollens which provoke an attack of hay fever. Because invading organisms, such as bacteria and viruses, are composed mainly of protein, our defence mechanisms are triggered when the body detects proteins which it cannot recognise as being part of its own structure (such as the proteins in food). In an allergic response, this process has gone out of control in some way: either by overreacting wildly, or by reacting to a protein which is not in itself any threat. Hay fever, eczema, urticaria and some forms of asthma are all typical of a classical allergic reaction.

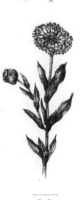

The aromatherapist's approach to allergy is to modify this overreaction by using essential oils which are calming and soothing. Camomile, Lavender and Melissa are the oils most often used successfully to help allergies. Baths, compresses, inhalations, skin lotions etc., are all appropriate methods, depending on the type of allergic response.

Stress is known to play a very important role in predisposing people to respond allergically. Quite often, a person who develops asthma, eczema or other allergic reactions to various irritants when under stress, can come into contact with the same allergen without any reaction when calmer and happier. So, one of the most important things the aromatherapist can do is to help decrease the levels of stress. We are fortunate in that massage itself is one of the most effective ways to reduce stress, and that there are so many essential oils which help to do so too. The three oils mentioned above as being most used for allergies are also de-stressors, which is undoubtedly why they are so effective in treating allergies. Bergamot, Clary, Neroli, Rose, Jasmine, Sandalwood and Ylang Ylang are some of the other oils that are most often used to help with stress. Massage is certainly the best method of use, but aromatic baths in between massage treatments are a real help too.

The number of people suffering from allergies has increased vastly in recent years, and the increasingly stressful conditions under which many of us live have much to do with this, as well as the proliferation of chemical pollutants in our food, air, water and in the environment. The term allergy is now often used to describe reactions which do not fall strictly within the original definition and some people prefer to use the term sensitivity to describe these reactions, particularly if the offending substance is not a protein. Some of the conditions which have been identified as occuring as a result of adverse reactions to foreign substances, include catarrh, headaches, hyperactivity, fluid retention and a variety of skin problems.

The role of food allergy is much better understood than a few years ago, though it is debatable whether in many instances it is the food itself which is responsible, or the conditions under which the food was produced, the feeding of hormones and antibiotics to farm animals, and the use of chemical fertilisers, pesticides and herbicides on fruit and vegetable crops being obvious examples. Pressure on food manufacturers to remove many chemical additives has resulted from observation of the range of allergic reactions, or sensitivities, which they provoke.

In all these reactions, as in classical allergy, stress is a major factor, so the role of the aromatherapist will be the same, whatever the cause and whatever the form of allergy – to soothe, calm and comfort, to reduce stress, while alleviating the immediate symptoms. Dietary advice is often necessary, but the factors involved may be so complicated that it could be advisable to refer the client to a trained nutritionist or a clinical ecologist.

see also entries for **ASTHMA, ECZEMA, HAY FEVER** *and* **NETTLERASH,** *also* **STRESS** *because of the connection between* **STRESS** *and* **ALLERGIES.**

Allopathy

Allopathy is a term devised by Samuel Hahnemann to describe orthodox drug treatment or, 'treatment by opposites', as opposed to homoeopathy, or 'treatment by like'. It is often used, somewhat incorrectly, to describe the whole system of orthodox medicine.

Alopecia

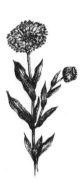

This term is usually used to describe temporary baldness, to distinguish between this and male pattern baldness, which is permanent, progressive, and unlikely to be influenced by any treatment. Temporary baldness, or severe hair loss, can often be helped considerably by aromatherapy and other means.

Temporary baldness may follow illness, or be a symptom of it: for example, hair loss may be a sign of thyroid or pituitary deficiency, or defective functioning of the ovaries. Hair loss in such cases is gradual and general, causing thinning more or less evenly from all parts of the scalp. There are many well-documented cases of partial or complete loss of hair following shock, bereavement, accidents or a period of extreme stress. This is usually sudden and patchy, with one or more completely bald patches appearing, and is called alopecia areata. The hair may suddenly start growing again just as mysteriously as it stopped, but the very fact of becoming bald, or partly so, can create an extra element of stress which delays recovery.

Stress, shock and other mental and emotional problems are areas in which aromatherapy is particularly effective, and hair will often start growing again when the therapist has been able to help with the underlying cause. Local treatments to the scalp should concentrate on massage to increase the circulation and the general health of the skin of the scalp, since each hair grows from a 'root' or follicle in the inner layer of the skin. Rosemary, Lavender and Thyme have been found to stimulate hair growth, both where the loss is total, or where there is severe thinning. If there is some hair remaining, any one of these oils, in a base of almond or jojoba oil can be rubbed gently into it once or twice a week and left on for two hours or more before washing out with a gentle, natural shampoo. Hot towels can be wrapped round the head to aid absorption. This kind of treatment will improve the appearance of the remaining hair, giving an illusion of greater bulk, and this in itself can be a big boost to morale. While these treatments are being carried out by the therapist, the person suffering hair loss should be shown how to massage his or her own scalp daily.

Aromatherapy treatments to help with stress and many kinds of trauma are discussed in other parts of this book, so I will only say here that massage is very important, and can be backed up by aromatic baths.

If physical illness seems to be a cause of hair loss, it may be necessary to combine aromatherapy treatments with help from a doctor, naturopath, acupuncturist or other suitably trained and qualified person. The actual treatment of the scalp should be as I have described above.

Complete or partial loss of hair is sometimes caused by a food allergy, or by a chemical irritant, such as hair dyes, perms, industrial chemicals or fumes, and then obviously the avoidance of the irritant food or chemical is the first necessity; but essential oils can often be used to encourage hair growth once the irritant has been identified and removed.

The loss of hair is a side effect of some drugs, most notably those used in the treatment of cancer; aromatherapists in Norway have reported success in encouraging cancer patients' hair to grow again, particularly when using oil of Lavender.

Good general nutrition is important to the health of the head and hair, in particular adequate protein, vegetable fats in small amounts, and vitamins of the B family.

see also **BALDNESS.**

Amenorrhoea

ᨠ

absence of **PERIODS.** (*see under* **MENSTRUATION.**)

Angelica
Angelica archangelica or A. officinalis

ᨠ

Angelica is a vigourous plant of the Umbelliferae family, rapidly growing to six feet or more in height and crowned during the flowering period with great umbels of greeny-white flowers. The whole plant is strongly aromatic and the flowers have a honey-like smell. It is native to Northern Europe, but cultivated throughout the continent.

Angelica

Essential oil can be distilled from the root or the seeds and is virtually colourless when freshly distilled, gradually darkening to a yellowish-brown. It has a very rich, pleasant aroma and is used commercially in many liqueurs and aperitifs including Chartreuse and Benedictine. The main constituent is phellandrene, which accounts for up to 70% of the oil, with angelicine, bergaptene, various acids, etc. The proportions vary somewhat between the oil from the root and that from the seeds.

Angelica has been renowned as a medicinal plant since antiquity, and probably got its name because its healing powers were so great as to seem of divine origin. (An alternative name was 'Holy Spirit Root'.) Writers from Paracelsus to Gerard credited it with the ability to give protection from the Plague. It is, in fact, an excellent tonic and stimulant and appears to strengthen the immune system, so it would be of genuine value

CAUTION
Angelica root oil has a photosensitising action similar to Bergamot. Do not use on any area of skin that will be exposed to sunlight.

in epidemics of all kinds. Traditionally, Angelica has been used to restore strength and stamina during convalescence, anaemia or whenever a patient is generally weak, which leads me to think it could be valuable in M.E.

It is an excellent tonic for the digestive system, as we might deduce from its use in liqueurs, etc., and helps with loss of appetite. Fabrice Bardeau in 'La Medicine Aromatique' cites Angelica for anorexia. It is particularly valuable for digestive problems originating from stress.

It can be used for all kinds of respiratory infections, from the common cold to bronchitis, and is specially helpful for dry, irritating coughs. It has a very soothing action on the skin and is used a great deal in commercial skin preparations.

Another important use of Angelica is as a detoxifier and diuretic. It helps all the organs of elimination (liver, kidneys, skin) and improves lymph drainage and for that reason is particularly valuable as a massage oil for rheumatism, arthritis, fluid retention and cellulite. Its pleasant aroma makes it easy to incorporate in blends with many other oils.

There are thirty or more varieties of Angelica growing around the world, at least ten of them in China which are all used for various medicinal purposes. Increasing use is being made in the West of a variety known as Dong Kwai which can be used as an alternative to artificial hormones during menopause.

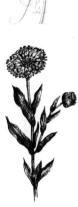

Aniseed
Pimpinella anisum

The essential oil of Aniseed is seldom used, on account of its relatively high toxicity. It contains up to 90% trans-anethol and in high doses, or taken over a long period of time, it is a narcotic which slows the circulation, damages the brain and is addictive (c.f. the addiction to absinthe which was common in 19th century France). The effects are cumulative. It can also cause dermatitis in some people.

Theoretically, it can be used to calm digestive or menstrual pain, stimulate the flow of breast milk, or treat heart and lung disease, but as there are other safe essential oils with the same properties, it is better to leave this one well alone.

Anorexia Nervosa

The dictionary definition of anorexia is, simply, loss of appetite, but we usually use this term to refer to a dramatic inability to eat, allied to serious psychological disturbances, and usually seen in young girls and women, although the number of anorexic males has increased in the last few years. Aromatherapy alone is almost certainly not enough to help an anorexic, but can be very valuable when allied to skilled counselling or psychotherapy. Massage helps to bring the receiver into contact with her own body. This is important, since so many sufferers are alienated from their physical body and even develop a strong self-loathing. The Bach remedy Crab Apple can be helpful here. Anorexic girls have a distorted self-image and may perceive themselves as being overweight when they are, in fact, emaciated.

The choice of oils depends very much on the individual needs and preferences of the person receiving treatment, but will almost always need to be selected from among the calming, soothing antidepressants such as Lavender, Camomile, Neroli, Ylang-Ylang and Clary Sage. Bergamot is important, not only because it is a powerfully uplifting oil, but it may help to regulate appetite. A number of authors describe Bergamot as increasing the appetite, though in the case of anorexia, I feel that the action of Bergamot on an emotional level, leading to some reduction in the stresses that underlie the inability to eat, is probably more important. Angelica is another oil that is thought to stimulate appetite, and is particularly recommended for people who are weak, underweight, nervous or debilitated which makes it very appropriate for helping in anorexia.

Very often, an anorexic girl is afraid of growing up, and cannot come to terms with her own potential sexuality and having an adult woman's body. Rose oil cries out to be used here. It relates to women's sexuality on every level, physical and emotional, and creates a wonderful feeling of being pampered, which is also a great help in restoring self esteem. Jasmine might be useful as a confidence-boosting alternative.

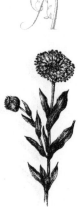

Once the therapist has some idea of which oils the girl really responds to, she can prepare some bath oils using these favourites and perhaps add some of the same oils to a body lotion for use after bathing.

Baths with essential oils are very helpful in between massage sessions, and here again, the idea of pampering and nurturing comes in. Emphasis should be on the 'luxurious' oils (providing that their perfume is appreciated). Applying the lotion to her own body is also a form of therapy for an anorexic girl, and as progress is made, this might even be extended into some self-massage with oils mixed by the therapist for use at home.

A high level of vitamin and mineral supplementation is advisable, especially Vitamin B complex and zinc. Initially, very small, but frequent, meals should be made up of fruits, raw vegetables, tiny amounts of dried fruits and nuts. These foods are full of vital nutrients and are not seen as a threat by most anorexics, as they are often thought of as 'slimming'. Gradually, a simple wholefood diet can be introduced.

This is obviously an area where enormous sensitivity is needed and trust needs to be built up between the therapist and the client before there can be any hope of seeing any signs of improvement.

Anosmia

Loss of the sense of smell.

---

see under **SMELL, SENSE OF.**

Antibiotics

Drugs which attack bacteria and kill them within the body.

While the discovery of modern antibiotics has done much to reduce mortality from infectious illnesses, and has almost eradicated certain diseases, the over-prescription and unwise use of these powerful drugs has done more harm than good. Antibiotics are often prescribed for viral infections (the common cold and 'flu for example) which they can do nothing to help (though they may help avert a secondary infection from bacteria). Overworked doctors give antibiotics for minor ailments which would clear up with an antiseptic or simply with time and rest, or 'old fashioned' treatments, such as compresses or poultices. Taking an antibiotic for minor illness will often build up an immunity to that drug, which will then be ineffective when needed in a crisis.

In the body, antibiotics aren't particularly discriminating, and will kill 'friendly' bacteria along with those causing illness so we very often find acute diarrhoea occurring when antibiotics are taken, as a result of the helpful bacteria in the intestines being killed by the million. Women on antibiotics often suffer an outbreak of vaginal thrush when the bacteria normally present in the vagina are affected.

It is often safer to use essential oils to combat infection. All essential oils will kill some bacteria, while a number of oils are powerful bactericides affecting a wide range of infectious organisms. Ti-tree, Lavender, Eucalyptus, Bergamot and Juniper are the most important of these.

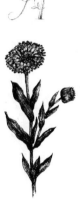

Perhaps even more important than their bactericidal action, is the fact that these oils stimulate the body's own immune response to infection. The amount of essential oil taken into the body would certainly not be sufficient to destroy the disease-causing bacteria present, but the stimulus to the body's defence mechanisms does not seem to be dependent on the amount of essential oil involved. Indeed, as Dr. Jean Valnet has written, without actually going so far as using homoeopathic doses, the smaller the amount of oil used, the greater the effect seems to be on the body.

An antibiotic may be really necessary in a crisis – pneumonia, for example, or severe cystitis when blood or pus are present in the urine, or pain affects the kidneys. It would be irresponsible to depend on self-help in such cases, or when a young child or an elderly person is involved, but you can do a lot to offset the harmful side effects of antibiotics by taking at the same time large amounts of live natural yoghurt, or taking acidophilus tablets.

The wisest course, though, would be to tackle infections in the earliest stages of their potential development with essential oils, rest and fasting where indicated, and avoid them ever reaching the acute, crisis condition.

see also entries under the individual oils mentioned, and under various illnesses.

Antidepressants

Many essential oils have marked antidepressant properties and this is probably one of the areas where aromatherapy is most valuable in present day society, offering a safe, natural and non-addictive alternative to the millions of tablets prescribed annually for depression and anxiety.

The oil of Bergamot is perhaps the most widely known of the antidepressant oils, with its fresh lively smell and uplifting effects, but there are many others, including Basil, Camomile, Clary, Geranium, Jasmine, Lavender, Melissa, Neroli, Patchouli, Rose, Sandalwood and Ylang-Ylang.

Each of these oils is subtly different in its action, and in its appeal to the individual, and the aromatherapist needs to use his/her intuition and skill in carefully choosing the best oil, or blend of oils, for each person. Preference for a certain aroma may tell us much about a person's mental/emotional state at the time, and as the causes of depression are many and varied, so must be the choice of treatment oils. The sympathetic understanding of the therapist, and the human touch involved in massage, is an important part of the therapy. Massage almost always forms the core of the treatment, but aromatic baths are a very valuable way of prolonging the effect between treatments. If the person seeking help likes the aroma of the essential oil(s) used for the massage (and they certainly should, as this enjoyment enhances the value of the massage) they may be given some to use every day as a skin perfume, so that the helpful, healing aroma is constantly about them. Essential oils can be used as a room spray to influence mood, too, or a drop or two evaporated by placing them on an electric light bulb.

see also entries under **MASSAGE, DEPRESSION, ANXIETY, STRESS** *and each of the oils named above.*

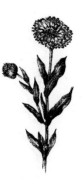

Antidote

Essential oils, like all strong-smelling substances, will antidote homoeopathic remedies, and for this reason it is not always wise to try to combine these two modes of treatment.

Homoeopaths recommend that no strongly scented substance – in particular peppermint, camphor and coffee – should be consumed, or used, within a certain time of using a homoeopathic remedy. The time that must elapse to avoid antidoting the remedy varies according to the speed with which the remedy is expected to take effect. Standard homoeopathic remedies sold in chemists and healthfood shops generally state half-an-hour, but many homoeopaths would disagree with this. Three hours is often given as a minimum, and if the remedy being used is a very slow working one, it may be necessary to avoid scented substances for weeks, or even months.

Should you wish to use aromatic baths, or receive massage with essential oils, for example, while taking a homoeopathic remedy, you should find out which of these categories your remedy falls into. If you take Nux Vomica for a stomach upset and your stomach is quickly relieved, there is no reason why you should not have a comforting massage later in the same day, but if you are receiving treatment for a long-standing condition which is expected to respond only gradually to the remedy, then you should talk with your homoeopath before using essential oils in any form.

Obviously, essential oils should be stored far away from homoeopathic remedies.

A few essential oils (or the plants from which they are obtained) have had a reputation since ancient times for being antidotes to various poisons. Fennel is the most noted of these, and is certainly a valuable aid to eliminating toxins from the body, though whether it will really counteract poisoning from snake bites, poisonous plants or mushrooms as claimed in the old herbals, nobody has put to the test in modern times.

Anxiety

Anxiety in some circumstances is a perfectly healthy response. It is normal, for example, to feel a little anxious before a demanding interview or examination, and the anxiety may even be useful – spurring us on to complete revision or preparation. It is normal for a parent to feel anxious if a child is late returning from some outing, but not normal to feel anxious every moment that the child is out of sight.

Anxiety only becomes a problem when it is excessive – i.e., when the response is prolonged, or out of proportion to the threatening situation, or where anxiety is experienced when there is no objective, external reasons for it. Unfortunately, twentieth century life gives rise to many genuine sources of anxiety, whether it be motorway driving, unemployment or the ultimate fate of our planet. Anxiety can give rise to many physical symptoms, ranging from tight muscles, through digestive problems, migraine, allergies and insomnia to heart disease, and is a predisposing factor in many other serious illnesses.

In aromatherapy we have a valuable alternative to the psychotropic drugs and muscle relaxants that are commonly used to treat anxiety allopathically. Any of the sedative oils may be helpful, and there are many for the therapist to choose from: Benzoin, Bergamot, Camomile, Cedarwood, Clary Sage, Cypress, Frankincense, Geranium, Hyssop, Jasmine, Juniper, Lavender, Marjoram, Melissa, Neroli, Patchouli, Rose, Sandalwood, Verbena and Ylang-Ylang. In choosing from such a wide range the therapist will be guided by what he/she knows about the personality, lifestyle and background of the person needing help, the source of anxiety and also their individual preference for the smell of different oils. The personal choice of a person you want to help is often very revealing. They will often pick instinctively the very oil that most closely corresponds to their present state, and this can sometimes tell the aroma-therapist more than a whole chapter of talk. For, although all these oils fall under the heading of sedative, there are subtle differences in their properties and effects which may make one more appropriate than another in any situation.

Obviously, the caring approach of the therapist counts for a great deal in helping with anxiety, and massage with essential oils should be the basis of treatment because it will allow reassurance, love and concern to be expressed in the most direct, non-verbal way. Aromatic baths with essential oils are very valuable between treatments, especially if insomnia is part of the picture, as is so often the case. If the person concerned has a special liking for any of the essential oils used in treatment, they might be encouraged to use tiny amounts of that oil as a personal perfume and/or as a room spray so that the effect of the treatment can be prolonged.

Aromatherapy works harmoniously with such de-stressing techniques as autogenics, yoga, meditation, or simple relaxation exercises. An aromatherapist working on holistic principles may often be able to teach one or more of these techniques, or will know other teachers from whom they can be learnt.

Jasmine

Aphrodisiacs

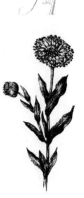

Yes, a number of essential oils DO have aphrodisiac properties and they deserve to be taken seriously, for they can be of great value in easing marital disharmony and helping people who suffer from impotence or frigidity. Physical reasons for these conditions are rare indeed, but should be checked before essential oils are used. The root of such problems is nearly always mental/emotional, and aromatherapy has been found again and again to be most effective when helping on the emotional plane.

Aphrodisiac oils fall – rather roughly – into three categories: those which are calming and soothing, and which create the desired (!) effect by reducing anxieties and stresses in the relationship; those which are directly stimulant (and these need to be used with great circumspection); and those which may possibly have a hormonal effect.

The most notable oils in the first category are Rose and Neroli (orange-flower). Rose petals were strewn on marriage beds by the Romans, and brides crowned with orange blossoms because the perfume of these flowers was found to allay any nervousness about the wedding night. (Plastic orange blossoms and crepe paper confetti rose petals, both derived from these ancient customs, will not, alas, have the same effect.) Clary Sage, Patchouli – if you can stand the smell – and Ylang-Ylang are in the same category. All of these are oils which are relaxing in general, and it is important to remember that external stresses – money, work, accommodation, etc. – can as frequently be a cause of sexual difficulties as problems arising within a relationship. Help with underlying tension may be what is needed, and the therapist has to be very sensitive to all the circumstances of each individual. Any of these oils, or combinations of them, can be used as aromatic baths before bedtime, or in massage oils. If a loving partner can be taught to use the oils in a gentle massage, they will obviously have the maximum effect. Essential oils should NEVER be applied directly to the genitals, even when diluted.

The oils of Jasmine and Sandalwood can be included with those that are calming and relaxing, as they are both wonderfully sedative oils, but I prefer to consider them apart, as it is possible that they have an actual hormonal effect on the body. Although this is speculation on my part it arises from observation of their effects. Certainly, both these oils have a heady, almost irresistible attraction for both men and women (and cats too, in the case of Jasmine). People using these oils for reasons totally unconnected with any sexual problem – such as Sandalwood for a chest complaint – have often reported erotic 'side-effects'. This in itself is enough to refute the allegation that 'They only work because you think they are going to.' None of the people I have in mind had the slightest idea that the oil(s) in question were reputedly aphrodisiac.

There are one or two oils – Black Pepper, Cardamon and possibly some of the other warming spices – which have a directly stimulating effect. These can be useful where fatigue underlies a sexual problem, but must never be abused, as over-use can cause urinary, digestive and other problems. They can be used in a low concentration in massage oils over the lower spine but the safest way to use these plants is as the powdered spice in food or drink, rather than as an essential oil.

None of these oils should be regarded as more than a temporary help during a difficult time. Even when there is no danger of chronic toxicity, it is possible for people to use the oils as an emotional 'crutch', though physical dependence is unknown. If sexual problems persist over a long time, help in the form of counselling, psychotherapy, etc., might be needed as well as aromatherapy.

Appetite

Appetite is a curious phenomenon, working on various levels. On the one hand, there is the physical sensation when the stomach has well digested the last meal, and is ready for another – though this should more properly be called hunger. Appetite is a function of the mind, and is affected by many factors other than the fullness or emptiness of the stomach. For example, the sight or smell of food can stimulate appetite even when we are not hungry (just try walking past a baker's in the early morning!). Even reading about food can do the same. At a deeper level, appetite can be affected by mental/emotional factors such as stress, anxiety, depression and shock. This is not surprising when we take into account that appetite is regulated by the hypothalamus, at the base of the brain, which is closely linked with those areas of the brain associated with the emotions, and in many respects acts as a link between the mind and body.

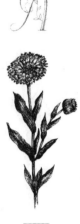

What is harder to understand is why such diverse mental states can have the same effect on the appetite, or why similar emotional or mental states can have directly opposite effects on different individuals. A young girl may 'go off her food' because she is deliriously in love, or because her boyfriend has jilted her. Her father may be pushing his plate away untouched because he is desperately worried about the threat of redundancy, while his wife is secretly stuffing cream buns and chocolate to allay her anxiety about the same threat.

The aromatherapist's response to an individual with a disturbed eating pattern must be holistic. It is important to look at the whole person and his/her deeper needs, and to try to help him/her to work through the feelings of insecurity, depression, anxiety or whatever seems to be causing the abnormal shift in appetite. Any of the antidepressant oils may be appropriate, depending on the individual's personality and needs, and sensitive use of massage can help to restore the individual to a comfortable relationship with his or her body, if a disturbed self-image is at the root of the trouble.

If the appetite is temporarily decreased, such as in convalescence, it is a relatively simple matter to stimulate it by using essential oils. Camomile, Cardamom, Hyssop and Bergamot are all known to help with loss of appetite. Fennel is given by some authorities as a stimulator of appetite, while others state the opposite. Roman soldiers used to chew Fennel seeds to stave off hunger pangs on long marches, when they had no time to stop and eat, and I have done the same thing when dieting. The answer to this apparent contradiction, I am sure, is that Fennel, like many essential oils, has a normalising effect, rather than specifically decreasing or increasing appetite.

A similar situation is seen with Bergamot. I have already mentioned that it is used to stimulate appetite, but I have also used it to help compulsive eaters. Bergamot is one of our most powerful allies in helping people with depression and anxiety. As well as being antidepressant, it is described, very accurately, as being 'uplifting'. So, if we use Bergamot as a massage oil, personal perfume or bath oil we can gently work on the underlying causes of the disturbed eating pattern.

Just occasionally, loss of appetite may be linked to previous bad eating habits, and a fast to rid the body of toxins might be a good start to the treatment, followed by dietary advice and appetite stimulating essential oils for a very short period.

see also **ANOREXIA, BULIMIA** *and* **OBESITY.**

Armoise

❧

see **MUGWORT.**

Arnica
Arnica montana

❧

This is another highly toxic essential oil, and is never used in aromatherapy. However, several other Arnica extractions have valuable uses.

The infused oil of Arnica is valuable for bruises and sprains, and as a massage oil for muscular aches, especially after sport or any heavy exertion. It is sometimes recommended for nappy rash but much care would be needed if using it for this purpose as no Arnica product should ever be used if the skin is broken. It is also possible to get an Arnica hydrolat, which can be used for the same purposes, with the advantage of being non-oily in situations where an oil base would not be suitable.

Arnica is of great value in homoeopathy, where it is used both internally and externally in miniscule doses (see **HOMOEOPATHY**) for shock, bruising and sprains. A tube of arnica cream is a 'must' for any plant-based medicine chest. Remember to store it well away from essential oils as all strong smells antidote homoeopathic remedies.

Arthritis

❧

Arthritis is a disease of imbalanced body chemistry. Whatever the immediate factor that heralds the onset of arthritis, the body is not eliminating uric acid efficiently. Some people's bodies get rid of toxins more efficiently than others, and all of us do so better at some times than at others. Stress and anxiety reduce our ability to deal with toxic wastes; incorrect diet gives the body more toxins to deal with and environmental pollution adds to the total burden the body has to cope with. Once a toxic accumulation has built up, it will eventually manifest itself as disease, taking varying forms in different individuals.

In arthritis, uric acid is deposited as crystals in joint spaces, causing inflammation, pain, stiffness, loss of mobility and eventually damage to the joint surfaces. The joints affected are often those that have been most heavily used: in sports, dance and physically demanding occupations, for example, or through incorrect posture and where extra loads are imposed on the major weight-bearing joints (hips, knees and ankles) in people who are seriously overweight. The site of an earlier injury may be a vulnerable point. In gout (which is a form of arthritis) the joints of the toes are most commonly affected, though the fingers may be, too. Attacks are intensely painful, with acute inflammation of the joint. After repeated attacks, large deposits of uric acid crystals (known as tophi) cause permanent swelling and deformity of joints, particularly noticeable in the knuckles.

Inflammation, sometimes acute but quite often of a 'grumbling' nature, is also a feature of rheumatoid arthritis. The onset of rheumatoid arthritis may be caused by infection – possibly by a virus – but recent evidence suggests that a form of auto-immunity is involved, i.e., that the sufferer has an allergic reaction to some of his or her own body tissues.

Osteo-arthritis is less likely to be inflammatory in nature, but is characterised by degeneration of the smooth gliding surfaces of the joints, and occurs more often in middle-aged and elderly people as the result of 'wear and tear'.

The accepted medical view is that arthritis is incurable and treatment is confined to pain relief with analgesic and anti-inflammatory drugs (often with undesirable side effects). Joint replacement surgery may be offered where there is very serious degeneration of the joint, but this can only be used for the largest joints, such as the hip and knee, and involves far more major surgery than most people realise.

Natural therapies, particularly aromatherapy and naturopathy, aim at altering the body chemistry. First, the toxic build up must be eliminated, and then new accumulations of uric acid must be prevented. The body's own resources need to be stimulated to repair damaged surfaces as far as possible. Circulation to the affected joints must be improved, both to drain off the wastes and to improve nutrition to the affected tissues.

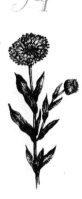

Essential oils can be used in a variety of ways to achieve these results. Detoxifying oils, such as Cypress, Fennel, Juniper and Lemon are used in baths and massage to help the body throw off poisons. Painkilling oils, such as Benzoin, Camomile, Lavender and Rosemary are used in baths, local massage or compresses on the affected joints, and local circulation can be improved by the use of rubefacient oils – Black Pepper, Ginger and Marjoram, for example. Whenever heat is applied to a stiffened joint in the form of baths, hot compresses or warming massage, the joint should be moved as much as possible immediately afterwards, otherwise the heating can cause congestion which will make the condition worse rather than better. Any of these forms of treatment will reduce pain in the joint and make some movement possible. If very little unaided movement is possible, the therapist can gently manipulate the joint through as wide a range of movement as possible at the end of the massage. Gentle exercise is very helpful, yoga undoubtedly being the most valuable.

41

A holistic aromatherapist will obviously not 'treat' arthritis simply by trying to relieve symptoms. She/he will look at the whole person, and all the circumstances of that person's life. Often, a complex association of factors is involved. Bad nutrition, stress and obesity may all be found in one person, or poor nutrition allied to old injuries. In my experience, arthritis often afflicts people who are 'bottling up' grief, rage or hatred, or who are unable to express a creative talent. The aromatherapist needs to look at all these subtle factors and decide on essential oils and the form of treatment according to the personality and needs of the person.

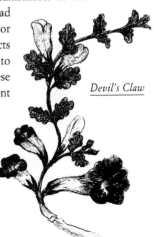

Devil's Claw

If the arthritis is of long standing, it may not be possible to undo all the damage to joint surfaces, but in all cases pain can be reduced a great deal, mobility improved and further damage prevented. If arthritis is treated early enough complete rehabilitation is possible.

Dietary advice is an important part of any treatment. A cleansing fast will help elimination of toxins and mobilise the body's own powers of recuperation. A restricted diet may be needed until pain and inflammation have been reduced, and some permanent adjustments made to the diet – usually excluding red meats (especially pork and all pig products), tea and coffee and reducing or excluding alcohol. Some people may discover other foods that aggravate their condition. Vitamin and mineral supplementation is often helpful during the early stages of treatment, especially of Vitamin A, the B complex and E, also calcium pantothenate. A herbal extract, 'Devil's Claw' has been found helpful in a great many cases.

Asthma

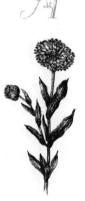

Asthma is characterised by difficulty in breathing, caused by muscle spasm in the small passages (bronchi) of the lungs. This narrows the space available for air to make its way out of the lungs, and breathing out is always more difficult than breathing in. This produces the wheezing sound associated with asthma attacks. Because the passages are narrowed and air flow reduced, mucus also builds up in the lungs, and this makes it even more difficult to breathe. The mucus is also a breeding-ground for bacteria, so attacks of bronchitis may arise as a complication of the asthma. Many asthma attacks are triggered by allergens, such as dust, mould spores, mites, animal hair or feathers but the onset may equally be caused by cold air, or it may be preceded by an infection such as a cold. The dramatic rise in the incidence of asthma in the past decade is almost certainly due to air pollution – in particular to traffic fumes. Certainly, stress and more specifically acute anxiety are known to be the immediate trigger for many attacks, and this can sometimes give rise to a vicious circle of asthma – anxiety about the asthma – further attacks.

Given those assorted facts, it is clear that the aromatherapist's approach needs to be flexible and varied according to the immediate circumstances of the asthma sufferer. During an actual crisis, inhaling an antispasmodic oil is the only practical help. Sniffing directly from the bottle, or some drops put on a tissue or hankie, is safer than a steam inhalation, as the heat of the latter may increase inflammation of the mucous membranes and make the congestion even worse. Moisture, however, is helpful, and a humidifier with a few drops of essential oil added is a good idea.

Unless the asthma sufferer is a member of the therapist's family or a close friend, treatment is more likely to be given between attacks. The whole thoracic area – back and chest – should be massaged, with particular emphasis on strokes which open out the chest and shoulders. The shiatsu pressure point Lung No. 1 should be gently pressed for a second or two at a time during the massage. The choice of essential oils will depend on many factors, such as whether or not there is an infection present, whether the asthma is known to be an allergic response, or whether emotional factors are involved. Bergamot, Camomile, Clary, Lavender, Neroli and Rose are all antispasmodic oils which happen also to be antidepressant, so they offer a wide choice if you know that stress and anxiety are factors to be considered.

Clary Sage

Of these, Bergamot and Lavender are also good for chest infections, and Camomile is always associated with the treatment of allergies. Another oil, which is not described by any of the standard reference works as being used for asthma, but which I have often found very helpful indeed, is Frankincense. Frankincense is often used for treating bronchitis and catarrh, so it can help where there is congestion and/or infection present, but I think that a more important factor is that it slows and deepens the breathing, which is why it is often used as an aid to meditation. This has a very calming effect, and I have found it one of the most beneficial oils of all for asthma sufferers.

Yoga and other forms of gentle exercise which improve posture and help to open the lungs are usually very helpful, and in many cases improved nutrition will reduce the number and severity of attacks.

Astrology

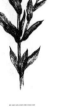

Many early physicians, from Avicenna right through to the renaissance herbalists, were astrologers as well. One of Nicolas Culpeper's many books was called 'The Astrological Judgement of the Sick'. Some modern aromatherapists also like to combine these two disciplines, making links between the essential oils chosen to treat an individual, and that individual's astrological chart. They use an astrological birth-chart to study areas of possible weakness in a person's physique or psyche, that might be assisted by the oils. For example, each sign of the Zodiac corresponds to a different area of the body and can alert the therapist to possible weaknesses. Planetary transits can highlight times when an individual may be more susceptible to illness or accidents.

The mediaeval and renaissance herbalists attributed a ruling planet to each medicinal herb, the character of the planet often being linked to the nature and properties of the herb concerned. For example 'fiery' or warming herbs such as Basil, Black Pepper, Garlic, Pine, etc., are seen as being governed by Mars, the fiery planet, and so forth. Venus rules cool and moist herbs: among the essential oils these are predominantly the flower oils such as Geranium and, above all, Rose. The Moon is the ruler of cold and moist herbs such as Camomile and the Sun of hot and dry ones like Angelica, Rosemary, Frankincense and Myrrh. Essential oils under the rulership of Mars are used at the physical level for cold, damp conditions or lack of stamina and at the mental/emotional level to give courage, combat inertia, etc. The Moon's oils are often good for heat and inflammation while Venus's oils often relate to female sexuality. If we compare these 'rulerships' with what we know about the properties of these oils, we can see many correspondences. This is perhaps a more poetic way of saying what we know to be from a scientific perspective.

Obviously, to work in this way requires either a detailed study of astrology on the part of the aromatherapist, or a close and sympathetic collaboration between an astrologer and the therapist. It is perhaps not an approach that would commend itself to everybody, but some very interesting and significant work has been done along these lines.

Athlete's Foot

Unfortunately, you don't need to be an athlete to suffer from this fungal infection, although the warm, damp conditions inside training shoes certainly favour its development, and changing rooms are a likely place to pick up the microscopic mould that is responsible. Several different types of mould or fungus which infect the outer layer of the skin can be the source and, even in orthodox medicine, treatment is often a matter of trial and error.

I have treated athlete's foot on various occasions with a combination of Lavender and Myrrh oils and with Ti-tree used on its own. All of these oils are fungicidal, and have other properties that help to soothe and heal the moist, itching and often cracked skin. If the skin is cracked and painful Calendula cream is very helpful. It is best to use the oils dissolved in alcohol for a few days until the moistness of the skin has dried out, and then continue treatment with an ointment or cream containing between 3% and 5% essential oils until the skin is completely clear.

It is important to clean repeatedly round toenails and fingernails, as the minute fungus often lodges under the nails and causes repeated infections.

Infection of this kind is not restricted to the feet, and may occur in the groin (common in hot climates, and nicknamed 'dhobie itch' by British troops in colonial times), between the fingers, and on the scalp – where it takes the form of ringworm (q.v.).

Aura

Also known as the etheric body, or subtle body. An area around the physical body, in which something of the person is still present. This is sometimes thought of as an energy field. Mystics have been aware of the existence of the aura for at least as long as we have records of human civilisation, and the haloes surrounding the Deity and saints in Western religious art, and round, oval or flame-like shapes surrounding the deities in Eastern religious art, are attempts to portray it. Twentieth century scientific discoveries offer explanations that some may find more acceptable. For example, we know that virtually all the body's activity is of an electro-chemical nature, and it seems likely that the energy generated extends beyond the body. Kirlian photography shows energy radiating as a visible pattern around human, animal and plant bodies alike. The aura can be seen by some sensitive people, but anybody can feel it, when giving massage, for example.

Aromatherapists take this into account when giving a massage, and may work in the aura as well as directly on the body, especially at the end of a 'hands-on' massage.

Avicenna

Abu Ali al-Husayn ibn Abd Allah ibn Sina, is understandably better known by the Latinised version of his name, Avicenna. He was one of the most outstanding of Arab physicians in an era when Arab medicine was the most advanced in the Western world.

He was born in 980 A.D. in the town of Bukhara in Persia (now in the Uzbeck state of the former Soviet Union). He was by all accounts an infant prodigy, and had memorised the Koran and quantities of Arab poetry by the time he was ten years old. His father provided him with tutors in logic, metaphysics, arithmetic and other sciences until he outgrew his tutors, and continued to educate himself, in subjects including Islamic law, astronomy and medicine until he was 18.

By the age of 21 he was already famed for his mastery of all branches of formal learning, and for his medical prowess, and became physician-in-chief to the hospital at Bhagdad. Inevitably, such a brilliant young man was invited to become personal physician to a succession of Caliphs, and almost equally inevitably, he attracted jealousy and intrigue, as a result of which he spent several periods in prison.

Even in prison he continued to study and to write, and he is said to have had such a strong physique that he withstood ordeals that would have killed a lesser man.

His two most important books were the 'Kitab ash-shifa' – 'The Book of Healing', which dealt with natural sciences, psychology, astronomy and music as well as purely medical matters; and the great 'Canon of Medicine' in which he summarised the medical knowledge of his Greek, Roman and Arab predecessors and added to it from his own experience. These books were translated into Latin in the 12th century, at the same period when mediaeval scholars were also rediscovering the work of Hippocrates, Galen and Dioscorides, and in this way Avicenna became a very important influence on European medical thought for several centuries.

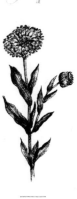

The importance of Avicenna to the history of aromatherapy is threefold, for he not only described accurately many hundreds of plants and their uses, and set down such accurate instructions on giving massage that they could be used today as a teaching manual now, but he is often credited with having discovered the method of distilling essential oils from flowers.

Archaeological finds indicate that a form of distillation existed before Avicenna's time, but it does seem probable that he considerably improved the technique by adding a cooling coil to the basic still. What is certain is that Rose Attar was produced in Persia during his lifetime, and there are some persuasive arguments for attributing this to him. Apart from his all-round brilliance as a scientist, poet, doctor and scholar, Avicenna was an alchemist, and roses had a very specific significance in alchemical experiments. White roses and red roses held different symbolic importance and were used at different stages of the work. They were placed in a flask, or alembic, and heated with other materials, the vapour so produced being collected in another flask as it cooled. Roses heated in this way produce rosewater, with a very small amount of rose oil, or attar, floating on the surface. Such an attribution is, of course, somewhat speculative, but it fits the known facts about Avicenna.

The medicinal plants described in his various writings amount to over 800, but we are not able to identify all of them accurately, as he used their vernacular names from India, Tibet and China, as well as the Middle East. Among those that we can identify, we find Lavender, Camomile and, of course, the ubiquitous Rose, all of them very valuable aromatherapy oils.

Avicenna wrote lucid descriptions of massage techniques, describing, for example, brisk friction to produce localised warmth and redness, and more gentle strokes which he prescribed for 'the softening of hard bodies'. Writing about massage for athletes he said, 'There is a friction of preparation, which comes before exercise . . . Then there is a friction of restoration, which comes after exercise and is called rest-inducing friction. The object of this is the resolution of superfluities retained in the muscles, not evacuated by exercise, that they may be evaporated, and that fatigue may not occur. This . . . must be done smoothly and gently.' It would be hard to better this advice, which corresponds almost to the letter to the regime followed today by some Olympic teams.

Some of Avicenna's medical thinking is astonishingly modern, and encompasses much that is valued in alternative medicine. As well as using massage, plants and plant oils, he originated various forms of manipulation for spinal problems (and traction for broken limbs), and either introduced, or at least popularised, the all-fruit diet as a cleansing process, using fruits rich in natural sugars, such as melons and grapes.

Avicenna died in 1037 A.D. from colic, when he was in a state of exhaustion after accompanying the Caliph on a military campaign.

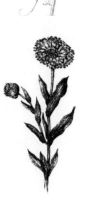

Ayurvedic Medicine

Many of the essential oils which we use in aromatherapy today are obtained from plants which have been used as part of traditional Indian herbal medicine, or Ayurveda, for thousands of years.

Ayurveda means 'laws of health' and is at least 3,000 years old. Like acupuncture in China, it is based on an underlying philosophy which relates man to the whole of nature and the cosmos, and in particular to the three elements of air, fire and water. These three elements are seen as influencing mental and physical health, and man is seen as a fusion of body, soul and psyche, three aspects, none of which can be treated without taking the others into consideration.

There has been increasing interest in traditional Ayurvedic practices in the West in recent years, and lectures, courses and seminars on this form of medicine are given from time to time, which any aromatherapist who wishes to extend his or her knowledge of the plants from which our oils are derived, would undoubtedly find interesting.

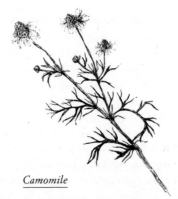

Camomile

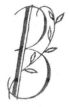

Babies

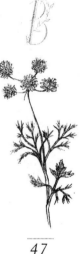

Aromatherapy can be used to advantage from the moment of birth (and indeed even before that – see the entry for **PREGNANCY**) provided that one or two commonsense precautions are borne in mind.

The oils and methods which are most helpful in infancy are described fairly fully under **CHILDREN**, but when thinking about babies, there are one or two additional factors to be considered. You will see in the entry for **CHILDREN** that essential oils should always be diluted before adding to the bath, and when we are thinking about young babies, this becomes even more important, because babies so often suck their thumbs or hands, and rub their fists into their eyes. Undiluted essential oil will stay on the surface of the water in an ultra-fine film, and this can very easily be transferred from the baby's hand to the mouth or eyes, with dangerous consequences. Essential oil should always be kept away from the eyes, even when dealing with adults, as it can irritate the cornea; and whereas in an adult this may be merely unpleasant, in a young baby it could cause permanent damage to the eye and possible deterioration of vision. Undiluted oils in the mouth could be damaging to the sensitive tissue inside the mouth, or more important, may be swallowed and cause damage to the stomach lining.

Before putting essential oils in the bath, they should be added either to a few teaspoons of almond, soya or other bland oil, or to a cup of milk (not skimmed) and well mixed before adding to the bath. A single drop of oil of Camomile or Lavender will be sufficient in a baby bath to ease minor discomforts and promote sleep. Regular addition of the oils to the bath is a good preventative measure against nappy-rash, as almost all essential oils will prevent bacteria developing on the skin for some time.

If nappy-rash does become a problem, creams containing oil of Calendula or Camomile are very healing, and Benzoin or Myrrh might be added if the skin is cracked and slow to heal.

A safe and effective way of using essential oils to help with coughs, colds and other respiratory ailments of young babies, is to simply place a drop of an appropriate oil on the sheet in the cot, so that the baby will continually inhale the vaporised oil. This method can safely be used for babies from a few days old. Another helpful method is to spray or vaporise essential oils in the baby's room, either to help a cold or a cough, or to encourage sleep.

A single drop of Lavender oil on the nightie or pyjamas of a restless baby or toddler will often work like magic. I have known babies to sleep for up to 14 hours after this was done, giving a great deal of relief to the mother and the rest of the family too.

If a baby is in pain due to colic, gentle massage on the tummy will help to ease the discomfort. Put 2 drops of oil of Camomile or Lavender in a teaspoon of almond, soya or other bland oil (you might like to warm it a little first) and oil your hand with it, then work, always in a clockwise direction, with firm but gentle movements on the baby's abdomen for about five minutes. If the baby does not respond to this, you could also try lying him or her across your knees face down and gently massaging the lower back.

Many babies suffer earache when they are teething, or when they have a cold. The safest way to ease the pain is to massage gently round the outside of the ear, and maybe a little down the neck, using diluted oil of Camomile (see entry for Otitis for details of dilution, etc.). If the earache persists, do not hesitate to consult your doctor.

see also entries for **CHILDREN, EARACHE, TEETHING, COLDS,** *and* **BATHS.**

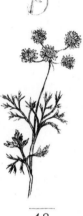

Bach Flower Remedies

Bach Flower Remedies are sometime confused with aromatherapy, because both are prepared from plants. Although they are, in fact, rather different ways of using the energy of plants in healing, they are totally compatible with each other, and I quite often suggest Bach remedies to be used at the same time as essential oils.

The remedies are prepared in a completely different way from essential oils. Whereas the latter are highly concentrated substances usually extracted from the plant by distillation, the Bach remedies are made by floating the flowers on clear spring water and exposing them to sunshine until the flower's healing energies have been transferred into the water. This is then put into clean bottles, with an equal amount of brandy to act as a preservative, and this forms the 'Stock Bottle'. A few drops of this mixture can be put into another clean bottle, filled with half spring water and half brandy as before and used as a remedy. You will see that the dilution begins to resemble that of homoeopathic remedies, and in fact Dr. Bach was a homoeopath before he began to develop this system of healing.

The remedies work at an extremely subtle level. Each of them is associated with a certain mental/emotional state, or a personality trait, which, in the experience of Dr. Bach, affected the way that different people reacted to physical illness. By healing the mind, the body could be healed too. There are thirty-eight remedies in all and one person may have need of a variety of them in different circumstances and at different times in his or her life. Some practitioners develop such an intimate knowledge of the properties and appropriate uses of each remedy that they can 'match' each one to a person's needs intuitively, while others dowse with a pendulum to find the most appropriate one. Alternatively, there are several excellent reference books which act as guides to the most appropriate remedy.

By far the best known of the Bach remedies is the Rescue Remedy, which is a mixture of several plants. It can be used in every kind of emergency, both physical and emotional, and does not need any special knowledge. It is one of the best antidotes to shock that I have ever known, and can also be used before a traumatic event, such as a surgical operation, or a particularly important interview or examination, to minimise bad reactions. I am never without a bottle of

Rose

Rescue Remedy in my handbag. It is simple to use – simply put a few drops on the tongue, and if somebody is unconscious or unable to swallow, it is equally effective to moisten the lips with the remedy.

In recent years, healers using Dr. Bach's methods have found many more plants to prepare in the same way and the number of flower remedies now available totals several hundreds. These newer remedies are often known as 'flower essences' which sometimes causes confusion with aromatherapy.

Dr. Edward Bach

Dr. Edward Bach, the discoverer of the thirty-eight flower remedies that bear his name, was born in 1886 in Warwickshire. His family had Welsh roots and he was always very fond of Wales, where he later discovered the first of the remedies.

He was trained initially in orthodox medicine at University College Hospital, where he also held several important posts, but later turned to homoeopathy as a way to treat the whole person, which was nearer to his own ideals. He made several important developments based on Hahnneman's principles, but eventually even this was not a sensitive enough way for him to heal the sick, and he began to seek out other methods.

He left London and began to wander in the countryside, often sleeping out of doors, very close to nature, and developing a great sensitivity towards plants and their energy. Without his medical appointments and private practice, he found himself living on very little money: at times he was quite literally penniless, but friends and grateful former patients more than once came to the rescue unasked.

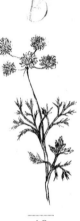

His sensitivity was such that when he was seeking the right plant to cure a particular condition, he would himself develop symptoms of that condition, which would get more intense as he came nearer to finding the plant he was looking for. Because of this, and his poverty and vagrant lifestyle, his own health suffered, but this did not deter him from continuing his work and making it known in various books and pamphlets. He died in November 1936, exhausted by his work and by the persecutions he had suffered from the General Medical Council.

Backache

More people consult alternative therapists about back pain than for any other reason, and the causes of their pain are very diverse. The right form of treatment – chiropractice or osteopathy, acupuncture, Alexander technique, massage with or without essential oils – needs to be carefully chosen in relation to the source of the back pain.

Aromatherapy massage is a very effective form of treatment where the pain is due to muscular fatigue, spasm or tension, and there are a large number of essential oils that will help both to reduce pain in the short term and treat the muscular problem in the longer term. Lavender, Marjoram and Rosemary are the essential oils most often used, sometimes with an oil from one of the warming spices, such as Black Pepper or Ginger where there is acute pain.

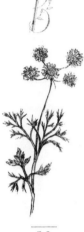

Rosem

A well trained aromatherapist will have a good knowledge of anatomy and will be able to decide whether to refer a patient to an osteopath or chiropractor for manipulation. Even if there is no apparent displacement in the spine or other joints, back pain that is not improved after three or four massages with essential oils needs to be investigated further. Apart from such obvious causes as sporting injury, domestic or industrial strains such as heavy lifting, bad posture, faulty seating at work or in a car, back pain can arise from a number of mental, emotional or physical problems. Backache may be a symptom of kidney infection or disease, of various gynaecological problems or of degenerative conditions of the spine itself, and these possibilities must be investigated by a properly qualified specialist in that field.

A great deal of back pain arises from stress. Many people respond to stress by tensing muscles, usually without realising that they are doing so, and the back is one of the areas most often affected. The upper back, neck and shoulders are very often the site of such tensions, and tension in the neck can often affect the lower (sacral) area of the back as well. Aromatherapy is one of the best forms of treatment, since massage with the oils not only relieves the physical pain but can reduce the stress which has given rise to it. Massage is a valuable way of re-educating tense muscles. Many people are not aware of just how much tension they are holding in some areas of the body, and the degree of relaxation that can be achieved through massage is a very good way of learning to let go of that physical tension. Essential oils can be sensitively chosen to help with the mental/emotional stress that has given rise to the physical tension.

Aromatic baths are a very useful form of self-help when backache is caused by tension, using relaxing, painkilling and antidepressant oils, either between visits to a therapist for massage, or to prevent tensions building up to the state where help is needed.

When manipulation for any spinal or other displacement is needed, massage with essential oils both before and after the manipulation can reduce pain and increase the effectiveness of the treatment. An increasing number of osteopaths insist on a thorough massage of the affected area before they begin manipulation. Some carry this out themselves, while others employ masseurs in their clinics to do this for them. Some stretching of the muscles is inevitable in any manipulation, but if the muscles are warmed and relaxed beforehand this can be minimised. Following manipulation, this stretching can give rise to some surface soreness but massaging with analgesic oils will reduce this. It will also help the muscles to recover strength and tone, and essential oils such as Rosemary will make the progress more effective.

Many back injuries which require manipulation arise because of poor muscle tone, when the muscles are no longer capable of doing their job of supporting the individual vertebrae of the spine, or the various joints associated with it, such as the fixed joint where the sacrum (part of the lower spine) meets the ilium (part of the massive hip-bone). In the long run, the best way to increase muscle tone is exercise, but the exercise must be carefully chosen to improve the condition of the back without placing further strain on it. Osteopaths will often give advice on suitable exercise, and yoga teachers will be able to give expert advice, too. In the short term, exercise is usually best avoided and the back rested until the injury or displacement has been successfully treated.

The best form of treatment for backache is prevention, and regular aromatic baths and massage with essential oils can help to prevent pain by reducing stress, improving muscle tone, relaxing tight muscles and improving the general level of well-being.

Bacteriostatics

A bacteriostatic is any substance which inhibits the growth of bacteria. It may not destroy bacteria, but it will help to halt the growth of the organisms so that they do not present a threat to health.

The human body can deal efficiently with the many different bacteria that it encounters at every moment of each day, and it is only when a particular strain of bacteria begin to multiply rapidly that the body's defences may not be adequate, so restricting the spread of bacteria is a valuable aspect of preventative medicine.

All essential oils are bacteriostatic to a greater or lesser degree. Some are effective against a limited group of bacteria, and others against a very wide range, and the amount of essential oil needed to produce a bacteriostatic effect is very small indeed. Among the most effective oils for this purpose are Clove, Lavender, Rosemary, Sage and Thyme, and indeed all the herbs which have been traditionally used in cooking have this property, even in very low concentrations.

Baldness

It is important to distinguish between permanent, progressive baldness in men – which is described as 'male pattern baldness' and is usually hereditary and thought to be linked to levels of the male hormone, testosterone – and various forms of temporary hair loss which may occur in men, women and children and can be due to illness, stress, poor nutrition, drugs or other causes.

Whatever claims have been made on behalf of various 'cures' for baldness, there is no evidence that anything can restore hair once it has stopped growing, though it is just possible that treatment of the scalp to improve the health of follicles from which the hairs grow, may be effective if applied at the very first signs of hair loss.

Of all the essential oils, the one that is particularly associated with the health of the hair and scalp is Rosemary, and regular vigorous massage of the scalp with Rosemary may help. Massage will, in any case, increase local circulation, which will bring a greater volume of oxygenated blood to the scalp and may help the hair follicles that way. Such traditional treatments as rubbing a freshly cut onion on the scalp, or laying stinging nettles on it, are in fact based on the same principle of increasing the local circulation.

Temporary baldness can often be treated very effectively. The Latin term ALOPECIA is used to denote this kind of baldness, in order to make clear the distinction between it and male pattern baldness, and aromatherapy treatments are described under that heading.

51

Basil

Ocimum basilicum

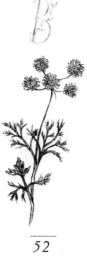

The Basil plant takes its name from the Greek word for a king – 'basileum', possibly because the plant was so highly prized that it was considered a King among plants, or maybe because it was an ingredient of an oil for anointing kings. Sir John Parkinson in his herbal says, 'The smell thereof is so excellent that it is fit for a king's house.' The plant is still greatly valued in present-day Greece, both for cooking and as a medicinal herb, and has various popular names, such as 'Joy of the Mountains' and 'Boy's Joy'. Pots of it may be found placed at the foot of the pulpit in Greek churches.

The plant grows wild all over the Mediterranean, especially on sunny hillsides, and there are a number of varieties, varying in height, colour of leaves, etc. The leaves may be a very dark green, or may be lighter and hairy, narrow or straight. The scent also varies, in some cases resembling Fennel or Tarragon, but the variety used in aromatherapy has pale pink flowers, hairy oval leaves and its own characteristic scent which is a little like that of Thyme, but hotter and more spicy. Although the plant has naturalised in the Mediterranean and many other parts of Europe, it is a native of Asia, and has a long history of use in Indian traditional medicine.

The essential oil is yellowish, and its active principles include methylchavicol (40% to 50%) with linalol, cineol, eugenol, pinene and camphor.

Basil has been used since antiquity for chest infections, digestive problems and jaundice and some writers consider it an aphrodisiac. By the 16th century it was widely used for headaches, migraines and head-colds, being made into a powder and inhaled like snuff to clear the head! We may find inhaling the essential oil a more civilised method, but it is still used for the same problems. It is also an excellent cephalic, second only to Rosemary in its clarifying effect on the brain, so it is good for mental fatigue. It is certainly an oil that can be described as uplifting and one early herbalist said that Basil 'expels melancholy vapours from the heart'.

Major uses include treating all kinds of respiratory infections, including bronchitis and whooping cough, and many feverish conditions. It is also antispasmodic, and massage over the stomach with Basil will ease many digestive difficulties. It can be used, again in gentle massage over the abdomen, to assist scanty and painful periods.

As a massage oil, Basil may perhaps not be a popular choice used alone, but blends well with other oils, especially Lavender, and is very good for tired, tight, overworked muscles. It is especially good for athletes, dancers and other people engaged in strenuous physical activities.

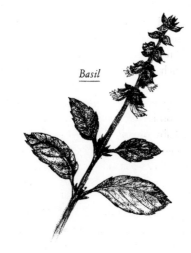

Basil

Some lesser, but welcome uses include compresses to reduce engorgement of the breasts, and as a mouthwash which is very effective for mouth ulcers and gum infections.

Basil is a generally tonic and stimulating oil, but if used to excess has the opposite effect.

When used in the bath it makes the skin tingle, and could be irritant to people with sensitive skins. Used in dilution it is good for the skin, and improves the tone and appearance.

Baths

Bathing is as old as civilisation, and archaeological remains show that as soon as people began to live together in towns they built baths, which were usually communal, and became a focus of social life – at least for the more leisured. References to aromatic baths are found in the early records of many civilisations. Hippocrates wrote that 'a perfumed bath and a scented massage every day is the way to good health' indicating that the medicinal and the pleasurable aspects of bathing overlapped to a great extent, then as now.

The earliest and simplest method of perfuming a bath was to tie a bundle of aromatic herbs or sweet-smelling flowers in a cloth and place this in the water. Liquid extracts from the plants, made by boiling or steeping, are another way of adding the scent and medicinal properties of a plant to bath water, but essential oils offer an extremely easy and attractive way of adding the properties of healing plants to the therapeutic power of water itself.

Aromatic baths are one of the most important and versatile forms of treatment in aromatherapy. A bath with essential oils can be relaxing or sedative, stimulating, tonic, aphrodisiac, warming or cooling. It can give relief from muscular pain and skin conditions and act as a treatment or preventative measure for many physical conditions, depending simply on the choice of oils added to the bath. However, it is in reducing stress that aromatic baths are perhaps the most valuable in twentieth-century society. The incidence of stress-related illness makes such a simple technique for self-help a welcome one, and one of the most important aspects of aromatic baths is the fact that they can be taken at home, at will, either between visits to a therapist or (to a certain extent) taking the place of the other treatment, though it is wise to consult a trained aromatherapist about the most suitable oils to use. Baths can be combined with almost any other form of treatment, whether 'orthodox' or otherwise, except homoeopathy, as some strong scents can antidote homoeopathic remedies. If you are taking such a remedy, consult your homoeopath to find out whether the essential oils you would like to use in baths are likely to interfere with your treatment. For any given property, there will usually be a choice of several oils and some are less likely to act as an antidote than others.

The method of preparing an aromatic bath is very simple: fill the bath first with comfortably hot water, and just before getting into the bath, sprinkle about 6 drops of essential oil onto the water and stir it around with your hand to disperse the oil. Do not prepare the bath in advance, as you would then lose much of the value of the highly volatile oils.

You may prefer to add the essential oil to a carrier oil, or some other dilutant, such as milk or vodka, before adding it to the water, especially if you have sensitive skin. Dilution in this way is essential if you are making a bath for a baby or young child.

The small amount of essential oil in relation to the amount of water in an average bath may surprise you, but this is quite enough. The oil spreads out to form a very thin film on the surface of the water, and some of this will adhere to your skin as you get into the bath. The heat of the water aids absorption of the oil through the skin, and some of the oil will also be released as an aromatic vapour and breathed in. Fifteen to twenty minutes in the bath is enough time to allow the oils to take effect.

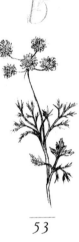

53

CAUTION
● Never use essential oils in their pure state in baths for babies or young children, but dilute them before adding to the bath water in a bland oil, such as almond, or in two or three tablespoons of full-fat milk. Essential oils are so highly concentrated that there is a risk of them irritating the delicate stomach lining if swallowed undiluted, and as babies often suck their thumbs or

put their fingers in their mouths, it is vital to ensure there is no risk of them picking up undiluted oil from the surface of the bath on their hands. Undiluted oil can also damage the cornea of the eye, and babies often rub their fingers in their eyes, too. A single drop of essential oil, suitably diluted, is enough to put in a baby-bath, and two or three drops can be used for a toddler who is being bathed in a full-sized bath.

● Some essential oils can irritate the skin, so should not be used in baths. See Appendix A for details of irritant oils. People with sensitive skins may experience irritation from oils that are not classed as such, and should always dilute the oils before putting them in a bath.

Angelica root oil has a photosensitising action similar to Bergamot. Do not use on any area of skin that will be exposed to sunlight.

The choice of oils will depend on the effect you hope to produce. The descriptions of individual oils in this book will help you to choose a suitable oil or combination, but some of the most valuable and frequently used are: Lavender, to relax, ease muscular tension and promote sound sleep; Camomile, also to help with sleep and to soothe allergic skin conditions; Marjoram, to counteract chilling and ease muscular pain; Rosemary, to stimulate, especially in morning baths and Grapefruit, for its cheering, uplifting effect and for its antiseptic and deodorant properties. Almost any essential oil can be used for bathing, with the exception of skin irritants and photosensitising oils. See **CAUTION** on this and previous page. The relaxation produced by a perfumed bath is as beneficial now as in Hippocrates' time, and you need not wait to be in pain or ill before allowing yourself this pleasure. In choosing oils simply for the enjoyment of their perfume, though, it is wise to check their major properties so you can avoid using a stimulating oil at night or a powerfully sedative one in the morning, for example.

---

see also **FOOTBATHS** *and the entries for individual oils. Some suggested bath blends are given in* **APPENDIX C.**

Beeswax

Beeswax is used in the making of creams and ointments which are used as carriers for essential oils, both for cosmetic purposes and in treating skin disorders.

The function of beeswax is to thicken the oils to a suitable consistency in creams that are made with oil alone, and also to act as an emulsifier in creams that include a flower-water or distilled or spring water.

Beeswax has therapeutic properties of its own – in common with honey, propolis and royal jelly – and this makes it a better choice for making creams than inert waxes of mineral origin. Natural unbleached beeswax is preferable to the bleached white kind, as the latter may contain some traces of chemical bleaching agents.

Benzoin
Styrax benzoin

Benzoin is derived from a tree which grows in Thailand and adjacent islands. It is not, strictly speaking, an essential oil, as pure Benzoin is a resin, and has to be melted by heating over hot water before it can be used. When you buy Benzoin from an essential oil supplier it is usually dissolved in ethyl glycol, but this product is not very satisfactory from the point of view of a natural therapy using plant products, so it is worth finding a supplier who dissolves the Benzoin resin in wood alcohol, or buying it in the solid state and melting it when needed.

The granulated gum, called 'gum Benjamin' in old herbals, is a dark reddish-brown, and is often used as a fixative in pot pourris, but the form in which Benzoin is probably best known is as 'Friar's Balsam' or compound tincture of benzoin. The active constituents of pure Benzoin include benzoic acid, benzoresinol, siaresinotannol and vanillin, which gives it its characteristic 'ice cream' aroma.

Like Myrrh and Frankincense, Benzoin has been used for thousands of years as an ingredient of incense, and to drive out evil spirits, and like these two it is both soothing and stimulating. It is also very warming, and this makes it particularly helpful for colds, 'flu, coughs and sore throats. Its use in the form of Friar's Balsam, as an inhalation for sore throats and loss of voice, is probably its best known virtue. Because of its ability to stimulate at the same time as soothing, it seems to 'get things moving' in the body, whether it is clearing mucus, stimulating the circulation, expelling gas or increasing the flow of urine. It is very comforting for griping pains in the stomach, and for urinary tract infections.

Benzoin is used for healing many kinds of skin lesions, from cracked and chapped hands to chilblains. Friar's Balsam has long been used by ballet dancers to heal cracked toes and prevent further cracking. I often put Benzoin into hand creams for people who work in the open – gardeners, foresters, builders, etc., usually adding Lemon and/or Lavender, to mask the vanilla smell and contribute their own healing properties.

On the psychological plane, as with many essential oils, we find a parallel with its physical properties – warming, soothing and stimulating. I use Benzoin to help people who are sad and lonely, depressed or anxious. It combines well with Rose, and I can recall being greatly helped through several crises in my own life by receiving massage with this blend, as well as being able to help many other people in the same way. We might perhaps see here an echo of its former use to 'cast out devils', for what are the devils of our time, if not such psychological states as these.

Bergamot
Citrus bergamia

The Bergamot tree takes its name from the small town of Bergamo in Northern Italy, around which it was originally cultivated. The fruit (like a miniature orange), has been used for hundreds of years in Italian folk medicine, but not in that of other countries, as the tree was almost unknown outside Italy, and the fruit was not exported until relatively recent times.

The oil is obtained by simple pressure from the rind of the fruit, and although various attempts to mechanise the process have been tried, the best oil is still that which is hand-pressed. As you might expect, it has a delightfully fresh, citrussy aroma, which is almost universally liked. The active constituents include linalyl acetate, limonene and linalol, and the essential oil is of a delicate green colour.

The three main areas in which the oil is uniquely valuable are: urinary tract infection, depression and anxiety, and skin care.

Bergamot oil has a strong affinity for the urino-genital tract, and is one of the most valuable oils (along with Camomile, Sandalwood and Ti-tree) in treating cystitis and urethritis. Many cases of cystitis begin as urethritis, and the infection travels up the urethra to the bladder. Bergamot oil, used in the very early stages, can often prevent the infection from spreading upwards in this way. It should be added to the bath, and used as a local wash (diluted to 1% or even 0.5%). As a local wash, it is also valuable for the relief of vaginal itching and mild discharges (though it is important to ensure that the cause of any discharge is investigated). If an attack of cystitis does not respond to treatment, particularly if there is fever, medical help should be sought without delay.

Bergamot is especially valuable to people who suffer from recurrent attacks of cystitis, as it is a powerful disinfectant of the urinary system.

Many people with recurrent cystitis are also tense, anxious or depressed, and this can become a vicious circle, in which the tension sparks off an attack, and the lowering effects of the illness lead to even greater depression. Although Camomile and Ti-tree are both valuable for the physical treatment of this debilitating condition, there is nothing better than Bergamot to break this chain reaction, by relieving the tension and depression, whilst actively treating the physical causes.

In helping with mental and psychological states, Bergamot is almost the most valuable oil at the aromatherapist's disposal. It is often described as 'uplifting' and I cannot improve on this description. My own experience has verified this quality of Bergamot again and again. (I have come across a lot of people who confuse 'uplifting' with 'stimulant', so I would point out here that Bergamot is not a stimulant oil – it lifts the spirits but is relatively relaxing.) For all tense, anxious or depressed people, Bergamot should be used in a massage oil (either alone or in a variety of blends) as the human contact with the therapist is an important factor in such situations; but daily use as a bath oil, room fragrance or personal perfume can be very valuable additions to the treatment. The fragrance is equally acceptable to men and women, and it blends with almost any flower oil, giving it considerable versatility. Lavender/Bergamot, Geranium/Bergamot or all three of these oils together, are some of the most pleasing combinations. It is particularly valuable for adding a sharper note to some of the oils which may be over-sweet to some people's tastes.

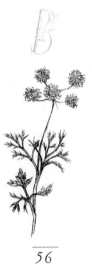

Dr. Jean Valnet mentions the use of Bergamot for loss of appetite, and this, combined with its powerful antidepressant properties, would seem to indicate a valuable possibility for helping in anorexia nervosa. However, my own experience suggests that its effect on the appetite is regulating rather than stimulant, and I have used it to help compulsive eaters. It may be that Bergamot directly influences the appetite-control centre in the brain, or that, by working with the underlying tensions that have provoked the under- or over-eating, it enables the sufferer to return to a normal weight and eating pattern. Perhaps it should be pointed out that this is not an overnight 'cure', but a process that involves great sensitivity on the part of the therapist, and a will to get better on the part of the person seeking help.

The antiseptic properties of Bergamot, allied to its really delicious fragrance, make it my first choice for treating acne, oily skins and all infected skin conditions. It can be used in a massage oil for facial treatments, or blended in creams, lotions or aromatic waters. A hot compress of Bergamot can be used on boils to draw out the infection and promote healing, though a person with boils should also be advised on dietary and other ways of eliminating toxins.

Bergamot is cooling in feverish conditions. It is an ingredient of Earl Grey tea, and of 'real' eau de cologne, both of which have a cooling and uplifting effect. It is an excellent deodorant, both for personal use and for rooms and buildings. It is also an effective insect repellent, and is used commercially for this purpose. It needs to be re-applied fairly often, and is probably more effective in a blend with Lavender and other oils.

Bergamot has been used with success in treating respiratory and digestive problems, but there is such a wealth of oils to choose from in these areas that I tend to keep Bergamot for the special uses in which it is unrivalled.

Bergamot inhibits certain viruses, in particular the herpes simplex I virus, which causes cold sores. Most people carry this virus all their lives, though blisters only appear when the individual is run down or has some other infection (typically, a cold).

Bergamot, either alone or combined with Eucalyptus, which is another powerful anti-viral agent, can be dabbed onto the site of the sore, either neat or, preferably, diluted in a little alcohol, at the first sign of an eruption. It may allay the pain of shingles, caused by the herpes zoster virus, the same organism responsible for chickenpox, and I have used the oil to considerably reduce the discomfort of chickenpox in children, and hasten the young patient's recovery.

Caution: Bergamot is a photosensitiser: that is to say, it increases the skin's reaction to sunlight and makes it more likely to burn. It used to be added to tanning preparations to speed up tanning but this was discontinued some years ago because it was thought to increase the risk of skin cancer. Thinning of the Ozone layer has greatly increased this risk. If using Bergamot in massage oils, bath oils or skin preparations during sunny weather it should be kept to less than 2% of the total as concentrations lower than 2% do not appear to have a photosensitising effect. Never use Bergamot undiluted on exposed areas of skin, as quite severe burning can result.

Remember that undiluted oil used in the bath makes a fine film on top of the water and can therefore deposit it over a large area of the body. Mix Bergamot in a carrier oil before adding to the bath to avoid this. Bear in mind that the photosensitising effect lasts for several days.

Birch
Betula lenta, and B. alleghaniensis

The Black Birch (Betula lenta) and Yellow Birch (B. alleghaniensis) are native to North America and both yield essential oils that have only one major constituent – methyl salicylate. Methyl salicylate was first identified in Willow trees, but is best known in its synthesized form as aspirin, which will immediately give you a good idea of the properties of Birch oil. It is analgesic, anti-inflammatory and reduces fever: all uses to which aspirin is put in conventional medicine. Birch oil is also a diuretic and blood-cleanser, and is rubefacient (locally warming). Although methyl salicylate may account for as much as 98% of the essential oil, the remaining 2% must not be disregarded: in aromatherapy, as in herbal medicine, tiny fractions of an oil contribute to its total action and often act as buffers which prevent the side effects seen in isolated or synthesized forms. The smell is very piercing and reminiscent of old-fashioned liniments.

Birch needs to be handled cautiously, as the analogy to aspirin suggests, but it has one or two valuable applications in aromatherapy and I have found it particularly useful in situations where other oils have been tried with little success. It is good for all kinds of muscular pain, being a very strong analgesic and a fairly mild rubefacient. In rheumatism and arthritis it helps to drain the toxins which are the cause of pain.

In treating cellulite, I have seen Birch give dramatic results when treatment with Rosemary, Geranium, Black Pepper and Juniper has not succeeded. It helps eliminate toxins, and the diuretic action reduces the oedema.

There is one group of inflammatory conditions for which Birch is my first choice of oil, rather than the last resource, namely tenosynovitis. Any tendon can become inflamed through over-use, usually due to repetitive tasks, but the tendons of the ankles and wrists are particularly susceptible. These tendons are enclosed in a slippery sheath which can also become inflamed. The condition is very painful and often takes a long time to get better. Birch helps to reduce both the pain and the inflammation.

CAUTION
Keep Birch oil tightly secured and away from children. Do not use during pregnancy.

Birch Bud
Betula alba

ॐ

White Birch is the Silver Birch native to Northern Europe. It yields a quite different oil to the N. American Birch species described above and is used mainly to treat chronic skin conditions, although some of its uses and properties overlap with those of Black and Yellow Birch.

The essential oil is extracted from the leaf-buds by steam distillation. It is pale yellow, with a woody scent and contains mainly betulenol. Birch-tar is produced by dry distillation from the bark and Birch-tar oil can then be obtained by steam distillation of the tar. It has a smoky, leathery aroma.

Birch has been used as a diuretic, blood-cleanser and skin treatment since at least the Middle Ages, especially in Northern Europe where the trees are native. As early as the 12th century, the Abbess Hildegard of Bingen mentioned Birch for healing ulcers, though it is not always certain whether these early writers are referring to the crude tar, an oil, the sap or an infusion of the leaves.

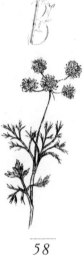

Birch bud oil is used for dermatitis, chronic eczema, boils and ulcers and may help psoriasis: this is always a difficult condition to treat and it is helpful to have another oil to add to the few that seem to help. It is sometimes used in alcohol-based frictions or in shampoo to treat dandruff.

It is a good diuretic for use in cellulite and all kinds of oedema and helps to eliminate uric acid accumulations in rheumatism and arthritis.

Birch-tar oil is used in perfumery, soap-manufacture, etc. and is the basis of all 'Russian leather' type perfumes.

Do take care when using any Birch oil that you are totally sure of the exact botanical origin because, despite some overlapping, the chemistry and properties are not the same.

Bleeding

ॐ

Several essential oils are haemostatic, i.e. they help to stop bleeding by speeding up the coagulation of the blood. The most useful of these is oil of Lemon, though Geranium and Rose have similar, though less powerful, effects.

Diluted oil of Lemon can be used on all cuts, grazes and minor injuries to stop bleeding. Either pour it simply over the wound, or if the cut is deep and bleeding continues, soak a wad of gauze in the dilute lemon and press it firmly against the wound. NEVER USE OIL OF LEMON UNDILUTED IN SUCH CIRCUMSTANCES. It is powerful enough to 'burn out' warts and verrucas, so dilute it in boiled and cooled water to 1% to 1.5%. Freshly squeezed lemon juice can be just as effective. Lemon is a good antiseptic which makes it doubly helpful for minor injuries, and it can be used mixed in equal proportions with Lavender to reinforce the antiseptic property. For more serious injuries, use Lemon as first aid until qualified help arrives.

Nosebleeds can be halted by soaking a pad of gauze in dilute Lemon oil, or lemon juice and pushing this as far up the nostril as possible. Let the person with the nosebleed lie down quietly until bleeding stops.

Bleeding following the extraction of a tooth can be minimised in the same way, by pressing a lemon-soaked swab over the gum or holding some lemon juice or dilute oil of Lemon in the mouth for a while. It should not be swilled around like a mouthwash, as the disturbance will prevent the blood clotting.

Oil of Cypress helps to reduce excessive menstrual bleeding (see also under Menstruation) and there are a number of oils recommended for haemorrhage, but they should be regarded as first-aid measures only, and the cause of any internal bleeding must be investigated by a doctor or other suitably qualified person. Anti-haemorrhage oils include the two already mentioned, and Geranium, Rose, Eucalyptus and possibly Myrrh.

Blisters

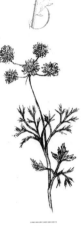

Blisters, of the kind that occur due to rubbing by shoes, are best dealt with by covering with a gauze that has had a few drops of Lavender oil sprinkled on it. If the blister is large, it may be more comfortable to puncture it with a thoroughly sterilised needle, and then apply neat Lavender oil and a gauze covering. Oil of Myrrh added in equal proportions to the Lavender is valuable if the blister remains very damp, and oil of Benzoin can be used after initial treatment with Lavender, to help the skin heal.

Do not cover the blister with a plaster that lets in little or no air, but anchor a gauze dressing in place with plaster strips so that the skin can 'breathe' and leave off shoes and socks for as much of each day as is possible until the blister has healed.

People who are particularly liable to get blisters – joggers, hikers, athletes and ballet dancers, for example – use tincture of Benzoin (Friar's Balsam) painted on the toes, or other vulnerable parts of the foot, both to prevent and to heal blisters.

Blood Pressure

The pressure at which blood is pumped by the heart into the major arteries. This pressure remains fairly constant in the major arteries, as they are wide enough not to slow down the flow from the heart. As the arteries sub-divide into minor arteries and arterioles they become narrow enough to reduce the flow and the original pressure is much lower. By the time the blood reaches the tiny capillaries, the pressure is only sufficient to resist back-pressure of tissue fluids and to carry the blood on into the veins. The blood pressure in the veins on the journey back to the heart is so low that it has to be helped along by pressure from surrounding muscles.

Blood pressure varies with the heartbeat, being higher on the systole when the heart contracts and pumps out blood, and lower on the diastole, when the heart relaxes and fills with blood from the veins. With some individual variations, normal blood pressure is about 2.4 lbs per square inch on the systole and 1.6 lbs per square inch on the diastole. This is usually measured by means of a sphygmomanometer which is is an inflatable cuff used for measuring the blood pressure in the brachial artery, where it is nearly the same as at the outlet from the heart. The pressure within the cuff raises the mercury in a tube (just as the atmospheric pressure does in a barometer) and the blood pressure is then read off in terms of the height of the column of mercury. The average normal reading is 120 millimetres of mercury at the systole and 80 millimetres at the diastole. This is written down as 120:80. Electronic measuring equipment is gradually superseding the sphygmomanometer.

The blood pressure, in fact, varies from moment to moment, according to the body's immediate requirements, and complicated chemical and nervous controls monitor the necessary adjustments all the time. The pressure is delicately balanced by constant adjustments between the rate of flow, i.e. the amount of blood being pumped out of the heart, and the resistance of the arteries. The rate of flow may vary from about 5 litres per minute when the body is at rest, to as much as 40 litres per minute during extreme exertion, so the pressure has to be adjusted by variations in the width of the blood vessels. Individual organs need greater or lesser amounts of blood at different times, for example the stomach after a meal, or the muscles of the legs when running a race, and this is governed by a widening of the arteries of the organ concerned, and a corresponding narrowing of other arteries. This widening and narrowing of the arteries is governed by the sympathetic nervous system and certain hormones.

The needs of the brain, though, are constant. Whether the body is working flat out or resting, the brain needs about 750 cubic centimetres of fresh blood every minute, and maintaining the supply to the brain is one of the most important functions of the blood pressure regulating mechanisms. Too little blood reaching the brain due to a drop in blood pressure, causes dizziness and possible loss of consciousness (fainting).

Too high a level of blood pressure is potentially damaging to the heart and blood vessels, so the body mechanisms work constantly to maintain the pressure within fairly narrow limits.

A number of essential oils are effective in lowering high blood pressure or raising low blood pressure and these are described under the entries for Hypertension (High blood pressure) and Hypotension (Low blood pressure).

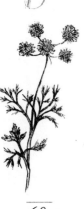

Boils

Hot compresses with essential oils can be used to 'draw out' a boil and speed healing, the most suitable being Ti-tree and Lavender because of their antiseptic properties, though Camomile is useful, too. The whole area around the boil should be washed several times a day with a 1% to 3% dilution of Lavender or Ti-tree.

A person suffering from boils, especially if they are numerous or recur frequently, needs help in reducing the level of toxicity in the body, and regular massage and/or baths, using purifying and detoxifying oils such as Juniper or Lavender are valuable. Garlic perles taken daily will help with the detoxifying process, and so will herbal teas or infusions, particularly fennel and nettle. Dietary advice may be needed, particularly to guide the sufferer away from over-refined foods, and towards a diet high in fresh fruit and vegetables. Vitamin and mineral supplements may be needed until the body returns to normal.

Boils often appear when a person's resistance has been lowered by illness or stress, and other essential oils and treatments might be needed to help with this state of lowered vitality that has contributed to the outbreak of boils.

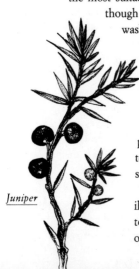

Juniper

Breastfeeding

Essential oils can be very helpful in easing some of the problems and discomforts which may arise during breastfeeding, and which might otherwise cause a mother to abandon this natural method and switch to bottle feeding. Cracked nipples and insufficiency of milk are the two major reasons mentioned by mothers for giving up breastfeeding, though too much milk, leading to painful engorgement of the breasts is sometimes a cause.

A number of plants, mostly of the Umbelliferae family, such as Aniseed, Caraway, Dill and Fennel have been known for centuries to promote the flow of breast milk, and have been widely used by nursing mothers, mostly in the form of herb teas or infusions. Jasmine is sometimes mentioned as having this property, but I do not know of sufficient evidence to substantiate this, while the various Umbelliferae have been extensively proved. Fennel tea is probably still the best choice here.

Cracked nipples can be extraordinarily painful, and slow to heal. Calendula is the most healing plant known for this condition, and a number of good firms make Calendula creams. However, it is very easy to make your own cream, or add a few drops of Calendula to a bought cream. It is very important to make sure that all traces of the cream have been washed off before the baby's next feed. Apply the cream immediately after each feed, so that the nipples have the maximum time to absorb the beneficial properties before the next feed.

To reduce the flow of milk, either because the breasts are painfully engorged, or because it is necessary to wean the baby, oil of Peppermint can be used in cold compresses. Various other oils have the same effect, but Peppermint is the safest, and this is, of course, very important if the baby is still feeding, though again it is necessary to wash off all traces of essential oil before each feed, as it is potentially dangerous to give the oils to a baby internally, even the relatively safe and mild oils.

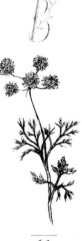

61

see under **COMPRESSES** *for the method of making and applying them.*

Breathing

see **RESPIRATORY SYSTEM**, *also entries for* **ASTHMA, COLDS, CATARRH**, *etc.*

Bronchitis

Bronchitis – like all other words ending in 'itis' – indicates a state of inflammation, in this case, an inflammation of the bronchi (bronchial tubes). Before considering the appropriate aromatherapy treatment, we need to distinguish between acute bronchitis and chronic bronchitis.

Acute bronchitis is a feverish condition, usually lasting a few days, with a harsh and painful cough. At first the cough is very dry, but as the lungs produce additional mucus in response to the infection, the cough becomes easier and less painful as the mucus lubricates the bronchi. Acute bronchitis usually originates with a viral infection of the upper respiratory tract, such as a cold or sore throat, spreading to the lungs.

Aromatherapy treatment aims at combating the infection, reducing fever, easing the cough and expelling mucus. In the first stages, when the cough is dry and painful, steam inhalation with Benzoin, Bergamot, Eucalyptus, Lavender or Sandalwood will give a great deal of relief. Bergamot and Eucalyptus oils are also effective in lowering fever, and all these oils will help to reinforce the body's own defence mechanism in response to the infection. In the latter stages of acute bronchitis, it is very important to clear all the mucus from the lungs, to prevent complications, and any of the essential oils described as expectorant will be helpful: Basil, Benzoin, Bergamot, Marjoram, Myrrh, Sandalwood or Thyme have all been used effectively, but of these I most often use Benzoin, Bergamot, Sandalwood or Thyme. The cough may persist for some time after the fever has subsided, but inhalations, baths and local massage to chest and throat with expectorant oils will shorten the time needed for full recovery.

A person suffering from acute bronchitis obviously needs to be kept warm and rested, preferably in bed. It is important to avoid anything which can aggravate the cough, such as smoke, and very dry air. If you have central heating which dries the air, vaporise some water in the patient's room to make breathing less painful and irritating. The old-

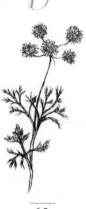

Marjoram

fashioned steam kettle was designed to do just this, but you can use a humidifier over a radiator, an ordinary electric kettle boiled in the room two or three times in the course of the day and last thing at night, or any of the various devices that use a candle or nightlight to evaporate water slowly. A few drops of any of the essential oils already mentioned can be added to the water for greater effect.

Most adults will recover from an attack of bronchitis fairly quickly and without complications, given this care and treatment, but the very elderly and frail, babies and young children, and people with heart conditions or a history of lung infections, are at much greater risk and must always be under properly qualified supervision. If antibiotics are necessary, you can safely, and in fact advantageously, continue with aromatherapy treatment as described, and you should also make sure that the patient eats plenty of live natural yoghurt, or takes lactobacillus tablets, to offset the damaging effects of antibiotics on the friendly bacteria in the gut.

Chronic bronchitis, as the word 'chronic' implies, is a long-term condition without fever. It is characterised by a permanent cough with sputum, due to continual over-production of mucus.

Healthy lungs normally produce a small amount of mucus all the time, and this is constantly swept up the bronchi by small hair-like projections called cilia. This process goes on all the time without us noticing it, as the amount of mucus is very small, and it is swallowed imperceptibly with our saliva. But when irritation of the bronchi, due to infection, air pollution, smoking, or other external irritants, provokes the production of abnormally large amounts of mucus, this literally swamps the minute cilia. The deep layer of mucus covers the cilia, so they can no longer propel it upwards. Then the body can only get rid of the mucus by coughing.

Chronic bronchitis is usually classified into three grades of severity – simple chronic bronchitis, which is mild but persistent with clear sputum; mucopurulent bronchitis, in which the sputum is occasionally or continually thick and often yellowish, due to the presence of pus caused by bacterial infection; and obstructive bronchitis, which occurs when structural damage has been caused by continual infection, inflammation and coughing. The bronchi become narrowed because the membrane that lines them gets thicker and scarred. The lungs lose some of their elasticity, so breathing becomes more difficult, as greater effort is needed to get a sufficient volume of air into the lungs. The amount of alveolar tissue is reduced, due to damage. This is the very thin membrane through which oxygen passes into the blood, and carbon dioxide and other waste material is extracted. Eventually the heart may be overstrained in trying to maintain sufficient circulation within the lungs.

The death rate from this form of bronchitis is higher in Great Britain than anywhere else in the world. Our climate and air pollution are serious contributing factors, especially when the two combine to produce fog. But the two most important factors are smoking and bad nutrition.

Smokers are still more likely to die from chronic bronchitis than from lung cancer, and to give up smoking is the first and most important preventative measure. The other is to improve the level of nutrition, and particularly to cut out or greatly reduce these foods which encourage the production of mucus. These are for most people, dairy products and refined starches. Of the two, dairy products seem to be the worse culprits, and cutting them right out of the diet for a time – maybe several weeks, or months if the bronchitis is of long standing – will often bring about an enormous improvement. After that, cheese, milk, etc., may be cautiously reintroduced but in very small amounts only. For some people, it may be necessary to omit them from the diet permanently. Goats milk is often found to be less mucus-forming than cows milk. Starches also provoke excessive mucus production, and refined starches (white flour and all products made from it) are far worse than unrefined grains. Additives, such as chemical flavourings, colourings and preservatives often trigger mucus excess as well, and should be avoided. The best and simplest rule is to eat foods in a state as near as possible to that in which they were grown, i.e., not processed, dried, frozen, packaged or pre-cooked, and as often as possible eat them raw or very lightly cooked.

Essential oils to help the detoxifying process should include Garlic, in capsule or tablet form, as well as fresh in the diet. Cedarwood, Frankincense, Juniper, Myrrh and Rosemary all help to reduce the amount of mucus produced, and one or more of the expectorant oils will need to be used to help clear it from the lungs. Of these, I find Benzoin one of the most helpful, and in fact a combination of three resins – Benzoin, Myrrh and Frankincense – used in baths and inhalations, is a very effective treatment. Another oil not often mentioned in connection with chronic bronchitis, but which I have found to be very valuable, is Ginger. In traditional Chinese medicine Ginger is used for any condition where the body is not coping effectively with moisture, whether internal or external, and chronic bronchitis is a perfect example of such a condition, for while the lungs are not dealing effectively with their internal moisture – mucus – the situation is aggravated by wet external conditions, such as the British climate or bad housing. Fresh root ginger can be sliced and made into an infusion (or 'tea') which is a very palatable and warming drink. About six thin slivers from a ginger root of average thickness should be simmered in a large cupful of water for about ten minutes, and then strained and drunk with half a teaspoon of honey. This drink can be taken two or three times a day, especially in winter.

Cedar

63

Although all these essential oils are valuable in treating chronic bronchitis, they will not be fully effective if the other factors involved are not taken into consideration. We can't do much about the climate, but landlords or local authorities can be pressed to improve damp housing, and the individual must be prepared to take responsibility for making any dietary changes that would help, and it goes without saying that smoking will render any treatment virtually useless.

Hyssop

Bruises

Several essential oils can be used to reduce bruising. Fennel, Hyssop or Lavender are effective if applied to the area as soon as possible after the bruising has occurred, preferably in an ice-cold compress. Lavender can be used later, too, to reduce pain. However, Arnica in a homoeopathic preparation is probably the most effective anti-bruising agent there is, and Arnica ointment should be in every natural first-aid kit.

In the latter stages of a bruise, when the colour turns green or yellowish, local massage with a stimulating oil such as Rosemary will help to disperse the bruising by increasing local circulation, which will help to drain away the blood that was released into the surrounding tissues by the original blow. In the case of severe bruising, such as that resulting from an accident, oils which stimulate the spleen, such as Black Pepper, Camomile and Lavender are helpful.

People who have a tendency to bruise easily may have a kidney disorder, and should seek help from a well-qualified person, such as an acupuncturist, homoeopath, doctor or medical herbalist, for diagnosis and treatment.

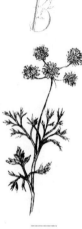

Bulimia

This severe eating disorder appears to be on the increase, perhaps because so much pressure is put on women to conform to standards of appearance that have little to do with reality. Comparing herself to media images of models, film stars, pop singers and the like, the bulimic woman feels that she is overweight, even when she is not. The condition has much in common with anorexia as far as distorted self-image is concerned, the important difference being that where the anorexic deprives herself of food, the bulimic eats compulsively and then forces herself to vomit and/or uses laxatives excessively. Because she does not retain food in her digestive system long enough for the body to extract vital nutrients, she may become severely under-nourished.

As with anorexia, aromatherapy alone is probably not enough to help a bulimia sufferer, but can be a great help when allied to psychotherapy. Bearing in mind that every case is different, the most appropriate oils and forms of treatment are likely to be those discussed under the heading of anorexia, so do please refer to that section.

Burners

There are a number of devices available for vaporising essential oils in a room, the simplest of which is a 'burner' with a lower compartment in which to place a nightlight, and a dish-shaped section to be filled with water, on which about a dozen drops of essential oil are placed. The heat of the nightlight gradually evaporates the water and essential oil(s) as a gentle steam. They may be made of glazed or unglazed pottery or ceramics. I do not recommend using metal burners as essential oils alter when in contact with metals other than stainless steel.

Another form is heated by a very small electric element, and the essential oil alone put on a small pad. Yet another kind also has an electric element heating a ceramic dish in which the oil is floated on water.

Burns

Essential oil of Lavender is one of the most effective treatments for burns, both major and minor, Ti-tree being a valuable alternative.

It can be applied neat to all minor burns, and if this is done very quickly after burning, blistering will not usually appear. Lavender is not only a very effective antiseptic, but is also analgesic (painkilling) and helps to reduce the pain of the burn. It promotes rapid healing, and will reduce eventual scarring. Lavender applied to a burn very quickly will often heal it with no scarring at all.

For larger burns, Lavender oil should be poured neat onto sterile gauze and applied to the burn, and renewed every few hours, though obviously if the burning is extensive qualified help will be needed. The patient may be in shock, and liquid loss may be severe, so do not lose time seeking help, but use Lavender oil as a very important first-aid measure until help arrives.

René-Maurice Gattefossé, who coined the word 'aromathérapie' and initiated the revival of interest in essential oils in the present century, began his research after he had burnt his hand in a laboratory explosion and experienced for himself how dramatically Lavender oil helped it heal.

Dr. Jean Valnet used oil of Lavender to treat serious battlefield burns during the French-Indo Chinese war, and more recently victims of the Kings Cross fire were treated with Lavender by aromatherapists who volunteered their services to the London hospital where they were being cared for.

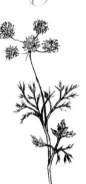

Lavender

Cajeput
Melaleuca leucodendron

ॐ

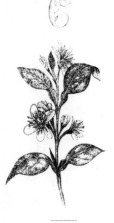

Cajeput (or Cajuput) gets its name from the Malaysian 'caju-puti' meaning 'white tree' referring to its whitish bark. It is one of the Melaleuca group, a sub-species of the Myrtaceae family which includes all the Eucalyptuses, Clove and Myrtle. The predominant property shared by all members of this family is the ability to combat and sometimes prevent infection.

The oil is extracted from the leaves and buds by steam distillation, and is a greenish-yellow colour which distinguishes it from several other closely related varieties of Melaleuca. The active principles of the oil include large proportions (between 45% and 65%) of cineol, with terpineol, pinene and various aldehydes. The odour is decidedly medicinal, camphorous and very penetrating.

Cajeput is best known as an inhalation for colds and other respiratory infections, and it is used in a number of proprietary cold treatments. Used in steam inhalations it effectively clears the nasal passages while inhibiting the bacteria that proliferate in the mucus formed during colds and 'flu, and which can lead to catarrh and sinusitis. It also has pain-killing properties which help to reduce the discomfort of sore throats and headaches that accompany colds.

Cajeput can irritate the skin, so it needs to be well diluted and must never be allowed to come into contact with the mucous membranes. For most situations where Cajeput might be used on the skin, one of the other Melaleucas, such as Niaouli or Ti-tree which are non-irritant would be safer.

see also the entries for **NIAOULI** *and* **TI-TREE** *to which* **CAJEPUT** *is closely related.*

CAUTION
Cajeput is a skin irritant. It is a powerful stimulant, and it is not advisable to use it in inhalations before bedtime unless it is mixed with a sedative oil to counteract this effect.

Camomiles
Anthemis nobilis (synonym: *Chamaemelum nobile*)
Matricaria chamomilla (synonym: *Chamomilla recutita*), *Anthemis mixta*

ॐ

Several varieties of Camomile are used in aromatherapy. Three or four kinds grow wild in the British Isles, and will be familiar to most people, with their daisy-like flowers and feather leaves, as well as the distinctive, apple-like scent. The varieties most used in aromatherapy are Anthemis nobilis, the Roman Camomile, and Matricaria Chamomilla, or German Camomile. A wild Camomile, Anthemis mixta – often called Camomile Maroc – is also used. Their medicinal properties overlap to a large extent.

Camomile has been recognised both in folk medicine and official pharmacopoeias. Camomile tea (or tisane) is one of the most widespread herbal remedies in popular use; for stomach upsets, cystitis, children's ailments or just as a refreshing and relaxing drink, and it can be drunk as a back-up to treatment with the essential oil.

The chemical composition of the essential oil varies between the different varieties. Roman Camomile is composed mainly of esters (angelic ester and tiglic ester account for over 80% of its composition) with isobutyl angelate, pinocarvone, chamazulene and other minor constituents. German Camomile is made up mainly of chamazulene and farnesene. Chamazulene is not found in the plant, but is produced during distillation when reactions take place between various plant constituents and the steam used in distilling. It gives the oil a beautiful blue colouration and is an excellent anti-inflammatory agent.

All the Camomiles are soothing, calming and anti-inflammatory, German Camomile being particularly anti-inflammatory because of the high proportion of chamazulene, so it is valuable in treating conditions where there is inflammation present, whether internal or external. It can be used in hot compresses on boils, abscesses, infected cuts, splinters, etc. and on tooth abscesses until the sufferer can get to a dentist. Camomile tea, and massage or compresses over the affected area should be used for internal inflammatory conditions, particularly of the digestive tract, such as colitis, gastritis and diarrhoea, especially if the latter is chronic. Tension and anxiety are often at the root of these conditions, and Camomile has a profoundly calming effect on the emotional level.

The properties and uses of Camomile often overlap with those of Lavender, and if you need to decide whether to use Lavender or Camomile in any particular situation, it may be useful to remember that as an analgesic Camomile is generally better for dull aches and pains, while Lavender may be better for a pain that is sharp and piercing.

Camomile is also a disinfectant, especially of the urinary tract. For all urinary infections, such as cystitis, copious amounts of Camomile tea should be taken and massage or compresses of Camomile applied to the lower abdomen. A few drops of essential oil in a warm bath will also help. The tea, taken daily, is also a good preventative measure against bladder or kidney stones.

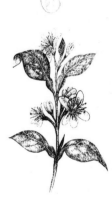

67

Menstrual pain and menopausal problems can, in many instances, be relieved by the same combination of compresses, massage, baths and teas. For premenstrual tension, Camomile's diuretic properties will reduce fluid retention, while its gently antidepressant action will help with the feelings of stress, depression and irritability that many women suffer premenstrually.

Camomile can be used in massage for muscular pain, and for inflamed joints in such conditions as arthritis. It is very effective in treating sprains, inflamed tendons, and swollen painful joints in bursitis (Housemaid's Knee, for example), always remembering that injuries and swellings must not be massaged, but a cold compress applied.

Camomile is very valuable for many skin problems, especially where the skin is very sensitive, red or dry. Its most important application is in the treatment of allergies, such as eczema, urticaria and all dry, flaky and itchy conditions, or those where patches of redness appear. It is used directly on the skin in
Camomile   aromatic waters, lotions and creams, but baths may be the simplest

approach if a very large area of the body is affected. Plenty of Camomile tea should be taken as well. Care must be taken to discover the cause of the rash, whether this is a physical irritant, emotional stress or very often a combination of the two. Otherwise, there is a danger that symptoms are merely being suppressed. Camomile is very calming on the mental/emotional level, and since many allergic reactions arise when the person concerned is under stress, it is far more valuable in treatment than in any preparation which attempts to deal with the problem only as a skin eruption. It is important, though, to remember that there may be a 'healing crisis' in which the skin appears to get worse before it shows any improvement. This phenomenon is common to many forms of natural healing.

The action of Camomile as a local vasoconstrictor (i.e., it causes small blood-vessels to shrink) can help reduce the redness of cheeks due to enlarged capillaries, though it may be months before any improvement is seen.

As suggested above, the mental and emotional effects of Camomile can be seen to parallel its physical effects, as with so many essential oils, for it is soothing, calming and antidepressant, and particularly helpful where stress and anxiety are inclined to make a person fretful, irritable or nervous. It is best used as a massage oil and in baths – perhaps blended with other oils.

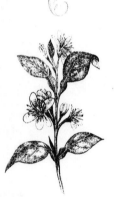

Camomile is one of the gentlest oils, and is particularly suitable for treating children. Teething infants can be soothed by rubbing a little Camomile, diluted to 1%, into the cheeks. You might try a few teaspoons of weak Camomile tea, sweetened with a little honey, in a spoon or bottle, especially just before bedtime.

Earache can be relieved by massaging around the ear, or applying hot compresses of Camomile. If the earache persists, or is recurrent, a doctor must be consulted.

For eye infections, use an infusion of Camomile flowers (NEVER PUT ESSENTIAL OILS IN THE EYES, EVEN WHEN DILUTED). I use Camomile tea bags, soaked in boiling water and allowed to cool, placed over the eyes as a treatment for conjunctivitis.

Camomile can be used as an alternative to Lavender, or blended with it, in baths to relieve insomnia, particularly if help is needed over a long period of time. It is never advisable to use one essential oil continuously for more than two or three weeks, so alternating and varying the oils is always a good policy.

NOTE: A variety of Mugwort (*Artemisia arborescens*) is often sold under the name of Blue Camomile. It is very rich in azulene and chamazulene and has the same anti-inflammatory properties as the Camomiles, but it is a powerful emmenagogue and must never be used during pregnancy.

Cancer

It must be stated straight away that aromatherapists do not 'treat' cancer. It would be both unethical and illegal for us to claim to do so. We can, though, offer immense comfort, support and reinforcement for cancer patients, within the framework of treatment that they have chosen. Whether that treatment follows the orthodox route of radiation, surgery and chemotherapy or one or more of the alternatives, such as dietary therapy, visualisation, healing, etc., is a decision that only the person with cancer can make, but whatever the choice, aromatherapy can be a valuable additional therapy provided that certain safeguards are followed.

The first safeguard is that both professional ethics and the safety and well-being of the patient require that no treatment is undertaken without the knowledge and consent of the doctor carrying out the principal treatment.

Some doctors are opposed to any massage for people with cancer, fearing that because of the stimulating effects that massage can have on the lymphatic system, it may accelerate the migration of cancer cells via that system, leading to the formation of secondary cancers. However, it would seem that these fears stem from a knowledge of the more vigorous forms of massage, and with the growth of 'soft' massage techniques such fears have diminished and many more doctors now feel that such gentle therapy cannot harm their patients, and can only do good in terms of relaxation and increased comfort. Massage should not, however, be used for patients with Hodgkin's Disease or bone cancer.

Since the development of chemotherapy for cancer, it has repeatedly been said that essential oils should not be used at the same time as chemotherapy or following a course of chemotherapy, at least until the body has been cleared of all residues of cytotoxic drugs. These drugs can lodge in the liver and other body tissues for a long time, being eliminated from the body very gradually. Opinions vary as to how long this might take, with estimates ranging from weeks to years. The ban on using essential oils is based on the fact that they can speed up all eliminative processes and could possibly trigger a rapid release of drug residues into the bloodstream. Great caution is needed when using any technique that increases elimination as this could have unpleasant side effects and possibly more serious consequences. The drugs used to treat cancer are so toxic that dosage has to be extremely carefully monitored when they are originally administered. The physician treads a tightrope between killing the cancer cells and poisoning the patient. After a course of chemotherapy it is impossible to calculate how much of a drug is left in a person's body, because some people will eliminate the residues faster and more efficiently than others.

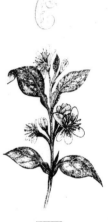

Some people are now querying this blanket prohibition of essential oils and feel that many factors need to be taken into consideration, including how many courses of chemotherapy have been given, in what dosage and for how long, also whether the patient has followed any detoxifying regime, such as a special diet, after their chemotherapy. The decision in each case must be based on a full knowledge of all the facts, plus observation of the patient's general state. One factor which may have reduced the risks inherent in too-rapid detoxification, is that the use of chemotherapy has been greatly refined in the past 20 years and very much lower doses of the drugs are used now than in the '70s. Many more aromatherapists are working with cancer patients, both within hospitals and in cancer support groups. A growing number of nurses are training in aromatherapy and incorporating this into their work.

Aromatherapists and nurses are increasingly using gentle massage with essential oils to help terminal patients in hospices. Aromatherapy helps to relieve pain and reduce the amount of oedema in limbs following operations. Lavender oil, in particular, can be used to prevent and treat pressure sores as well as to aid sleep. Many of these patients are too weak to take more than a brief, gentle massage to the face and head, or to the hands and feet, but the caring touch of the therapist, combined with the essential oils gives both physical and emotional comfort. Some cancer patients, especially if they have been mutilated by major surgery, or burnt by radiation treatment, feel that their bodies are repugnant or unclean, and for them human touch is even more important, as a way of assuring them that they are human with as much dignity and value as anybody else.

Certain essential oils have been described as anti-cancer agents, but their action has not been proved. Neither has it been disproved, and the traditional uses of plants have been shown to be valid often enough that we should consider using these oils in conjunction with the major forms of treatment. They include Bergamot, Cedar, Clove, Cypress, Eucalyptus, Garlic, Geranium, Hyssop, Onion and Violet leaf. However, any oil which will decrease pain, relieve the side effects of treatment or help the emotional trauma of cancer can be considered, with the proviso that oestrogenic oils should never be used for anybody with breast cancer or other oestrogen-related cancers (cancer of the endometrium, for example).

Two oils of the Melaleuca family, Niaouli and Ti-tree, have been used to reduce surface burning during cobalt radiation treatment. A thin film of essential oil is applied to the skin over the area to be treated before the radiation therapy and has been shown to give some protection. Lavender oil has been used in Norway to treat radiation burns, and has reduced scarring. It has also been used, with Rosemary oil, to stimulate regrowth of hair when the hair has fallen out after chemotherapy, subject, of course, to the safeguards already described.

However, valuable though these physical benefits of essential oils can be, it is on the emotional plane that aromatherapy perhaps has the most to offer as part of a holistic approach to cancer. The uplifting, calming, soothing and antidepressant oils, combined with caring support from a sensitive therapist, can add to the quality of life in a very special way, whatever the final outcome.

Candida

Candida albicans, a form of yeast, is present in all of us, probably from birth. Normally it is kept under control by friendly bacteria in the gut, and we remain unaware of its existence. Problems only arise when the candida organisms proliferate to a level where they migrate outside the gut, often following a course of antibiotics which kill some of the intestinal flora, along with the germs they are designed to attack.

The commonest symptom of candida proliferation is thrush, but if the organism really gets out of control it may lead to nausea, headaches, depression, abnormal fatigue and other problems. It is now thought that most people suffering from chronic fatigue syndrome, or M.E., are affected by candida.

Treatment with essential oils and diet is described in the entry for THRUSH.

Cardamon or Cardamom
Elettaria cardamomum

The Cardamon plant belongs to the same plant family as Ginger (Zingiberaceae) and they exhibit much of the same warming quality.

Several varieties of the plant are found growing in India, Sri Lanka, China and also parts of the Middle East. The oil may be colourless or yellow, and has a sweet, warm, aromatic aroma. Its main chemical constituents include terpineol and cineol, with a little limonene and zingiberene.

The plant has been used in Eastern traditional medicine for over 3,000 years, being mentioned in Vedic medicinal texts. Via the Middle East, Cardamon was imported into ancient Egypt, Greece and Rome, and the Egyptians used it in perfumes and incenses. Both Hippocrates and Dioscorides mention it, the latter describing it as good for sciatica, coughs, spasms, abdominal pains and retention of urine. In India, Cardamon is used as a digestive aid, both in the form of a spice added to food, and as a medicament. Indian use also confirms some of Dioscorides' descriptions, particularly for coughs, and as a diuretic. But the most widespread use in India is as an aphrodisiac. There is no real evidence that Cardamon has any physiological effect, but it is both tonic and stimulant so may act indirectly.

It is a good digestive aid, easing nausea, heartburn and flatulence, and is helpful for diarrhoea, easing the griping pains that often accompany it.

It can be used as a refreshing tonic and invigorating bath oil – perhaps better in a blend than alone. Although there is no evidence that Cardamon is a skin irritant, I would be inclined to exercise caution, as with all the spicy oils, and use small amounts, well diluted, for anybody with a sensitive skin.

Carrier Oils

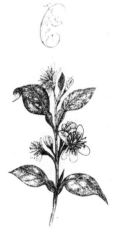

When essential oils are used for massage they need to be mixed into a base or 'carrier' oil (usually in the proportion of 3% essential oil to carrier oil) as they are far too powerful and concentrated to be used on the skin undiluted. Carrier oils also provide the lubrication needed for the therapist's hands to move freely over the patient's skin.

A carrier oil can be almost any unperfumed vegetable oil, such as soya, safflower or sunflower oil, though those used most often in aromatherapy are sweet almond and grape seed oils. Sesame seed oil is sometimes used, and has the advantage of washing out of sheets, towels and overalls easily.

Most carrier oils are simply used for lubrication, but a few have therapeutic properties of their own, which can be chosen to complement those of the essential oils used with them. For example, peach kernel, apricot kernel and particularly avocado oil are all rich and nourishing and help dry and ageing skins. Olive oil has many valuable healing properties, though its strong characteristic odour (which persists even when essential oils are added to it) is a disadvantage from the aromatherapist's point of view. Wheatgerm oil (rich in Vitamin E) is used to reduce scar tissue after injury or operations and also facial scarring caused by severe acne. It is a rather sticky oil which does not act as a lubricant and needs to be added to one of the more free-flowing oils, usually in the ratio of 25% wheatgerm to 75% almond or other oil. Wheatgerm is also a natural antioxidant which helps to prevent other oils from becoming rancid (i.e. oxidising). Small amounts (up to 10%) will improve the keeping ability of any other oil by a month or two.

All carrier oils oxidise sooner or later after being exposed to the air and become unfit for use, so it is not a good idea to blend essential oils into them in any quantity. The best method is to mix only as much as you will use for one treatment.

Most essential oil suppliers also stock carrier oils, though you can buy many of the more common ones from healthfood shops or grocers. If you do so, be certain that they are of good quality, cold-pressed and containing no additives of any kind.

71

Carrot
Daucus carrota

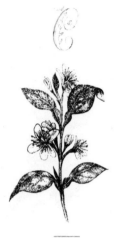

The humble carrot has been known as a medicinal plant, as well as a culinary one, at least since the time of Dioscorides (1st century A.D.). Many references to it occur in earlier Greek writings, but they are ambiguous about its name and description, whereas Dioscorides gives an accurate description of the modern domestic carrot.

The essential oil which is distilled from the seeds is pale yellow in colour, with the characteristic smell of carrots. Its active constituents include principally carotol, daucol, limonene and pinene. An oil is also obtained by solvent extraction from the roots, but this is not used in aromatherapy. A third product – an infused oil – is used in skin-care, especially for dry or mature skin, and for burns.

Carrot-seed oil has a powerful tonic action on the liver and gall-bladder, and is used in the treatment of jaundice and other liver disorders.

It has been used to treat eczema, psoriasis, ulcerative conditions of the skin and even skin cancers, which is extremely interesting, in the light of the use of large amounts of carrot juice, and/or raw carrots every day by pioneers in the 'gentle' treatment of cancer. Carrots contain a precursor of Vitamin A, which is valuable in cancer treatment and prevention, as well as Vitamins B1, B2 and C, and is one of the most useful forms of dietary fibre. (None of these are found in the essential oil.)

Carrot is a good aid to healthy skin. The essential oil, used in a cream or diluted in almond oil, restores tone and elasticity and may even reduce wrinkling. It is especially useful in spring, to undo some of the ravages of cold winds, over-heated homes and workplaces, and a diet that has perhaps been inadequate in vitamin content during the winter months. The infused oil can be used equally well for these purposes.

Catarrh

The production of excess mucus in the nose and other respiratory passages is a response to any inflammation of the mucous membrane that lines them. This can be caused by an infection, such as colds or 'flu, or by irritants like pollen and dust.

For the immediate relief of congestion, a steam inhalation with essential oil is very effective. Lavender, Peppermint, Rosemary, Eucalyptus, Thyme or Ti-tree will ease the congestion and also help to combat the infection which has caused it. For catarrh caused by pollen and other irritants, Lavender and Camomile are the best choice. (For method, see entry for **INHALATIONS**.)

Massage of the face, with special attention to the areas around the nose and over the sinuses, will help to drain away excessive mucus. With the exception of Lavender, most of the oils listed above are rather powerful so to use on the face they would need to be diluted to 1.5% or less in a carrier oil. Work around the nose and cheeks with circular movements: small on the nose itself and larger around the cheeks. Make some long, sweeping downward movements towards the neck.

Diet plays a part in many cases of catarrh. Dairy products and wheat are the most common culprits, and should be excluded for a period by anybody who suffers catarrh frequently, to see whether any improvement is noticed. If so, they may have to be excluded permanently from the diet, or included in very small amounts only. Other people are sensitive to other foods, and may need to experiment to find out what these are.

Cedarwood
Cedrus atlantica

Several trees yield essential oils which may be sold as Cedarwood, but you should ensure that you use only that obtained from *Cedrus atlantica*, the Atlas Cedar. This is closely related to the biblical Cedar of Lebanon and its therapeutic properties have been recognised since antiquity. Cedar was used by all the ancient civilisations in medicine, cosmetics and perfumery, and by the Egyptians in embalming. The wood itself is very aromatic, due to the high percentage of essential oil it contains, and was used for building and making storage chests, as the odour repels termites, ants, moths and other harmful insects. In common with other aromatic woods, it was widely used as an incense. It is still used as an incense in Tibet (and among Tibetan exiles) as well as having important uses in traditional Tibetan medicine.

The essential oil is yellowish, fairly viscous with a warm, woody fragrance. Its active principles include cedrol, cadinene and other sesquiterpenes, and several terpenic hydrocarbons.

Cedarwood is a powerful antiseptic, used particularly for bronchial and urinary tract infections. It is very effective for cystitis and vaginal infections and discharges (always remembering the need for medical investigation to identify the cause). It is mucolytic (i.e., it breaks down mucus) which makes it doubly useful in treating catarrhal conditions, especially chronic bronchitis.

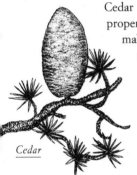

Cedar

Cedar is used in skincare as a mild astringent, and its antiseptic properties make it valuable in treating acne. Its 'masculine' odour makes it acceptable to young men and boys with acne, who might reject sweeter-smelling oils. It is used in men's toiletries, especially aftershaves where both the astringent and antiseptic properties are useful, though its popularity as a masculine perfume may be connected with its reputation as an aphrodisiac. It certainly has a tonic and stimulant action on the whole body, while at the same time reducing stress and tension, so there is some foundation for this belief.

Celery
Apium graveolens

Celery is a native of Southern Europe, but is now almost universally cultivated as a salad vegetable. It is grown specifically for essential oil extraction in India, China, Hungary and elsewhere. It has been known since antiquity as both a culinary and medicinal plant. Dioscorides and Hippocrates valued it highly as a diuretic and depurative. In the Middle Ages it was used, usually in the form of a decoction, to treat retention of urine, kidney stones, urinary infections, fevers and intestinal obstructions. One early writer also said that 'Wild Celery purges the melancholic humours that give rise to sadness' and it is fascinating to note that herbalists today use Celery very specifically for depression associated with rheumatoid arthritis. It is also used in herbal medicine as a tisane, decoction or tincture for urinary tract infections, kidney problems etc., just as in the past.

CAUTION
Cedarwood must not be used during pregnancy.

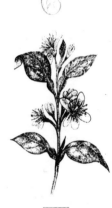

73

Essential oils can be obtained from all parts of the Celery plant but the most useful, and the only one generally used in aromatherapy, is produced by steam distillation from the seeds. It has a strong but pleasant, spicy scent and ranges from pale to dark yellow though some samples tend towards orange. The active principles include apigenol, apiol, limonene, selinene and others.

The use of Celery oil is very much what you might expect from its traditional, herbal use. It is one of the most effective diuretics at our disposal: in the words of Mme. Micheline Arcier, doyenne of aromatherapy in England, 'You use Celery . . . you run!' For kidney infections and urine retention, the best method would be hot compresses over the kidney area, replaced as soon as they began to cool (though I would add the caution that such conditions need medical attention and to use aromatherapy alone would be irresponsible). The same method is good for cystitis, putting the compresses over the bladder area.

Massage with Celery oil would benefit anybody with fluid retention but it does much more than just shift fluids: Celery helps the body throw off accumulated toxins, so it is particularly indicated in cellulitis and for arthritis, rheumatism and gout where accumulations of uric acid give rise to pain and inflammation.

Celery is a good tonic for the liver and the digestive system in general. In the past, the seeds were often chewed after a meal to help digestion and by nursing mothers to increase the flow of milk. (The seeds of many Umbelliferae have this property.) The crushed seeds were, and still are, used in cooking both for flavouring and to help digestion.

Perhaps more important than any of these fairly specific uses, is the fact that Celery stimulates the metabolism and is helpful for fatigue and exhaustion, especially if this is stress-induced. Perhaps this is another oil we might consider for M.E. or chronic fatigue syndrome? The same tonic and stimulant action is probably responsible for Celery's reputation as an aphrodisiac.

Celery is an emmenagogue and could be used to help absent, scanty or irregular menstruation.

74

Cellulitis (Cellulite)

The very word cellulitis, as well as the condition it is most often used to describe, is the subject of much debate, since the medical profession use this term to signify an inflammation of cellular tissue, generally as a result of infection from a septic wound, while beauticians, women's magazines and many alternative practitioners understand the term as meaning an infiltration of the subcutaneous fat cells by fluids and toxic wastes. Many doctors also state quite simply that this condition does not exist, and is just a fancy name for fat! To avoid such confusions, many people now use the French 'cellulite'. Some women with cellulite are overweight, but it can equally affect thin women, and I know of at least one case of cellulite associated with anorexia.

Cellulite affects women almost exclusively, and there is a definite connection with the hormonal balance. It is found most often on the outer side of the thighs, sometimes extending to the hips and buttocks and gives rise to the nickname 'jodhpur thighs' on account of the noticeable thickening. Another nickname is 'orange peel skin' due to the characteristic puckering which distinguishes cellulite from plain fat. The puckering is due to the fact that the walls of the subcutaneous fat cells gradually grow thicker, with deposits of fibrous collagen, so locking in the fluid and toxins.

Luckily, aromatherapy is one of the most successful forms of treatment for this condition – even more so if it is allied to advice about nutrition and exercise, since the condition is most often found in women with sedentary jobs. A woman with cellulite may often see it as a cosmetic problem, but the holistic practitioner will recognise it not only as a distressing condition in itself, but a sign of a more serious toxic state of the body, and an indication that the lymphatic system is sluggish and elimination in general less than efficient.

To help with the overall situation, we need essential oils with a variety of properties: detoxifying, stimulating to the lymphatic system, hormone balancing and diuretic. As treatment needs to be continued over some weeks, or months, depending on the severity of the cellulite, how long it has existed and how much the client helps herself with a cleansing diet, etc., it is also very important to vary the combination of oils used. I usually begin a course of treatment by using a blend of Geranium and Rosemary, and vary this by incorporating Black Pepper, Birch, Grapefruit or Juniper. I use these oils with a specialised form of massage to drain and stimulate the lymphatic system, and also give some to be used in baths. It speeds the treatment if the client uses a loofah, brush or massage glove on the affected areas between treatments. I suggest a cleansing diet of nothing but fresh fruit and spring water for 3 to 5 days, followed by a general wholefood diet with plenty of raw foods.

Stress is often a factor in cellulite, because the body accumulates toxins much more when stressed, and elimination may become less efficient. If this seems to be the case, it is a good idea to alternate the lymphatic massage with more general aromatherapy massage to help with the stress and its causes.

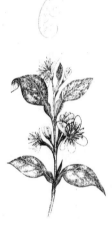

Juniper

see also **LYMPHATIC SYSTEM.**

75

Chemotype

You may sometimes find this term as part of the description of an essential oil. It is used to indicate oils of different chemical composition, even though they are obtained from plants which are botanically identical. Different soil conditions and climate can produce variations in the proportions of esters, alcohols, and other basic constituents of the oil, and slight variations of this kind, particularly from season to season, are quite usual. When such differences are sufficient to produce some variation in the properties of the oil, and this difference is constant, season after season, the resulting oil may be classed as a chemotype, in order to distinguish it from the 'standard' oil from the same plant.

A chemotype has not been altered in any way. Nothing has been added to or taken away from the natural oil distilled from the plant, and the chemical differences between the chemotype and the standard essential oil are those which arise within the plant itself.

Thyme is a plant which shows quite marked variations of this kind, and some suppliers list three of four chemotypes of this oil. Eucalyptus, Marjoram, Rosemary and Ti-tree chemotypes have been identified, and doubtless more oils will be classified in this way as techniques for identifying the differences become more widely used.

Chickenpox

Treatment with essential oils can considerably reduce the duration, severity and discomfort of an attack of chickenpox. Bergamot and Eucalyptus oils, which are both antiviral, were widely used against chickenpox before Ti-tree became readily available in this country. I now use and recommend Ti-tree for chickenpox, although it is also a good plan to alternate this with the other two.

If the child is old enough to be treated with essential oils (from about 4 years) you can use any of these oils in baths, sprays and dabbing lotions to reduce the itching. With a small child, it is easier to immerse the whole body in a tepid bath every few hours than to try to dab lotion on each blister. Use 2 drops of Ti-tree with 2 drops of Camomile to reduce itching or try 1 drop each of Bergamot, Eucalyptus, Camomile and Lavender.

For older children you can make a lotion with 5 drops each of Ti-tree, Camomile and Lavender added to 50 mls of witch hazel. Shake thoroughly and add to 50 mls of rosewater or distilled water and dab on the blisters as often as needed to reduce itching. Blisters treated in this way heal much faster than with the traditional remedy of calamine lotion which clogs the pores and in fact slows down healing.

Adults with chickenpox are often very ill indeed, with high fever at the outset, and acute pain while the blisters are appearing. In such cases, use 3 drops of Ti-tree with 1 drop each of Bergamot, Camomile and Lavender to each bath, and make a more pain-killing dabbing lotion with 6 drops of Ti-tree and 10 drops each of Bergamot, Camomile and Lavender to 50 mls each of witch hazel and water or rosewater. Shake well before each use. Bathing every few hours is strongly recommended if the patient does not feel too weak to do this. The dabbing lotion is particularly valuable in the latter stages of chickenpox, as it speeds healing and reduces the risk of scarring from the blisters.

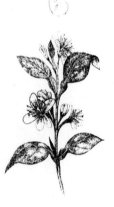

Childbirth

The value of massage with aromatic oils during childbirth has been known for many hundreds of years, and with the current trend away from 'hi-tech' hospital deliveries and towards a more gentle and natural way of giving birth, women are once again exploring ways in which essential oils can help them at this important point in their life.

Nicholas Culpeper in his 'Directory for Midwives' wrote 'If travail be hard, anoint the belly and sides with oil of sweet almonds, lilies and sweet wine' and almond oil is still the most commonly used carrier oil for massage. Lilies are not used in aromatherapy but there are a number of essential oils which can be of great help during childbirth, since they strengthen and deepen contractions while at the same time having an analgesic effect. The two which seem to be the greatest help are Jasmine and Lavender. Sage is sometimes recommended, but I have talked with women who found its action too powerful, and the resultant contractions rather hectic. Jean Valnet also mentions Clove, but I know no women who have tried this oil, so I cannot comment on it. Both Lavender and Jasmine are well-tried and known to be genuinely useful.

Either of these oils can be gently rubbed into the tummy and/or lower back from the beginning of labour and can indeed be used for a few days before the expected time of birth as a preparation. Whether to massage the back, the tummy or both will depend on what position the woman prefers and finds comfortable for her labour.

Some natural midwives will be able to do this, but it would generally be wiser to have somebody else ready to carry out the massage, or take over from the midwife when necessary. The baby's father might like to do this as a very practical way to help with the birth, or a close woman friend of the mother may offer her support. It needs to be decided well in advance who is going to do the massaging, so that they know exactly what to do and what is expected of them. It is by no means necessary to have a specialist trained in massage, but the volunteer should be shown how to apply oil in long smooth movements, preferably with a fairly firm pressure. Small circular movements on the lower back are often very comforting, and at all times the person carrying out the massage must be guided by the mother as to what kind of movement and what degree of pressure she finds most helpful.

It is a good idea to mix up the oils you plan to use some time beforehand as once labour starts there may not be time to measure accurately. Also, in the excitement of the moment it is very easy to knock over an oil bottle in the delivery room and a spilt bottle of undiluted essential oil could over-load the atmosphere to the point where the mother and her attendants would feel nauseated – quite apart from the expense of such a spillage (I know one young father who spilt a whole bottle of pure Jasmine!).

Gentle massage can be started in the week before the baby is due, but should not be tried much earlier than this, as there is some risk of triggering contractions and so inducing an early birth. This is even more important to observe if the woman has given birth prematurely in an earlier pregnancy. Warm baths with up to 6 drops of Jasmine or Lavender oil added can be taken during the last week of pregnancy, and if at all possible, at the onset of labour. This will help relax the woman and prepare the uterine muscles for the hard work ahead.

Lavender and Jasmine each offer slightly different advantages, although there is an overlap in their properties. Although both are analgesic, Jasmine is somewhat more effective at strengthening contractions, and so shortening labour, but some people find its heavy odour cloying during delivery, when the room will probably be kept fairly warm, and the mother herself feeling hot and sweaty from the efforts of her labour. The clean, fresh aroma of Lavender might be more acceptable and can be used in several other ways as well as massage. A few drops mixed in cool water will make a very refreshing mixture with which to sponge the mother's face and possibly her body if she is feeling very hot. A few drops on a light bulb or in a purpose made essential oil burner, or made into an air spray will cleanse and freshen the air of the room in which the baby is to be born.

Jasmine should be used immediately after the baby's birth, to help expel the afterbirth quickly and cleanly. It will also help to tone the uterine muscles and help them return faster to their pre-pregnancy condition. Jasmine is also a very good anti-depressant, and of great help to any woman who suffers from post-natal depression. It also has the reputation of promoting the flow of breast-milk, but this is not entirely substantiated. Oil of Fennel, fennel tea and preparations of dill-seed (a close relative of fennel) have been well-tried for hundreds of years and are known to be effective.

These oils which are so helpful during labour must be avoided during the first few months of pregnancy, because they can trigger contractions and therefore involve some risk of miscarriage. This is also true of some other oils which are discussed more fully in the entry for **PREGNANCY**.

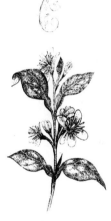

77

Children and Aromatherapy

Essential oils can be used safely and effectively for children, provided that certain precautions are observed. Children generally respond very well to aromatherapy and all natural forms of healing, partly because they have no preformed expectations or prejudices about what is involved, and partly because young bodies have excellent powers of recuperation. Their powers of self-healing have not yet been impaired by years of faulty diet, stress, unhealthy lifestyle, environmental pollution etc – which is not intended to imply that children are not affected by these factors. On the contrary, they are far more vulnerable to them on account of their smaller body-weight in relation to any potential poison, but they are able to quickly throw off poisons and infecting organisms, given the right healing environment, because their bodies have not been clogged by a toxic accumulation built up over many years.

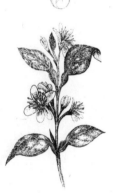

All the simple self-help uses of essential oils, such as baths, inhalations, compresses and air-sprays are valuable in treating childhood ailments, and babies and young children respond very well to simple massage. There is no need for any mother to have specialist massage training to be able to gently rub and soothe a child's pains away, although there are one or two excellent books suggesting ways of going about this. From birth onwards every mother touches her infant when bathing, changing, dressing, feeding and so forth, and this can be very easily extended into a gentle massage with diluted essential oils. As a child grows older, the amount of body-contact with the mother often decreases, but this can be avoided if children become accustomed to regular massages from mother right through from babyhood. Perhaps this can be incorporated as a regular part of bathing and bedtime?

The regular use of essential oils in the home, in baths, massages, air sprays or an essential oil burner is a very effective form of preventative medicine, and will often help children to avoid colds and other infections. However, young children have not yet fully developed their immune systems, and particularly when they begin school or playgroup and are in the company of other children (often in hot classrooms) they will inevitably develop colds and other infectious illnesses. When this happens, essential oil therapies can considerably reduce the discomfort of these illnesses and often help to shorten their duration and prevent secondary infections. The oils can also be used to treat minor injuries – the bruises, cuts, minor burns, grazes and insect stings that any normally active child is bound to suffer.

The safety precautions which must be observed when using essential oils for children are as follows:

- ✶ Never use an undiluted essential oil on a child (with the sole exception of small amounts of Lavender or Ti-tree on minor burns or injuries).
- ✶ Always dilute essential oils before adding them to a bath for a child and use less oil – up to 4 drops for a child – than you would in preparing a bath for an adult.
- ✶ Dilute the oil more when mixing a massage oil for a child: between 1% and 1.5% dilution, as opposed to the average 3% dilution used for an adult.
- ✶ Never leave a young child alone with a bowl of hot water when giving an inhalation, but supervise him or her the entire time.
- ✶ Give inhalations for only a few seconds initially – maybe half a minute – and increase this to a minute or two if the child tolerates the shorter inhalations.
- ✶ NEVER GIVE ESSENTIAL OILS BY MOUTH.

* Avoid all the essential oils described as toxic or slightly toxic (see the entries for each individual oil and **APPENDIX A**).
* Never attempt to treat serious illness without referring to a medically qualified practitioner – your G.P., a homoeopath or medical herbalist. Call your doctor or other qualified person immediately if your child is running a high temperature, is badly burnt, has convulsions or any other sign that he or she is in serious difficulty.
* Call your doctor or other qualified practitioner if minor conditions do not improve within 24 hours.

Apart from the occasions when children have a recognisable 'illness' there are many times when they are just a little off-colour, fractious, not sleeping, or over excited, and once again simple aromatherapy methods will do a great deal to smooth out these little 'hiccups'. The great panacea is a warm (not too hot) bath with 2 to 4 drops of pre-diluted oil of Camomile or Lavender added. Both of these oils have gently soothing, calming and sedative properties (among many others) which will help to dispel tears and tantrums, ease aches and promote gentle, natural sleep.

Camomile, in particular, is regarded as 'the children's oil' on account of its very gentle nature, absence of toxicity and appropriateness to so many of the problems of infancy and early childhood – teething, rashes, tummy upsets, and so forth. As mentioned above, it should never be used undiluted, but the dilute oil can be used in baths and massage and there are several excellent creams based on Camomile especially made for infant care, also Chamomilla pilules from homoeopathic chemists.

Other oils which are especially suitable for children are Lavender – already mentioned – Rose, Benzoin, Helichrysum and Mandarin. The properties and uses of each of these oils are described under their individual entries.

You should also refer to the entries for **BABIES**, **TEETHING**, and the various infectious illnesses of childhood – **CHICKENPOX**, **MEASLES**, etc., for a fuller description of the most helpful oils and the correct methods of use.

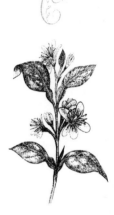

Cinnamon
Cinnamomum zeylanicum

The Cinnamon that is familiar as a cooking spice is the dried inner bark of a tropical evergreen tree, native to Madagascar and parts of S. E. Asia, also cultivated in Jamaica and parts of Africa. There are many species, varying according to the region, but the Madagascan is considered the best. Essential oil can be obtained from this bark by either water or steam distillation and also from the leaves. It is very important to distinguish between the two as the oil from the bark is a very strong skin irritant and should never be used on the skin. That from the leaf is an irritant, too, but not so powerful, and can be used on the skin with caution, i.e. in small amounts and very well diluted. If you are offered Cinnamon oil that is not labelled with the part of the tree from which it is obtained, don't buy it – you really do need to know which you are dealing with. The oil from the bark smells like the familiar spice, while that from the leaf smells more like cloves. Cinnamon Leaf oil is usually cheaper than Cinnamon Bark.

The difference between the two oils is due to their chemical constitution: the main constituent of Cinnamon Bark oil is cinnamaldehyde, which can vary from 40% to 70%,

CAUTION
Skin irritant. Do not use during pregnancy.

with eugenol, cinnamyl acetate and other minor constituents. Oil of Cinnamon Leaf has between 80% and 90% eugenol, eugenol acetate, benzyl benzoate, linalol, caryophyllene, cinnamaldehyde and small amounts of minor factors.

Cinnamon is antispasmodic and helps with many digestive problems, including sluggish digestion, stomach and intestinal cramps, colitis, flatulence, nausea and diarrhoea and is used in many commercial preparations. It is very helpful for menstrual cramps, too, used in a hot compress – perhaps blended with Clary. It is useful where the periods are scanty and painful and is also an emmenagogue (i.e. it can bring on the start of a period) so it must never be used during pregnancy.

It is traditionally considered an aphrodisiac, like many of the warming oils, but needs to be handled with caution. A very small proportion in a massage blend is pleasant and stimulating, but never allow it to come into direct contact with the genital area.

As you might guess, it is very warming, and helps to relieve aches and chilling in the early stages of colds and 'flu, and the feeling of debility that often remains after the initial feverish stage. It is helpful during convalescence after any illness, and Jean Valnet recommended giving Cinnamon to elderly people routinely during the winter to strengthen them and help them resist seasonal infections. Obviously, the essential oil must not be taken internally, and even greater care must be taken when using it on the skin of elderly folk if they are fragile. Use it as a minor ingredient in a blend of oils, with the Cinnamon making up not more than half of one percent of the whole. You might encourage the use of the spice in food, or look out for some of the spicy herbal teas that include Cinnamon.

Because of its warming qualities, Cinnamon is useful in massage blends for poor circulation, muscular aches and joint pain.

The risk of skin irritation is bypassed, of course, if we use the oil in burners or vaporisers, and it is a comforting one to use this way, especially in winter. It blends well with Benzoin, Cedarwood, Cypress, Orange and other citrus oils, and some of the other spice oils.

Circulation

The circulation of blood around the body is vital to the action of essential oils. Whether they are absorbed through the skin or inhaled (and of course, a certain amount will always be inhaled when oils are applied to the skin), aromatic molecules pass quite quickly into the bloodstream, and this is how they are transported to all parts of the body.

This is true of everything taken into the body, including nutrients from our food and oxygen from the air we breathe, which is essential to all the processes that maintain life. In the lungs, stomach, intestines and liver these substances are broken down into forms in which they can be assimilated. The circulatory system is the means by which they reach the individual cells.

Blood circulates in a system of tubes, or blood vessels, of various sizes, arranged in two separate but interconnected circuits, the smaller of which carries blood between the heart and the lungs, and the larger taking blood around all the rest of the body. In the lungs, oxygen from the air is absorbed into the blood. This bright red, oxygenated blood flows to the heart, and from there it is pumped out under pressure to make its circuit round the body. At the same time, the heart pumps blood from which most of the oxygen has been used up, back to the lungs.

The blood vessels carrying blood away from the heart are called arteries, and those returning it to the heart are veins. The major arteries and veins connect with a network of smaller vessels, and eventually with the smallest of all, capillaries, which are no wider than a hair. The walls of the arteries and veins are watertight, but those of the capillaries are extremely thin, and allow plasma (the watery part of the blood) and all the nutrients, oxygen and other substances dissolved in it (which may include particles of essential oil) to filter out into the fluid which surrounds the cells. This fluid can also filter in through the capillary walls, returning the waste products of bodily activities to the blood to be disposed of. It is at the level of the individual cells that the particles of essential oil exert their beneficial effect on the body.

Apart from acting as a transportation system for essential oils, the circulatory system can itself be affected by some oils. Disorders of the circulation, including high and low blood pressure and varicose veins, are discussed in entries of their own.

Rubefacient oils, such as Black Pepper, Juniper, Marjoram and Rosemary, stimulate circulation locally in the area to which they are applied. They cause the capillaries to widen, so a greater volume of blood can flow through them. The extra oxygen which this blood flow brings with it helps in many healing processes.

Other oils, most notably Camomile and Cypress, have the opposite effect, and bring about a contraction of the capillaries. This can be useful where there is heat, redness and swelling.

Garlic, in the form of tablets, capsules or eaten fresh, is beneficial to the health of the whole circulatory system, and so are Vitamins C and E.

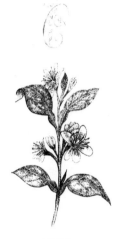

81

Citronella
Cymbopogon nardus

Citronella essential oil is obtained from a scented grass that grows wild and cultivated in Sri Lanka and other tropical areas. It is usually a yellowish-brown, with a very powerful lemony scent. The main chemical constituents are citronellal and geraniol, with traces of other chemicals which vary as several varieties of the grass are used.

It is little used in aromatherapy, though one possible therapeutic use which was suggested earlier this century is as a friction (diluted in alcohol) or massage oil for rheumatism. I have no evidence that this would be effective, but it seems possible, by comparison with similar uses of Lemon oil.

Its most widespread use is as an insect repellent and it is cultivated in large amounts for use in commercial insect-repellent preparations as well as the manufacture of soap, household disinfectants, etc. It is also used to adulterate more expensive essential oils.

I have used this oil to keep my cats away from plant tubs, and it also features in some preparations sold in garden shops for the same purpose. It does need to be re-applied every few days but will effectively keep animals away from small areas of soil.

Clary Sage
Salvia sclarea

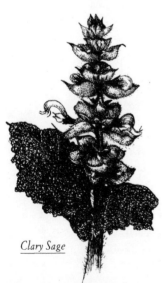

Clary Sage

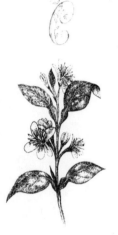

Clary Sage is used in aromatherapy in preference to Sage *(Salvia officinalis)* because, while Clary shares many of the properties of Sage, it does not present the risks of toxicity associated with the high level of thujone in Sage oil (up to 45% of some Sage oils).

The derivation of the name Clary is uncertain, some think it is a corruption of the Latin 'clarus' meaning clear, and others that the Latin 'sclarea' is itself derived from the Greek 'skleria', meaning hardness, because the petals end in a hard point. Mediaeval authors called the herb Clear Eye and attributed to it the property of healing all kinds of eye disorders. Nicholas Culpeper, more realistically, said that the sticky mucilage from the seeds, put into the eyes, would clear from it any small foreign objects 'gotten within the lids to offend them'.

The plant is native to Italy, Syria and southern France, but will grow wherever the soil is dry enough. Damp soil will rot the roots. It is a dramatic plant growing to 2 or 3 feet, with tall flower spikes rising above hairy leaves. The flowers themselves are not very significant, but they are supported by yellow and purple bracts. The essential oil is distilled from the flowers and flowering tips, and contains linalyl acetate, sclareol, linalol, salvene and salvone, etc. The exact composition varies according to the area where the plants were grown.

Essential oil of Clary has a wonderfully nutty aroma, which is in itself far more agreeable to use in treatments than oil of Sage. It used to be called Muscatel sage in Germany, as the taste was thought to resemble that of Muscatel wine. Dishonest merchants used Clary to adulterate cheaper wines to make them taste like true Muscatel – sometimes with disastrous results. Numerous writers have described how drinking wine or beer adulterated with Clary produced an exaggerated state of drunkenness followed by an equally exaggerated hangover! As one 18th century writer said, it was 'Fit to please drunkards who thereby, according to their several dispositions, became either dead drunke, or foolish drunke, or madde drunke.'

Amusing though this may seem, it is important to warn anybody using Clary oil not to take alcohol, as the combination can give rise to extremely severe nightmares, described by one person, who was unwise enough to combine the two, as being akin to a 'bad trip' on drugs. Clary alone I have found to induce very dramatic and colourful dreams, though these can be of a pleasant nature.

The effects of Clary have been described as 'euphoric' though not everybody experiences such a heightened state. Most will simply become very relaxed, possibly drowsy, so it is unwise to give massage with this oil to any patient who will have to drive home after the consultation. Better to give them a little of the oil for use in baths at home. From this it will be obvious that Clary is likely to be helpful in all kinds of stress and tension. It is a powerful muscle relaxant which, of course, is especially useful where muscular tension arises from mental or emotional stress.

Clary is valuable in treating asthma, as it both relaxes spasm in the bronchial tubes, and helps the anxiety and emotional tension often found in asthma sufferers. The same properties are potentially useful for migraine sufferers who often hold a lot of underlying tension. As well as being very relaxing, Clary is a powerful tonic, and this makes it very helpful in convalescence, especially after 'flu, when many people feel very debilitated, during depression and in the post-natal recovery period.

As it is warming and antispasmodic, it helps digestive problems, especially cramps or griping colicky pains. Either gentle massage over the stomach and abdomen, or hot compresses of Clary are very comforting.

Clary is an emmenagogue, and can help scanty or missing periods. It is best used during the first half of the menstrual cycle, as if used in the second half it can sometimes induce very heavy bleeding. It goes without saying that it should not be used during pregnancy.

One of the useful actions of Clary is in preventing excessive sweating. When tuberculosis was widespread, Clary was used to combat the night sweats experienced by patients, as well as to strengthen their defence systems in the fight against the tuberculosis bacillus. It may prove helpful to people with A.I.D.S in the same way.

Clary can help to reduce excessive production of sebum, especially on the scalp, and can be put in a final rinsing water after shampooing, for people with very greasy hair and dandruff.

Clary is one of the aphrodisiac oils and has proved very helpful for couples who are experiencing a 'bad patch' in their relationship, maybe because external stresses, such as financial or other worries, are creating tensions that affect the couple vis-à-vis each other.

However, whatever the physical benefits conferred by Clary, it is in the area of stress-related illness that it is most valuable. As one of the most powerful relaxants known to us in aromatherapy, it can be used with care and sensitivity to help the ever growing number of people whose suffering arises from the anxiety created by twentieth century life.

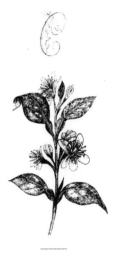

83

Clove

Eugenia caryophyllus

Clove oil is extracted from the dried, brown cloves familiar to cooks which are, in fact, the unopened buds of the tree *Eugenia caryophyllus*, originally native to Indonesia, and now grown in Madagascar, the West Indies, the Phillipines and other places with similar climates. Essential oils can be extracted from the buds, leaves and stalks, but that from the bud is the only one which should be used in aromatherapy as the others are powerful skin irritants. This is due to the high levels of eugenol (a phenol). Clove Stem oil can contain as much as 95% of eugenol with other minor ingredients and that oil from the leaves 80% to 88% with some minor constituents. The amount of eugenol in Clove Bud oil can vary from as little as 60% to as much as 90%, but it is to some extent 'buffered' by the presence of eugenol acetate, an ester, and beta caryophyllene, a sesquiterpene, which are calming and soothing in action. However, even the oil from the buds should be treated with caution and used on the skin only in dilutions of 1%. It is very important to be sure that the oil you are using is extracted from the bud: don't be tempted to buy any oil if you cannot identify the part of the tree from which it has been extracted.

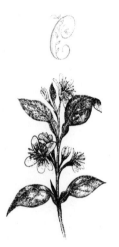

84

The tree belongs to the botanical family of Myrtaceae, which makes it a 'cousin' to Eucalyptus, Ti-tree and others that are noted for their anti-infectious action. Clove is no exception, and has been used for many thousands of years for the prevention of contagious illnesses, especially the plague. Jean Valnet records that when Dutch settlers cut down all the Clove trees in Ternate, the area was swept by wave after wave of epidemics, which had never happened before. Clove oil, cloves and pomanders made by sticking cloves into oranges are also effective insect repellents and help to keep disease-carrying insects away, as well as moths.

Lest we are tempted to think that these facts are of historical interest only, it is worth remembering that bubonic plague is still endemic in some parts of Asia, and that many bacteria have become resistant to modern antiseptics and antibiotics, due to mutation. Clove oil is a very powerful antiseptic – a 1% solution is four times more effective than phenol – and may well be of value in hospitals, old people's homes and other institutions where mutated bacteria are a serious problem. It is certainly well worth vaporising at home during epidemics of all kinds. It blends well with Orange, and I often use Clove, Orange and Cinnamon together to make a wonderful 'winter' fragrance that smells like a traditional pomander at the same time as giving some protection against winter epidemics.

Clove is also a good painkiller, and has long been used to ease toothache. It is still used as an antiseptic in modern dentistry as well as many commercial toothpastes, mouthwashes, etc.

It is occasionally used in ointments for the treatment of scabies (q.v.) and in lotions or alcohol-based solutions for infected ulcers and wounds, especially if they are slow and stubborn to heal, but care should always be taken when using Clove on the skin because of its irritant potential. Use only in very small amounts, and well diluted.

Clove is antispasmodic, and an infusion made from dried cloves (NOT the essential oil) helps to ease intestinal cramps and diarrhoea.

Traditionally, Clove has been used in midwifery as an antiseptic, and to prepare the uterus for childbirth. I do not know of anybody using it in this context at the present time, but pregnant women may well find it helpful to drink an infusion of dried cloves several times a day for a few days before the baby is due.

Colds

The common cold is a virus infection of the nose and throat. There are at least 30 different strains of virus which can cause cold symptoms, and these are constantly mutating. While the mucous membranes of the nose and throat are inflamed as a result of the infection, they are far more vulnerable to attack by bacteria, and this can give rise to secondary infections such as sinusitis, ear infections and bronchitis, which are more serious than the original cold.

Fortunately, there are quite a number of essential oils which not only diminish the discomfort of a cold, but help reduce the risk of secondary infections, partly because the oils themselves are bactericidal and partly because they stimulate the body's own

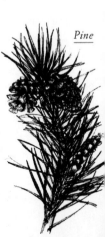

Pine

ability to fight off infection. Chief among these are Lavender, Eucalyptus, Ti-tree and the closely related Niaouli. Peppermint, Rosemary and Pine can also be used, and Thyme is a valuable inhalant for sore throats. Bathing with Marjoram will help to reduce shivers and aching, and also helps headaches associated with a cold.

The two most useful methods of use are inhalations and baths. Bathing with Ti-tree oil at the very first sign of a cold can often stop the cold developing. A steam inhalation with appropriate essential oils combines several beneficial effects. It clears the congested nasal passages and soothes the inflamed mucous membrane; at the same time the essential oil will kill many bacteria. Very hot steam, as hot as can be tolerated without actually burning the nose and throat, is, in itself, a hostile environment for viruses, and the addition of an antiviral oil such as Eucalyptus or Ti-tree, increases the effectiveness of the steam. Use either of these two oils for inhalations in the earlier part of the day (alternating with Rosemary and Peppermint if you want a change), as they are all somewhat stimulant, and could interfere with sleep. At night, use inhalations of Lavender, which will enhance sleep.

An evening bath with Lavender, alone or with Marjoram, will go a long way towards ensuring a good night's sleep, which in itself will help recovery. Some Lavender oil diffused in the bedroom is also good, especially if there is a cough.

Garlic tablets or capsules, and fresh garlic in the diet will not only help to clear an existing cold, but are valuable in preventing colds. A good level of nutrition with plenty of fresh fruit and vegetables to provide Vitamin C will also help to prevent infection, and a high intake of Vitamin C (up to 10 grams in a day) has been shown to shorten the duration of a cold. These measures can be combined with aromatherapy methods for maximum benefit.

see also entries for **COUGHS, INFLUENZA** *and* **SORE THROAT.**

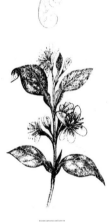

Cold Sores

see **HERPES.**

Comfrey
Symphytum officinale

Comfrey has a very long history of use in traditional medicine, especially for fractures, sprains, etc. An infused oil of Comfrey can be used in aromatherapy for sprains, muscular and joint strains. I have used it for deep massage of troublesome old injuries, sometimes with adhesions that were causing pain and restricting mobility. Comfrey oil contains allantoin, which aids healing, and is often helpful for itchy, rough skin and dry eczema. When using infused oils that have therapeutic properties of their own the proportion of essential oil in a massage blend should be lower than when using a bland carrier oil: between 1% and 2% is enough.

Compresses

Compresses are a very effective way of using essential oils to relieve pain and swelling and reduce inflammation. Hot compresses are most often used to treat pain of a chronic nature and cold compresses to treat acute pain, and as a first-aid for injuries such as sprains.

A hot compress is prepared by filling a bowl with water as hot as you can bear to put your hands in, and sprinkling 4 or 5 drops of essential oil on to the water. Fold a clean piece of absorbent fabric into several thicknesses and dip into the water, so that the cloth picks up as much as possible of the essential oil floating on the surface. Wring out the cloth to get rid of surplus water, and place it at once on the painful area. Suitable materials are lint, clean old sheeting or towelling, a face flannel, a clean handkerchief for a very small compress or a folded hand-towel for a larger one.

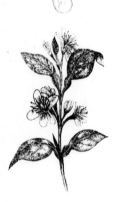

Cover the compress with a piece of cling-film or other plastic material to prevent soaking clothes and bandages. On ankles, knees, wrists, elbows etc. the compress can be held in position with a crepe bandage. For the back, abdomen or larger areas, it is usually more practical to wrap a large towel around the body over the compress and its plastic covering and encourage the patient to rest. The compress should be replaced with a fresh one when it has cooled to blood heat.

Hot compresses are particularly helpful in treating backache, fibrositis, rheumatic and arthritic pain, abscesses, earache and toothache.

Cold compresses are made and applied in exactly the same way, except that the water should be as cold as possible. If you have ice cubes available, put some in the water for a few minutes before making the compress. If not, run the cold tap for a few minutes to get the water as cool as you can. Cold compresses are helpful for headaches (apply to forehead or back of neck), sprains, tennis elbow, and other hot, swollen conditions. They should be renewed once they have warmed up to blood temperature, though there is no harm in leaving the compress in place overnight or during the day if circumstances do not allow frequent changing.

Very large cold compresses can be used to bring down a patient's fever if it is dangerously high, but this should only be done by people who are well trained in handling acute illness, and should never be applied to babies or elderly people, as their body-heat control mechanisms are less efficient than those of adults and older children, and it is possible to cause too rapid a swing from very hot to subnormally cold.

Alternate hot and cold compressing is a naturopathic technique which aids healing, and is very valuable for sprains and other conditions where massage cannot be used. Use cold compresses as a first-aid measure, but switch to hot and cold ones in the following days. Always start with a hot compress and finish with a cold one.

Concrete

A concrete is an aromatic substance extracted from plants by solvents.

Concretes contain fats and waxes as well as essential oil and need further treatment with alcohol to obtain an absolute. This method is used mainly where steam distillation would spoil the delicate fragrance of the plant material (Jasmine, for example).

Constipation

A number of essential oils are described as helpful for constipation, but I think such information should be approached with caution. Above all, do not fall into the mistake of thinking of essential oils as a 'dose'. Massaging the abdomen in a clockwise direction is very helpful and this is something that the patient can easily do daily at home. The best oils to use for this are Marjoram and Rosemary, together or singly, and I sometimes add a very small amount of Black Pepper or Fennel. Several cups of Fennel tea daily would be a good addition.

The most important part of any treatment for constipation must be dietary. Unrefined carbohydrates, raw vegetables, fruits and all foods high in fibre, and copious drinks of water, juices and herb teas should form the major part of the daily intake, with fats, dairy products and refined sugars and starches reduced to a minimum. A colon cleansing programme would be an effective way of re-educating the bowel for long-term health.

Sometimes, constipation is the result of stress, anxiety, shock or emotional problems, often suppressed. In such instances, aromatherapy can be used in a sensitive way to work on the underlying problems. Gentle full-body massage with carefully chosen oils and aromatic baths between visits will reduce stress or anxiety, though if the problem is an emotional one of long standing, it may be weeks or months before it can be resolved. Essential oils should be chosen for the immediate and long-term needs of the person involved, rather than to the physical state of the gut, though gentle tummy massage and some changes in diet can be introduced. An improvement in the physical condition will raise morale and help to create the conditions of trust and confidence in the therapist, in which work at a more subtle level can take place.

Fennel

Contagious Diseases

Contagion implies infection by direct person-to-person contact, as opposed to air-borne, water-borne or other sources of infection, although the term is very often used incorrectly to describe epidemics spread by these means. Essential oils in one's immediate environment, particularly when used regularly in the bath, are a measure of protection against contagious diseases. Clove, Eucalyptus, Lavender and Ti-tree are all good for this purpose.

Convalescence

The term convalescence may be used to describe anything from a few days of feeling rather fragile following a cold or 'flu, to a long period of recovery following an accident or major surgery.

Aromatherapy can be a particular help at such times in increasing the body's own powers of recovery and regeneration. A wide choice of essential oils can be called upon, according to the physical needs, mood and personal preferences of the person using them. Jean Valnet suggests Lemon and Thyme as strengthening and beneficial in convalescence, and any of the spice oils can be tried in very small amounts to stimulate appetite and increase energy, but the two oils which, in my experience, are the most helpful of all, are Rosemary and Grapefruit. Rosemary is tonic and gently stimulating, and Grapefruit is helpful in both increasing the appetite, which is so often lacking after an illness, and lifting the feeling of slight depression that is common during convalescence.

Regular massage, if possible, is a great boost to recovery, as well as being relaxing and enjoyable, but if there is nobody around to give a massage, or in the intervals between massage treatments, try aromatic baths with any of the oils mentioned, or indeed, virtually any oil that is found appealing.

If the period of convalescence is due to surgery or an accident, essential oils to minimise scarring might be useful. Lavender and Neroli in a base of almond (75%) and wheatgerm (25%) oils will help to reduce scars. They can be applied gently once or twice a day as soon as the actual wound has healed.

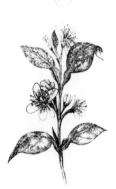

Adequate rest and really excellent nutrition are important, too. Most people who are recovering from illness will benefit from a multi-vitamin and mineral supplement, and this is one of the times that ginseng is very appropriate.

Coriander
Coriandrum sativum

Coriander is an attractive plant of the Umbelliferae family, which grows either wild or cultivated in the Far East, Spain, North Africa and the former U.S.S.R. Some plants are found growing wild in parts of England, where they have self-seeded from cultivated plants. The leaves, when crushed, give off an extremely unpleasant odour which the ancient Greeks found reminiscent of a squashed bedbug, hence the plant's name which is derived from 'koris', the Greek for bug! Fortunately, the seeds have an altogether different aroma, very pleasant, fresh and spicy, and the essential oil which is distilled from them is very true to the smell of a freshly crushed seed. The oil may be pale yellow or colourless, and its main chemical constituents include between 60% and 65% of coriandrol, pinene, geraniol and traces of phellandrene, dipentene, terpinene, cymene and borneol.

Like all the members of this big plant family (Caraway, Dill, Fennel, etc.) Coriander stimulates and aids digestion. For this reason, as well as the agreeable flavour, the seeds were used a great deal by the Egyptians and seeds have been discovered in various tombs. Because of its stimulating action on the appetite, Coriander has been used in the treatment of anorexia nervosa.

The oil is analgesic, and good for neuralgia and rheumatic pains. It is gently warming which is comforting in these conditions.

Commercially, Coriander is used in making liqueurs such as Chartreuse and Benedictine (having been originally incorporated in the formula for its digestive properties) and to flavour some brands of gin. It is used quite a lot in perfumery, soap and toiletries, and also as a raw material from which various of the chemical elements are extracted for use in manufacturing synthetic perfumes.

Coughs

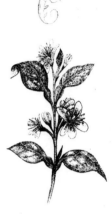

A cough is a reflex action of the bronchi (air passages) which is designed to clear these passages of obstructions such as dust, pollen or excessive mucus. As such, the cough is useful and should not be suppressed. Sometimes, though, the reflex is provoked by inflammation of the mucous membrane of the throat when there is nothing to expel, and this kind of cough can exhaust the patient to no useful end. Even a 'productive' cough (one which gets rid of mucus) can set up further non-productive irritation and perpetuate itself after it has ceased to be useful. Sometimes a cough can be triggered from pressures from outside the air passages, such as by enlarged lymph nodes in whooping cough.

The best form of aromatherapy treatment is a steam inhalation, since this will soothe the throat and bronchi, and also loosen any excessive mucus so that expelling it by coughing becomes easier. If the cough is due to a bacterial infection, bactericidal oils can be chosen to attack the root of the problem. Thyme is one of the most powerful of these, and others that combat coughs include Benzoin (extremely soothing to the throat), Eucalyptus, Frankincense, Lavender, Marjoram and Sandalwood.

The latter is particularly helpful for dry coughs that persist long after the original infection. Massage to the throat and chest, with any of these oils, is an alternative, or both methods can be used together. Oils in a burner, or other form of diffuser, will help, especially at night.

Such time-honoured remedies as hot lemon drinks with honey, or herb teas, also have the effect of soothing irritation in the throat.

Any cough which does not clear up after a few days with these simple self-help measures should be treated by a doctor, medical herbalist, etc.

see also **COLDS, BRONCHITIS** and **INFLUENZA.**

Coumarins

❧

Coumarins are a group of aromatic molecules that are not very volatile, so they are not easily extracted by distillation. They are found mainly in the Citrus oils, which are not distilled but extracted by simple pressure. Coumarins are sedative, antispasmodic and anticonvulsive. Examples include coumarin, small amounts in Lavender and some other oils; herniarin, in Helichrysum, Lavender, etc., and citroptene in various Citrus oils.

A sub-group of Coumarins, the Furocoumarins, cause photosensitisation of the skin. They include bergaptene and bergamotine, both in Bergamot and other Citrus oils, and Angelicine, in Angelica Root and other Umbelliferae oils.

Cracked Nipples

❧

see **BREASTFEEDING.**

Cracked Skin

❧

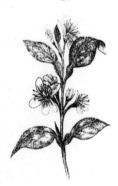

Cracked skin, for example the cracks which may occur in dry, hard skin on the heels, or cracking on the hands due to extreme weather, exposure to water, detergents, outdoor work and so forth, can be effectively treated with Benzoin, Calendula, Lavender or Myrrh.

If there is any sign of infection in the cracks, use Benzoin mixed with Lavender or Ti-tree, neat in very small amounts until the infection has cleared. Otherwise, the best method is to add the oils to a rich cream, which you may make yourself or buy, as the cream will help to restore suppleness to the skin and prevent more cracks appearing.

If you are treating cracks where the skin is damp, Myrrh is the best choice and can be combined with Benzoin or Lavender to promote healing. For cracked lips, Benzoin alone mixed into a salve can be applied several times a day.

Calendula

Creams

✍

Creams made from pure, natural plant products offer one of the most versatile ways in which to use essential oil. Essential oils can be chosen for a wide variety of therapeutic uses and added to an unperfumed cream base. Many people, especially those untrained in massage, find creams much easier to handle and apply than carrier oils, so if you wish a patient to continue using an oil at home between one visit and the next, a cream may be a better option than an oil mixture.

A characteristic of creams is that they stay on the surface of the skin longer than a carrier oil, and this is obviously helpful when you are dealing with any kind of skin problem, whether it is cosmetic, or a skin disorder. The heavier creams can provide a barrier between the skin and the outer environment which protects and promotes healing.

Simple creams can be made at home quite easily, usually using various combinations of oil, beeswax and flower waters. Almond oil is the classic base oil from which creams are made, and thicker, heavier creams can be made with coconut oil or cocoa butter added to the almond oil. Special base oils such as jojoba, avocado, peach kernel, etc. are usually added in relatively small amounts for their particular properties. To such a cream, any appropriate essential oil can be added. You will find some recipes for creams in **APPENDIX C**.

If you do not want to make your own creams, you can add essential oils to ready-made creams, but it is really important to be sure that they are made from pure plant substances and that no harmful chemicals have been added. It is not, as yet, obligatory for the makers of creams and other skin preparations to list all their ingredients, though some do so voluntarily, so do be certain that you buy only brands which are known to be trustworthy in this respect. Some of the better essential oil suppliers also sell excellent base creams to which you can add your own essential oils.

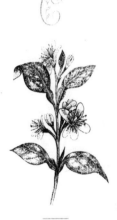

---

see **APPENDIX C** *for* **CREAM RECIPES.**

Culpeper, Nicholas

✍

Nicholas Culpeper was born in 1616, the son of a clergyman related to the Culpeper family who owned Wakehurst Place, Sussex.* After early schooling at home he went to Cambridge University at the age of 16, and studied in particular the medical writers of antiquity. After leaving the University he was apprenticed to an apothecary in Bishopsgate.

[Footnote:] * *Wakehurst Place is administered by the National Trust, and its gardens come under the care of Kew. Anybody interested in aromatherapy or plant medicine in general, would be likely to enjoy a visit to the walled garden, where many of the plants that furnish us with essential oils can be found. Clary Sage and Hyssop rub shoulders with Thyme and Marjoram and many different varieties of Rosemary. There are more kinds of Lavender than I ever knew existed, and old fashioned climbing roses clothe the walls. A visit in early summer when most the of the plants are in flower is a delight to the nose as well as the eye.*

In 1640 he set up on his own as an astrologer and physician, and managed to keep his medical practice going throughout the Civil War, in spite of fighting in Cromwell's army in at least one battle, when he was seriously wounded in the chest. His injuries left his lung function permanently impaired, and weakened him for the rest of his life.

In 1649 Culpeper fell foul of the College of Physicians, by publishing his translation of their 'Pharmacopoeia' under the title 'A Physical Directory'. All medical texts at that time were written in Latin, the language of scholars, and this restricted access to the information in them to a small section of society. Culpeper wanted to make medical information available to anyone who could read, by translating it into English, but in doing so he infringed the monopoly of the doctors and aroused their wrath. The College of Physicians attacked Culpeper in various periodicals, accusing him of drunkenness, lechery, heresy and atheism – quite apart from having made a bad and miserable translation! (which, in fact, he had not: it was meticulously accurate).

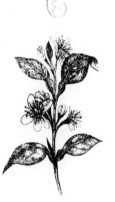

Culpeper replied with an attack on the secrecy, exclusivity and mercenary nature of the organised physicians and, more seriously, questioned the use of toxic chemicals, such as mercury, which they were increasingly prescribing, despite the fact that it killed the patient almost as often as it cured.

Altogether he wrote or translated 79 books, including second and third editions of 'The Physical Directory' and translations from the Greek and Latin works of Galen and other early writers, as well as his own original works such as 'The Anatomy of the Body of Man' published in 1653, and a 'Directory for Midwives'. The hours he spent in writing and research, in addition to his medical practice, and his responsibilities as the father of a large family (he had seven children) undermined his health. He contracted tuberculosis and, with his lung already damaged by his earlier battle wound, was unable to fight it. He died in 1654, aged only 38.

Throughout his brief career, Culpeper strove to make medicine more accessible to ordinary people, whether by translating previously obscure texts, or by giving treatment free to poor people, even though he never had a great deal of money himself. He chose to practice in a poor district, rather than one of the fashionable areas where he could have attracted wealthy patients, and put a lot of his own money into publishing his books.

The book for which we now revere him, generally known simply as 'Culpeper's Herbal' was published in 1653 under the title 'The English Physician, with 369 Medicines Made of English Herbs that were not in any Impression Until This'. The title was intended to make clear that this was an original work, rather than another translation, though following in the tradition of John Gerard a generation earlier, he did draw quite heavily on the writings of Galen and other early doctors. Also like Gerard, Culpeper added many comments and observations of his own, including an astrological classification of the plants according to the planet by which each one was ruled. He distinguished between the botanical and medicinal facts set out by the classical writers, and certain elements of myth which sometimes crept into the ancient texts, by setting out the opinions of the earlier authors but adding his own wry comments, such as 'It is marvellous (if it not be fabulous)' on some of their wilder claims. He gave clear descriptions of the plants and places where

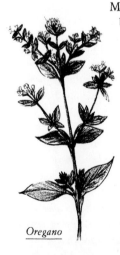

Oregano

they could be found, for he intended the book to be used by

ordinary people as a practical aid to finding medicinal plants for their own use. He wanted, he said, to make it as easy to find and use these plants as those commonly used for food.

Culpeper distinguished clearly between the use of plant 'simples' which he encouraged untrained people to use, and essential oils, which were known as 'chymical oils' and prescribed by apothecaries. 'Such country people as know not how to draw the chymical oil, may content themselves by eating ten or twelve of the ripe berries every morning fasting.' He gave clear and practical instructions on how to prepare various types of remedy from the basic plant material, including infusions, poultices, aromatic wines and infused oils, which he often suggested should be used to 'anoint', i.e. massage, an afflicted person.

The book is of far more than historical interest, and any aromatherapist can find in it useful indications on the properties and uses of many oils. Among the 369 plants described are many used in modern practice by medical herbalists, as well as a score or more of those we use in aromatherapy, including Basil, Camomile, Clary, Fennel, Garlic, Hyssop, Juniper, several of the Mints, Lavender, Marjoram, Rosemary, three different kinds of Roses, Sage, Thyme and several others.

Hyssop

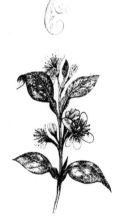

Cumin
Cuminum cyminum

Cumin is a close relative of Coriander, Dill, Fennel etc., and is a native of Egypt which now grows all round the Mediterranean and in the Far East. The seeds are used to distil the essential oil, which is colourless initially but yellows with age. The aroma is slightly bitter, musky and aromatic, with a slight resemblance to aniseed. The chief chemical constituents are cuminol, varying from about 35% to 50%, with cymene, pinene and terpineol.

Cumin is another of the spices which has been used since antiquity. Both the Egyptians and the Hebrews used large quantities for flavouring food as a digestive aid. Nowadays, it is probably best known as an ingredient of curry.

In common with almost all of the Umbelliferae family, Cumin is a good aperitive, a digestive aid and carminative. The essential oil is a digestive, stimulant and tonic, and helpful when the digestion is sluggish. It is antispasmodic and using it for gentle massage of the abdomen will relieve griping pains caused by flatulence and diarrhoea.

Cumin is also a more general tonic and stimulant, acting particularly on the heart and nervous system, and it may possibly have some aphrodisiac action.

It needs, however, to be used with great care, as it may cause sensitisation of the skin in some people. In most cases it would be wiser to use Coriander which has very similar properties.

93

Cypress

Cupressus sempervirens

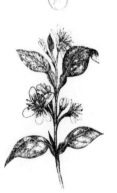

This is the familiar Cypress which is such an inextricable feature of the Mediterranean landscape, familiar through the paintings of Cezanne and Van Gogh. The tree is associated with cemeteries, a use which may derive from the fact that both the ancient Egyptians and Romans dedicated the tree to their gods of death and the underworld. The word 'sempervirens' in its name means 'ever-living' – referring to the evergreen nature of the leaves, but the perpetual greenness of the trees may also have been used as a symbol of life after death.

The essential oil is distilled from the leaves and the cones, and contains d-pinene, d-camphene, d-sylvestrene, cymene, sabinol, terpenic alcohol and camphor of Cypress. The oil varies from colourless to yellowy, and has a pleasantly smoky, woody smell, reminiscent of turpentine but less so than the oil of Juniper.

It is very astringent, and is used wherever there is an excess of fluid, from oedema, incontinence and excessive perspiration to bleeding gums, bilious attacks and over-heavy menstruation. It is also very useful in skin care, for oily and over-hydrated skins. It is used quite often in men's toiletries for its antiseptic and astringent properties – useful in an aftershave, for example – and its woody smell. It is a good deodorant, too.

The astringent action is also helpful for piles, used as a local wash or in an ointment. Haemorrhoids are symptomatic of a poor circulation, and Cypress is a tonic to the circulatory system. This makes it helpful in treating varicose veins. It can be applied locally to varicosed areas – very gently. Never massage directly over varicose veins, and apply oils or creams with light strokes in an upward direction.

Cypress is antispasmodic, acting especially on the bronchi, so it is one of the oils to think of when treating asthma. A drop or two inhaled from a hankie or tissue will help to relieve an asthma attack and the spasmodic coughing of whooping cough. As a preventative measure, a few drops of Cypress can be put on a saucer of water in the bedroom, or in an essential oil burner. This is specially valuable for asthmatic children, because many of them are very frightened when an attack happens during the night.

Another important use of Cypress is in regulating the menstrual cycle. It helps to relieve painful periods and reduces abnormally heavy loss, particularly when this happens in the early stages of the menopause.

Valnet suggests that Cypress might be of help in some forms of cancer, but he places a query after this information, indicating that he has no proof of this possible use. It is an area that might be rewarding to investigate.

A humble but very welcome use of Cypress is for excessive sweating of the feet. It is both deodorant and astringent and reduces both the amount of perspiration and unpleasant odour. Use it in footbaths as needed.

This is another insect-repelling oil. I have in the past used it to keep a dog free from fleas; and because it is deodorant, too, it helped to reduce doggy odours, particularly in summer when these can be rather noxious.

Cystic Fibrosis

In cystic fibrosis, several areas of body chemistry malfunction, affecting principally the lungs and the digestive system. The digestive problems (mainly inability to digest fats) can be helped with a carefully chosen diet and digestive enzymes and the area where aromatherapy can be of greatest value is in alleviating the respiratory problems.

In cystic fibrosis the lungs constantly produce too much mucus, which leads to congestion, breathing difficulties and frequent infections, because the excess mucus forms a breeding ground for bacteria. The parents of children with cystic fibrosis are taught to carry out physiotherapy on their child several times each day to help the draining of mucus. Using essential oils greatly increases the effectiveness of this treatment, as well as helping to prevent and treat lung infections.

To alleviate this condition we need oils which are mucolytic, expectorant and anti-infectious, and because treatment will be needed constantly, the widest possible range of oils must be included, to avoid the dangers implicit in using any oil continually over a long period of time. The oils which I think of as the prime choice are the resins: Benzoin, Elemi, Frankincense and Myrrh, which can be used in rotation. To them I would add Lavender, Manuka, Niaouli, Ravensara and Ti-tree for their anti-infectious and immuno-stimulant action, plus Bergamot, Cedar, Eucalyptus *(globulus, radiata* and *citriodora)*, Inula, Pine and Sandalwood. If these are combined in blends consisting of one resin, one immunostimulant and one other oil, a great many different permutations are possible and should be varied every week or so. The longest any one blend should be used without a break is three weeks.

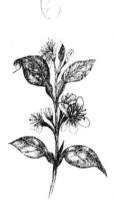

For young children, do not exceed 1% of essential oil to carrier, increasing this to 2% as they get older. Massaging the oils into the chest and back as part of the daily physiotherapy sessions is the most important aspect of treatment: it makes it much easier for the child to cough up mucus, and reduces the risk of bronchial infections and other complications. I suggest to aromatherapists helping children with cystic fibrosis that they give ready-mixed blends to the parents to use between visits.

Steam inhalations are another effective way to get the oils into the lungs, and baths will help to reduce the risk of infection and strengthen the immune system. Even better would be an aerosol diffuser that projects minute droplets of essential oil into the air: this form of treatment has been proved highly effective for respiratory problems of all kinds.

Finally, looking after somebody with cystic fibrosis can be physically and emotionally demanding, so we need to ask 'Who cares for the carers?' and try to see that they get relaxing bath oils and massage as often as possible.

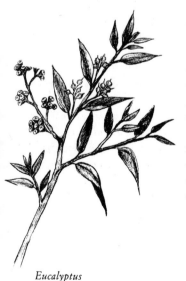

Eucalyptus

Cystitis

Cystitis, or inflammation of the bladder, is most often caused by bacterial infection, though occasionally it is due to irritants such as crystalline deposits in the urine. It is far more common in women than in men because infection frequently spreads upwards from the urethra (the tube that carries urine from the bladder to the exterior of the body) and this is only about 1.5 inches long in women and four to five times that length in men, giving the bladder greater protection. The use of essential oils at the first sign of irritation of the urethra will often prevent a full-blown attack of cystitis from developing.

The most valuable oils in treating this painful and depressing condition are Bergamot, Camomile, Eucalyptus, Garlic, Lavender, Sandalwood and Ti-tree. Of these, those I find most effective, and think of as the first line of defence, are Bergamot and Ti-tree used externally as a local wash and in the bath, Camomile in the form of Camomile tea, and Garlic taken in perles or capsules. Camomile can be added to external washes, too, to ease the painful stinging and irritation. As with all use of essential oils on delicate mucous membranes the essential oils should be diluted to

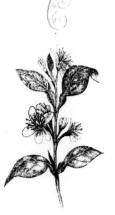

1% or less in boiled and cooled water and the opening of the urethra swabbed with this at frequent intervals. At the same time, as much Camomile tea as possible should be drunk, alternating with pure spring water or lemon barley water (home-made). Bergamot or Ti-tree should be added to the bath – about 6 drops, and used at least once every day, more often if possible.

A massage oil containing Bergamot and Lavender or Camomile can be massaged gently over the lower abdomen, and if there is a lot of pain, a hot Camomile compress may be helpful. Full body massage with any of the oils I have mentioned helps to combat the infection and relieve the depression that often goes with it.

Camomile

If there is blood or pus in the urine, or the temperature is very high, do not delay in consulting a doctor, because cystitis can quickly lead to serious infections of the kidneys. This is one of the situations in which antibiotics should not be rejected, and it is also important to get a proper analysis of a urine specimen carried out to identify which strain of bacteria is involved, since different ones respond to different antibiotics. If treatment with antibiotics does become necessary, the aromatherapy treatment can beneficially be continued at the same time.

The bacteria most commonly responsible for bladder infections are normally present in the gut, but are kept under control by the helpful bacteria found there. One of the disadvantages of antibiotics is that they kill many of the 'friendly' bacteria in the intestines along with the invading ones, and this can lead to the debilitating cycle of cystitis-antibiotics-cystitis which many women dread. Eating a good quantity of live yoghurt while taking antibiotics helps to counteract this effect and re-establish a healthy intestinal flora. Regular use of essential oils, especially in the bath, can break this cycle and prevent frequent recurrence of cystitis. Avoiding synthetic underwear and tights, and close-fitting trousers helps, too.

Sandalwood has been used as a urinary antiseptic in India for many centuries and is a valuable alternative to Bergamot, Ti-tree, etc. if repeated treatment is needed.

Dehydrated Skin

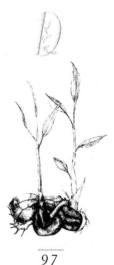

This type of skin, which lacks moisture, is often confused with the 'dry' skin that lacks natural oils (sebum), though a shortage of oils may contribute to dehydration, since the surface layer of sebum helps to conserve whatever moisture is present in the skin.

Dehydrated skin often feels tight and cold, and wrinkles easily. You are most likely to observe this type of skin in older people, but central heating and air conditioning are making it far more common.

Lack of oil and lack of moisture are both concerned with endocrine imbalance, and essential oils which help to correct such imbalances should be used. Geranium and Lavender are among the best to use. Gentle oils to soothe the surface of the skin are Camomile, Neroli and Rose. Fluid lotions are more helpful for such skin than creams and any of these essential oils can be added to the lotion. The skin needs protection all the time to prevent loss of fluids, and lotions can be applied several times a day, especially before going out in hot, or very dry and windy weather.

The diet should include plenty of fresh raw fruits and vegetables, fruit juices and natural mineral water. Alcohol has a really damaging effect as it causes further dehydration, not only of the skin but of the whole body, so it should be avoided or kept to a very small amount. Smoking is very damaging too.

Massage needs to be very, very gentle indeed. Face-packs containing honey are really beneficial for dehydrated skin. The honey can be patted onto the skin on its own, or mixed with mashed avocado pulp or banana.

Deodorants

Several essential oils are effective deodorising agents, and can be used in room sprays to neutralise cooking, smoking or other domestic odours, as well as in baths for personal hygiene. One or two firms making plant-based products offer deodorant sprays made with essential oils. The most effective deodorising essential oil is Bergamot, though Lavender, Neroli, Juniper, Cypress, Thyme and Sage can be used. Bergamot has the advantage of a delicious fragrance of its own, which is fresh and citrussy and acceptable in use to both men and women. However, great care should be taken when using Bergamot in sunny weather as it increases the risk of the skin burning. If the skin is likely to be exposed to sunshine, use one of the alternative oils.

Depression

Depression can take many forms, and stem from different causes, and Mother Earth in her generosity has given us a great number of plants to help alleviate it. The antidepressant essential oils are as diverse as the ways in which depression can manifest itself, and part of the aromatherapist's skill must lie in selecting the most appropriate oil or blend for the client at any given moment – for the client's needs may also change from day to day and even from hour to hour.

It would be worse than useless, for example, to use a very sedative oil when the depressed person feels abnormally fatigued or lethargic. On the other hand, if the depression is taking the form of restlessness, irritability and inability to sleep, such an oil may be exactly what is needed. Camomile, Clary Sage, Lavender, Sandalwood and Ylang-Ylang are oils that are both sedative and antidepressant, while Bergamot, Geranium, Melissa and Rose can help to lift the mood without sedating.

Where anxiety is associated with depression, Neroli is one of the most valuable of oils, and Jasmine is traditionally held to increase confidence, both in one's self and in the likelihood of overcoming difficult circumstances.

Massage is obviously very important, because of the contact with the therapist, but baths can be valuable too, partly because they can be taken every day, or whenever the client feels inclined, and partly because they involve the depressed person doing something for him or herself.

In helping people who are depressed, perhaps more than in any other aspect of aromatherapy, it is important to pay attention to the client's preferences in regard to the oil or oils to be used, since this will often instinctively be the right choice at that particular time. Changing preferences as the treatment progresses can give the therapist valuable clues to the changing moods and needs of the client.

When helping a depressed client, the 'listening' aspect of aromatherapy becomes very important. Some aromatherapists are also trained in counselling and feel able to offer this in addition to essential oil treatments, while others may want to refer clients to a counsellor or psychotherapist. This may need to be done with great sensitivity, as many people still think that psychotherapy is only for people who are 'crazy'!

Melissa

see also entries for **ANXIETY** and **STRESS**.

Dermatitis

Dermatitis means, literally, inflammation or irritation of the skin, and is not so much the name of a specific skin condition as of a group of conditions, characterised by redness and itching, often intense.

Sensitivity to one or more substances with which the skin has come into contact is often the immediate cause, though stress is a predisposing factor.

All essential oils and treatments described under **ECZEMA** are appropriate.

Devil's Claw
Harpagophytum procumbens

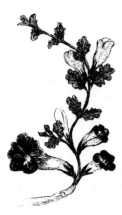

Devil's Claw

I have known Devil's Claw for over thirty years as a herbal remedy, taken internally for rheumatism, arthritis and other inflammatory conditions, so I was delighted to find that it also prepared as an infused oil, which can be used in massage for the same conditions. The oil is highly anti-inflammatory and analgesic, and I have been using it for muscular strain and repetitive strain injury with very good results. Essential oils can be added in small amounts – 1% to 2% at most – bearing in mind that the infused oil has considerable therapeutic properties of its own. Some people will be helped by taking Devil's Claw internally as well: most health food stores stock it as tablets.

Diarrhoea

As food waste passes through the large intestine, much of the water contained in it is reabsorbed through the intestinal walls, so that the final state of the faeces is moderately soft without being watery. Disruptions of the normal passage of food through the large and small intestines will disturb this pattern. Too slow a passage through the gut (as in diets which are lacking in fibre) allows a greater amount of water to be absorbed, leading to hard faeces and constipation. Too fast a passage will not allow enough water to be absorbed, and gives rise to diarrhoea.

Rapid passage of food through the intestines is most often due to an inflammation of the intestines, though the causes may be various. Viruses and bacteria, irritant drugs, poisons, and allergic reactions are among the commonest. The muscles of the intestinal wall become over-active when irritated, and this adds to the problem of diarrhoea, as the increased peristalsis propels the food mass faster through the gut.

The intestines are influenced in their functioning by the endocrine and nervous systems, and anything – such as shock, fear, anxiety or continued stress – that disturbs either of these two systems, will often result in diarrhoea.

Some essential oils are useful in helping diarrhoea because of their calming and soothing effect on the intestinal lining, some because they have an antispasmodic action on the intestinal muscles, some because of their astringent properties and yet others because they calm the nervous system. The choice of essential oil for helping with any case of diarrhoea will, therefore, depend on identifying the cause though the various actions often overlap in a single oil. Camomile, Cypress, Eucalyptus, Lavender, Neroli and Peppermint are among the most effective antispasmodics and are all used to allay attacks of diarrhoea.

Eucalyptus might be the best choice if there is any suspicion that a viral infection is the cause of the diarrhoea, as it is a potent antiviral agent. Camomile is an anti-allergic oil, and would be my first choice if a food allergy was involved though the food responsible should obviously be avoided, too. Sometimes warming and carminative essential oils, such as Benzoin, Ginger, Fennel or Black Pepper are used to relieve the pain in diarrhoea. Massaged gently over the abdomen, these can be helpful in easing the griping pains caused by spasmodic contraction of the intestinal muscles.

When diarrhoea is provoked by fear, anxiety or stress, whether in the short or long term, Camomile, Lavender or Neroli will help. Neroli is especially helpful for the prevention of diarrhoea in stressful circumstances which a person fears may provoke an upset tummy. The very fear of having diarrhoea is often enough to bring on an attack, and in these situations bathing or massaging the abdomen with Neroli, and inhaling it shortly before the feared event, will all help to soothe both the fears and the intestine. I am thinking particularly of situations such as exams, interviews, auditions and other short-term stressful occasions. Sometimes diarrhoea becomes persistent in people who are anxious, fearful or stressed over a period of time. Here, we should try to help the underlying stress, as well as giving immediate help with the diarrhoea.

Most attacks of diarrhoea clear up within a day or two, but anything that persists for longer must be investigated in order to be sure that there is no serious disorder of the intestine. Prolonged diarrhoea is dangerous because of the risk of dehydration from the loss of water – especially if there is also vomiting. This is particularly so in young children, who become dehydrated much faster than adults, and must be treated without delay.

During any attack of diarrhoea, plenty of fluids should be given to prevent the risk of dehydration. Food will delay the healing process by adding to the bulk of waste matter in the intestines, and giving invading organisms the kind of environment in which they can multiply. Most people suffering from diarrhoea will not feel like eating, in any case.

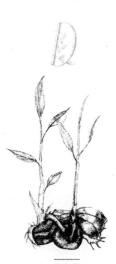

Dilutions

Essential oils are highly concentrated materials, and are hardly ever used neat, with the exception of tiny amounts of Lavender or Ti-tree on burns, cuts and grazes, insect bites and stings. For most other purposes the oil must be diluted in a carrier oil.

The most usual dilution for massage is 3% – 3 drops of essential oil to each 100 drops of carrier oil. 100 drops roughly equals 5 mls, so the simplest way to calculate your dilution is to add 3 drops of essential oil to each 5 mls of carrier oil, using a measuring spoon or glass.

When working with babies and children, with pregnant women, the frail, elderly and people with very sensitive skins the oils should be even more dilute, to 1.5%, 1% and sometimes even as little as 0.5%. The same simple method of measuring can be used. (As it is not possible to measure half a drop of essential oil, add 3 drops to 10 mls of carrier to get a 1.5% dilution, 1 drop to 10 mls for 0.5%, and so on.)

When essential oils are added to water THIS DOES NOT DILUTE THEM because water and oil do not mix. So, for example, when you put essential oil in your bath, it is not diluted, even though you have added it to many gallons of water. Most of the oil will float in a fine film on top of the water and some of it will settle on your skin in undiluted form. It is important to remember this when dealing with skin irritant or photosensitising oils.

To dilute essential oil which is to be added to water, mix it first in alcohol or a commercial dispersant, then add to the water and shake well before each use.

Disinfectants

All essential oils will either kill bacteria or inhibit their growth to a certain extent, some of them acting on one or two organisms only, and others on a very wide spectrum. A small number of oils will also kill or inhibit viruses. Some of these are very much more powerful than chemical disinfectants, such as phenol (which is used as a standard of comparison in laboratory tests). Among the most useful are Bergamot, Clove, Eucalyptus, Juniper, Lavender, Ti-Tree and Thyme.

Any of these can be used very effectively to disinfect rooms, especially during or following infectious illness. A fairly strong solution with water can be used for swabbing down all washable surfaces, but the best method is to diffuse the oil in the air. This can be done by means of air sprays, an essential oil burner, putting some oil on a light bulb or radiator or, most effectively of all, with aerosol generating equipment.

see also **BACTERIOSTATICS, EPIDEMICS** *and* **INFECTIOUS ILLNESSES,** *and* **AIRSPRAYS, BURNERS** *and* **AEROSOLS** *for details of how to use the oils.*

Dispersants

A dispersant (in the context of aromatherapy) is any substance that helps essential oils to mix with water. Alcohol is a readily-available but not terribly effective dispersant. Dispersants based on an alcoholic extract of plant cells are much more effective, and can be used for bathing, preparing lotions, etc. They can be obtained under various brand names from essential oil suppliers.

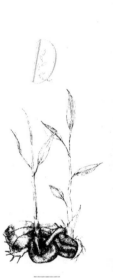

Distillation

Distillation is the main method by which essential oils are extracted from plants. Indeed, according to some authorities, it is the only method that produces essential oils as correctly defined – those obtained by other methods being known as essences or absolutes.

Distillation involves heating the plant material, either by placing it in water, which is then brought to the boil, or placing the plant material on a rack or grid and heating the water beneath it, so that steam passes up through it. Leaves, twigs, berries, petals and other parts of the plant may be used. If the plant material is placed in the water, the process is known as direct distillation, and if it is put on a grid and the steam passed through it, the system is known as steam distillation.

In either method, the heat and steam cause the walls of the specialised plant cells in which the plant essence is stored, to break down and release the essence in the form of a vapour. This vapour, together with the steam involved in the distilling process, is gathered into a pipe which passes through cooling tanks, and this causes the mixed vapours to return to liquid form so that they can be collected in vats at the end of the process. The steam condenses into a watery distillate, while the essence from the plant becomes an essential oil. This, being lighter than water, collects in the upper part of the vats and can easily be separated from the watery part. In some cases, the watery distillate is also a valuable product, and is sold as flower-water or herbal water. In France these distillates are usually described as a hydrolat.

With one or two plants, the amount of essential oil that can be obtained by distilling is insignificant, and is regarded as a by-product of the production of rosewater, or orange-flower water, for example. Other methods, such as enfleurage or solvent extraction are used to obtain the essences from these and other delicate flower petals.

The process of distillation has been known and used for obtaining essential oils since at least the 10th century A.D. and is thought to have originated in Persia, where the oils were highly prized as perfumes (Shakespeare's 'perfumes of Arabia'). However, recent archaeological digs in Italy have uncovered simple stills which suggest the Romans already knew this technique and the Persians merely improved upon it.

Some of the stills in use today, especially in less developed countries, and at small-scale rural distilleries in Europe, differ very little from the earliest stills known, but in areas where essential oil production is an important industry, they may be very large and complex, though the basic principles of production involved are identical. Stainless steel is often used in the construction of modern stills to avoid any contamination of the distillate, and this may produce better quality oils, though it is non-proven.

The distiller's role is vital in producing good quality essential oils suitable for therapeutic use, as variations in heat or the length of time the process takes have a direct influence on the final product.

see also ENFLEURAGE, ESSENCES, ESSENTIAL OILS, EXPRESSION, EXTRACTION and PERCOLATION.

Diuretics

Any substance which increases the flow of urine is called a diuretic. They are frequently used to treat conditions where water is retained in the body, and also, in conventional medicine, to reduce high blood pressure, and in the treatment of heart-failure. (See the entry under BLOOD PRESSURE for the relationship between blood pressure and the kidneys.)

The kidneys normally process very large amounts of water from the blood. The greater part of this fluid is returned to the blood with salt and other vital minerals, and the waste products which are extracted by the kidney are then passed as urine with a small amount of the water. The level of salt and other minerals in the blood is delicately balanced during this process, and diuretic drugs, used in orthodox medicine, mostly operate by interfering with the reabsorption of salt and minerals. The kidneys are then stimulated into passing through extra water in order to carry this extra load away in the urine.

There are some dangers in prolonged use of diuretics, particularly the loss of important minerals. If diuretics are self-administered, there is the added danger of overlooking kidney malfunction, or other serious illness, which is leading to water retention and which should be urgently treated.

However, there are some situations in which a diuretic can be helpful, especially in premenstrual fluid retention for example, and some of the plant diuretics are gentle and relatively safe to use. They are also valuable in attacks of cystitis, in order to keep large amounts of fairly dilute urine flowing to the bladder, to reduce pain and wash out the infecting bacteria.

A surprisingly large number of essential oils have a diuretic effect. The most important are Camomile, Cedarwood, Celery, Fennel and Juniper, but Eucalyptus, Frankincense, Geranium, Hyssop and Sandalwood also have this effect.

I always suggest the use of infusions (teas) of the corresponding herb, in particular Camomile and Fennel teas as mild and safe diuretics. Never use any diuretic for more than a few days at a time, unless properly qualified medical advice has been sought.

Douches

It is possible to use essential oils to make douches to treat vaginal infections, especially thrush, but remember that the oils are very concentrated substances, and need to be very much diluted before using on the delicate mucous lining of the vagina.

The best way is to dilute the oil in vodka (2 drops of essential oil to a 5 ml teaspoon of vodka) and then add one teaspoon of the oil/vodka mixture to one pint of boiled and cooled water. The water should be just below blood heat.

Large chemists sell douche equipment. It is not a good idea to use a douche unless it is really necessary, as constant douching interferes with the vagina's own secretions, which are a natural protection.

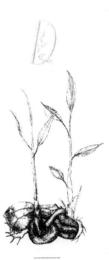

Dowsing

Dowsing involves using a pendulum, which will move in different directions in response to questions. For many people, a clockwise swing indicates 'Yes' and anticlockwise 'No' but this is not universal, and everybody who wants to use a pendulum needs first to find out what the appropriate movement is for themselves, by asking a simple question with a known answer, such as 'Is this Lavender oil?'.

Some aromatherapists employ dowsing as an aid to choosing the right essential oil to use for a particular purpose. My own feeling is that with a thorough knowledge of the oils and their properties and an intuitive response to the person you are treating, dowsing is not really necessary. It often confirms what you already know intellectually, or have felt to be right intuitively. However, even this confirmation can be valuable for a beginner at aromatherapy.

Another area of use, which I do employ quite often, is to check on the purity and origin of a sample of essential oil, if I am not entirely certain about its quality. It is possible to ask such questions as 'Is the oil in this bottle completely pure?' or 'Are there chemical residues in this oil?'

Dowsing is also used extensively to check on foods for allergy sufferers. This is a really useful 'spot-check', as it can be done in a few moments, in a small space and unobtrusively, which is very useful when eating out or shopping. More comprehensive tests can be done later if necessary.

How does dowsing 'work'? If we take the analogy of a clock, the hands don't tell the time; the inner mechanism of the clock does that, but the hands make it possible for us to see what the time is. A pendulum doesn't 'know' anything, but it makes it easier for us to get in touch with our own intuitive knowledge, perhaps even with the collective unconscious.

No special knowledge or skill is needed to dowse. Everybody can do it if they wish to. You can buy a pendulum ready made, or improvise with any small, heavy object, such as a doorkey or ring, threaded on a cord.

Dry Skin

The surface of the skin will appear dry if the glands just beneath the surface do not produce enough of the natural lubricant, sebum, which protects the skin from extremes of cold and heat, wind and other environmental factors. This type of skin is usually of a fine and close-grained appearance, very attractive in youth but deteriorating and wrinkling much more rapidly than an oily or balanced skin. Commercial skin preparations concentrate on adding lubricating oils externally, but the aromatherapy approach is to combine such oils (almond, avocado, cocoa-butter etc.) with essential oils that gently stimulate the sebaceous glands to function more efficiently. Anything which improves the general health of the skin and the blood supply to its growing layers will also help.

This kind of skin is often very delicate and sensitive, so gentle flower oils such as Camomile, Jasmine, Neroli or, best of all, Rose are the most suitable. Oils which have a balancing effect on sebum production are also good. These include Geranium, Lavender and Sandalwood. You will see elsewhere that these three oils are also used in treating oily skin, and this is because they have a normalising effect, and will reduce or increase the amount of sebum secreted by the little glands beneath the skin, according to what is needed.

Regular massage will increase the circulation in the tiny blood-vessels (capillaries) that feed the growing layer of the skin, and this in turn will improve the whole health of the skin. Nourishing and lubricating creams made from pure plant oils, beeswax and essential oils should be used regularly, and especially before going out in damaging weather.

The skin can also become rather dry if the diet is deficient in fats. As little as a teaspoon per day of good quality oil (preferably olive) added to the diet can make a difference.

see also **SKIN** and **SKINCARE.**

Dysmenorrhoea

see **MENSTRUATION.**

Dyspepsia

see **INDIGESTION.**

104

Thyme

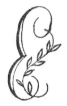

Earache

൧

---

see OTITIS.

Eau de Cologne

൧

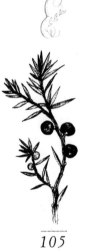

Real eau de cologne is made from essential oils, usually Bergamot, Neroli, Lavender and Rosemary, though other citrus oils (Orange, Lemon and Petitgrain) may be included, and occasionally Thyme is used in place of Rosemary.

The formula was originally devised in the first decade of the eighteenth century by Johann-Maria Farina, a German-naturalised Italian who lived in Cologne, and called his aromatic blend 'Kolnisches Wasser' after the town. It rapidly became well-known for its cooling, refreshing, deodorant and antiseptic properties. It is not quite certain whether Farina or one of his descendants later changed the name to the French equivalent to make it sound more elegant, and possibly give the product a wider appeal, or whether this came about when French soldiers, stationed in Cologne during the Seven Years' War, took samples home with them. With the change of name, the maker's signature on the labels was also Gallicised to Jean-Marie Farina. The head of the firm was called Johann-Maria, or Jean-Marie, for many generations, as each successive son or nephew christened his eldest son after the founder.

By the end of the eighteenth century many perfumiers throughout Europe were making their own versions of eau de cologne, among them several Farinas who had no connection with the originator (Farina is not an uncommon name in Italy) but who benefited from the resulting confusion. The original firm in Cologne has remained in the same family right into the present century, though many colognes labelled 'J.M. Farina' originate elsewhere.

Napoleon used vast quantities of eau de cologne – in the region of 600 bottles a year – and never travelled without it, even on military campaigns. When we consider the properties of the essential oils used in making the toilet water, it is easy to understand how valuable it would have been to a fastidious person in the insanitary conditions of a military encampment. In Napoleon's time, cologne was often called 'Aqua Admirabilis' in recognition of its many virtues.

The quality of an eau de cologne depends as much on the alcohol used as a base as on the essential oils blended with it. The original Kolnisches Wasser was made with highly rectified potato alcohol, in plentiful supply in Germany, but modern colognes are usually based on perfume-grade ethyl alcohol. The blend of alcohol and essential oils is left to rest for at least six months and really good colognes are matured for a year. Perfumery alcohol cannot be bought without a Customs and Excise licence, and is never available in small quantities, but you can make a cologne-scented bath or body oil by blending the appropriate essential oils in a bland oil base. Or you might try using a high-proof vodka as a substitute for ethyl alcohol.

There are many versions of the eau de cologne formula, but a typical one is:

Essential oil of Bergamot 100 drops
Essential oil of Lemon 50 drops
Essential oil of Neroli 30 drops
Essential oil of Lavender 50 drops
Essential oil of Rosemary 10 drops

Add this to 150 mls of high-proof vodka to make a toilet-water strength, or to 100 mls of almond or other oils as a bath oil. For a body or massage oil double the amount of carrier oil to 300 mls. You could also use this blend as a bath oil without further mixing, using 6 to 8 drops for an average bath. Leave it in a dark and cool place for as long as you can, to mature before using. If you want to experiment with a small quantity, divide all the amounts by ten. This makes a very citrussy cologne, but you might like to vary the proportions of the oils to make your own favourite version.

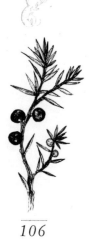

Echinacea
Echinacea purpurea

Echinacea is very well known and widely used as a herbal remedy with antiviral, fungicidal, bactericidal and immunostimulant properties. It is perhaps less familiar as an oil, but a valuable infused oil is made by macerating the roots and rhizomes, usually in sunflower oil. It is a very healing oil, especially for the skin, and can be used for acne, dry skin, minor burns and wounds. It helps to minimise wrinkles, stretchmarks and old scars. As with all infused oils, it can be used alone or with a small proportion (1% to 2%) of essential oil added.

Eczema

Eczema is so varied in the way it manifests, and in the underlying causes, that it should scarcely be considered as a single condition. Consequently, the aromatherapist's approach needs to be very flexible. A number of essential oils are described as being useful for eczema, but by no means all of them will be helpful in every case, and not all of them are suitable for use directly on affected skin. Correct diagnosis is extremely important, for several reasons: firstly because if the condition is incorrectly diagnosed, treatment with essential oils may cause irritation or inflammation. More seriously, misdiagnosis may lead to potentially dangerous situations being overlooked: for example, various forms of keratosis, which can become malignant, are easily mistaken for eczema and dermatitis. If in any doubt, consult a doctor and ask for referral to a dermatologist. *Any* skin lesion which does not heal over a period of time should be investigated in this way.

Stress is involved in almost all cases of eczema, and a very important part of the aromatherapist's task is to try to reduce the level of stress, without which direct treatment of the skin is merely palliative. Oils such as Camomile, Lavender, Melissa and Neroli are very important here, and should be used in massage and in baths that can be used every day at home, or when the person with eczema is feeling particularly fraught. In the case of infantile eczema, a child may often be reacting to the parents' tensions, and it is often helpful to treat one or both parents as well as the child.

Some, though by no means all, eczema is allergic in origin, and because of what we know about the relationship between stress and allergy, it is again important to do everything possible to lower the level of stress, as well as determining what allergens seem to aggravate the skin and making sure that they are avoided as far as possible. These may be contact irritants, such as soaps, cosmetics, detergents and other household chemicals, dust, plants, etc. or the reaction may involve one or more foodstuffs and help from an allergy clinic or clinical ecologist might be needed to identify them.

Sometimes, eczema can be seen as an attempt by the body to throw off accumulated toxins through the skin, especially where the diet has been very poor, or high in additive-laden foods. In these circumstances, detoxifying essential oils need to be used in massage and baths, and perhaps a short fast or cleansing diet undertaken. When this is done, the eczema may get temporarily worse as the body begins to throw off more toxic waste, and the person with eczema needs to be encouraged and supported through this healing crisis before real improvement is seen. Juniper is perhaps the most important oil to use in detoxifying, and it is significant that it is emotionally detoxifying too.

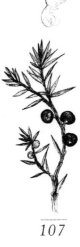

For direct treatment of the skin, I have found Camomile to be the most helpful oil in the great majority of cases, though for a small handful of people Melissa turns out to be a better choice. Some therapists like to blend these two oils together, but I prefer to use one at a time, so that I know which is actually helping most in each instance. If you use Melissa direct on the skin, dilute it to very low proportions, perhaps 1% or even 0.5%, as it is a very strong oil and can set up a worse irritation than was present already. In tiny amounts, though, it can have an almost magical effect on even stubborn eczema.

I like to mix essential oils in a purchased non-perfumed lotion or a light aqueous cream, as many people with eczema find that carrier oils and fatty ointments make the condition worse. You might also consider using the corresponding hydrolat instead of an essential oil: dabbed on or used in cold compresses this can be extremely soothing when the eczema is very itchy. It is also the most effective way, other than bathing, of treating the skin if a large area is affected.

Geranium and Lavender are other oils that can be used to help, but in each case a little trial-and-error may be necessary, since this is such an individual and unpredictable condition. In every case, use the oil diluted to 1% to 1.5% initially.

Effleurage

This term is used to describe a number of light and fairly superficial massage strokes. It is included here in order to clarify any confusion with the term enfleurage, used to describe a method of extracting absolutes from the petals of flowers.

see **ENFLEURAGE** *overleaf.*

107

Elderly, the

Aromatherapy is ideally suited to help with many of the problems that beset us as we grow older: joint pains, respiratory problems, digestive difficulties, poor memory, lack of energy, increased susceptibility to minor ailments and much else. It is also valuable as an adjunct to other therapies, both 'alternative' and 'conventional' in treating more serious illness but a certain amount of caution may be needed in adapting treatments to suit the special needs of older people. In particular, oils for massage need to be diluted more when working with a frail, elderly person. I would suggest 1% to 2% at most. The more 'aggressive' oils are often inappropriate, and gentle oils such as Benzoin, Camomile, Helichrysum, Mandarin, Lavender and Rose will usually be more useful. Where Eucalyptus is indicated, Eucalyptus radiata would be preferable to the commoner, but more robust Eucalyptus globulus, or you might substitute Myrtle, which belongs to the same botanical family, and is even more gentle in its action. Either of these oils would be helpful for the bronchial problems that beset many older people. Similarly, if you wish to use Thyme, try the Linalol chemotype.

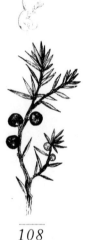

An element of commonsense is needed here! Some people in their 70s and even 80s are as physically robust and mentally alert as others in their 40s, and can tolerate, indeed enjoy, full massage and the usual dilutions of essential oils perfectly well. Others may need to have the treatment sensitively adapted to their individual needs.

One of the problems which may need to be addressed is joint pain, arthritis or impaired mobility which could prevent your client lying flat on a massage table in the usual way. You may need to use extra padding or cushions to make your client comfortable, or experiment with various positions such as sitting on a stool or facing backwards on a chair for a back massage. Some elderly people may have difficulty getting on and off a massage table – a small stool or block could make this easier.

Remember that a person with reduced mobility – regardless of their age – may need longer for dressing and undressing, and allow time for this when planning your appointments. Some older people may be reticent about removing clothing: respect their wishes and massage as best you can. A partial massage with a relaxed client will do far more good than a full massage if your client feels uneasy.

Indeed, full body massage will often be more than a frail person can tolerate: many find it too tiring. A simple back massage can do almost as much good as a full sequence, and will often be more appropriate. In other cases, massaging a painful limb or joint may be all that the client would like. This may go against all that we are taught about holism, but in the end, the client's wellbeing is what matters most. Sometimes just massaging the hands, or the face is all that can be tolerated, and all that is needed. This can be done with the patient sitting in a chair, or indeed a wheelchair, and without removing any clothing, so it is possible to go into a retirement home, for example, and give a great deal of comfort to the residents with the minimum amount of fuss.

Whether you give a full or partial massage, you may well need to omit some of the more vigorous strokes and use far lighter pressure than you would for somebody more robust. Strokes that would be enjoyable for a sturdy, well-muscled person could be quite painful if the client is extremely thin, frail, or has poor muscle tone. There could even be a risk of causing fractures in clients with fragile bones due to osteoporosis – do be certain to ask about this in your preliminary consultation.

Another reason for taking a gentle approach to massage is that the skin often becomes more delicate with age, dry, papery-looking and easily damaged. You will obviously avoid any oils that might cause skin irritation and use greater dilutions, as described above.

It is also advisable to dilute oils in a carrier before adding to the bath, and if there is any risk of a client being mentally confused or forgetful, this should be done before giving any oil to them for home use.

Provided these considerations are borne in mind, older people can derive much benefit from aromatherapy. An increasing number of aromatherapists are, in fact, working with older people and reporting how much benefit and pleasure this brings to thier elderly clients.

Elemi
Canarium luzonicum

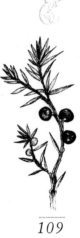

Elemi is a tropical tree native to the Phillipines and neighbouring islands, though it has been known and used in the Middle East for thousands of years. The tree is closely related to those that give us Frankincense and Myrrh and, like them, it exudes a resin that is steam distilled to produce the essential oil.

The oil is yellowish with a very pleasant aroma, somewhat like Frankincense with a slight hint of lemon. Its main constituents are elemol, elemicine, dipentene, terpineol, limonene and phellandrene.

The Egyptians used Elemi resin for embalming, and it has a very long history of use in skin care and for respiratory complaints. It first came to my notice some years ago when Frankincense was becoming scarcer and more expensive. (War and drought in the producing regions are responsible for this.) I was offered some Elemi to try as a possible substitute, and have since come to value this oil in its own right, not just as a 'poor man's Frankincense' though it does, in fact, have many of the same properties.

It is very effective for all chest infections, especially where there is a lot of phlegm, such as in chronic bronchitis. Catarrh and sinusitis, too, are helped by steam inhalations of Elemi.

It is an excellent skin-care oil, especially for mature skin. It has a general rejuvenating effect and reduces wrinkles. It is also antiseptic and speeds healing, and I have used it with good results for sore, chapped skin and allergic rashes.

The name Elemi is derived from an Arabic phrase meaning 'above and below', an abbreviation of 'As above, so below' and this tells us something about its action on the emotional and spiritual planes. It is a harmonising oil, bringing mind, body and spirit into alignment with each other. I find it a wonderful oil to burn during meditation, whether sitting alone or in a group: it induces a deep calm without any drowsiness.

The same properties make Elemi helpful for anybody who is stressed, especially when stress has led to exhaustion, for it has a tonic and stimulant action, too.

It is a completely safe oil in use, being non-toxic, non-irritant and non-sensitizing.

Enfleurage

Enfleurage is the traditional method used to extract the finest quality essences from delicate flowers, such as Rose and Jasmine. It is a laborious and therefore costly process, which accounts for the high price of these oils, or absolutes.

Sheets of glass are coated with fat, usually purified lard or beef fat, and freshly picked petals are sprinkled over the fat. The glass sheets are stacked in tiers in wooden frames, and the essence from the petals is absorbed into the fat. The faded petals are removed and fresh ones spread over the fat for many days, sometimes as long as three weeks in the case of Jasmine, until the fat can absorb no more essential oil.

The fat is then collected and cleaned of any debris, such as stale petals or stalks. At this stage it is called a pomade. The pomade is then diluted in alcohol and shaken vigorously for twenty-four hours to separate the fat from the essential oil.

Oils produced by this method are known as 'absolutes', and are very concentrated in character. Their perfuming power and therapeutic properties are very strong indeed, and far smaller amounts are needed to give the same effect as with distilled oils. Some absolutes, such as Rose, solidify at normal room temperature and return to a liquid state when the bottle is gently warmed by being held in the hand for a few moments.

An alternative method of enfleurage employs sheets of muslin saturated with olive oil. These are stretched on wooden frames, and stacked in racks in the same way as the glass sheets. Flower petals are spread over the oil-soaked cloths and renewed each day until the olive oil has absorbed as much essence as it can hold. It is then technically known as 'huile antique' or 'huile Francaise' and can then either be used as it stands as a perfumed body oil, or treated with alcohol to separate the absolute.

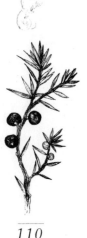

These two methods have been used traditionally in the perfume industry, especially around Grasse, to produce the very highest quality aromatic oils, but only about 10% of absolutes are now produced by this method, as it is so time consuming and expensive. About 80% of Rose and Jasmine absolutes are now extracted by means of volatile solvents, the remaining 10% being essential oils extracted by distillation.

see also **ABSOLUTE** *and* **EXTRACTION.**

Epidemics

Aromatic plants have been used since antiquity as a protection against infectious illnesses, the most notable example being the great waves of plague which swept across Europe from the middle ages to the late 17th century. There are many records of people who worked with aromatic plants or oils, escaping the plague, while others all around them were dying; most notably labourers working in the lavender fields, gardeners tending herb gardens and tanners and glove-makers who used essential oils to perfume fine leather. For many centuries, bad smells themselves were thought to be responsible for infection, and sweet smells used to counteract them, but we know now that these aromatic plants are all powerful bactericides and that some of them are also antiviral agents.

Vaporising some of the most powerfully bactericidal and antiviral essential oils in your home, offers a real protection against infection during epidemics. (See the entries for **AEROSOLS**, **AIRSPRAYS** and **BURNERS** for simple methods of doing this.) If you are in contact with people outside your home during an epidemic, it is a good idea to put a few drops of one of these oils on a tissue, or on your clothes, where you can inhale it frequently. Daily baths, with essential oils added, are an extra protection.

For burning or spraying in the air, Clove, Eucalyptus and Ti-tree are among the best protectors. (Interestingly, they all belong to the same large botanical family of Myrtaceae.) Jean Valnet recounts how the Molucca islands were swept by waves of previously unknown epidemics after Dutch settlers destroyed all the Clove trees, and Australian aboriginal people have used Eucalyptus as a protection for longer than anybody knows. I always vaporise Ti-tree during 'flu epidemics, and stay remarkably healthy most winters. I also burn a mixture of Clove and Orange a great deal in winter time, recalling the pleasing smell and anti-infectious properties of the traditional pomander.

Clove is a skin irritant, and so is Orange, so do not use these in the bath. Rather use Lavender, Rosemary, Ti-tree or Thyme, any of which will give you a high level of protection from infection.

If you have a sick person in your home, you can protect the other members of the household by constantly spraying the sickroom and surrounding areas.

---

see also **INFECTIOUS ILLNESS, INFLUENZA** *and* **CHICKEN-POX, MEASLES, WHOOPING COUGH.**

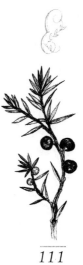

Epilepsy

111

There are a number of essential oils which can provoke an epileptic-type fit in people who are susceptible, so it is extremely important to be certain that a person does not suffer from epilepsy before beginning any treatment. A properly trained aromatherapist will always include this in the questions asked before the first treatment.

If you are using essential oils at home, the oils to avoid are Sage, Fennel, Hyssop, Wormwood and Rosemary. Classic aromatherapy literature often states that extremely small amounts of Rosemary may be beneficial to epilepsy sufferers. Until recently, I knew of nobody who had applied this in practice, but recently I talked with a friend who had worked in a residential village for handicapped children, many of whom suffered from epilepsy, and he told me that the helpers carried a bottle of Weleda Rosemary Bath at all times, and whenever a child had a fit, they would rub a little under the child's nose or on the cheeks, which quickly brought them out of the fit. This bath preparation contains essential oil of Rosemary in almond oil and a soft soap base: in other words, the amount of Rosemary applied to the child would be very, very small indeed. Any well-diluted Rosemary solution could safely be tried in the same way.

Some oils are anti-convulsive, most notably Lavender, but I would counsel against attempting to treat epilepsy by aromatherapy alone. The only aromatherapists who might consider this should be those who already have a medical qualification.

hyme

Essences

Essential oils are sometimes referred to as essences, but this is, strictly speaking, incorrect.

The essence is what is produced by the plant, and it only becomes an essential oil after distillation. Certain chemical changes take place in the essence during this process, due to the effects of heat and contact with the air and steam, but these changes are not harmful, and do not spoil the therapeutic value of the essence. In a sense, they seem even to subtly enhance it.

Essences are produced in the plant in highly specialised secretory cells. These may be in the leaf, bark, or other parts of the plant. The essence may be stored within the same cell in which it is made, or it may pass into a storage sac or duct. These cells are often just below the surface of the leaf, and the essence is released if the leaf is crushed, giving off its characteristic perfume. In other plants, storage ducts are in minute hairs on the leaf. These plants are highly aromatic and release their perfume when simply brushed against, since the tiny hairs break and let the essence into the air. In some woody plants and trees, the essence is stored in ducts in the fibrous parts of the wood or bark. Extraction is much more difficult, as the woody material must be crushed and broken down before the essence can be extracted. In citrus fruits, the essence is found in relatively large storage sacs in the peel, and is very easy to extract by means of pressure. If you crack a piece of orange peel, holding a lighted match nearby, you can see the oily essence ignite, and burn for a few seconds.

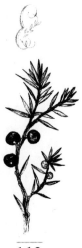

The proportion of essence in the plant varies a great deal from species to species, and this accounts in part for the varying prices of essential oils. The amount of essence in an individual plant also varies to a lesser degree according to the growing conditions (soil, moisture, amount of sunshine, etc.) and according to the time of year, so the time for harvesting must be carefully chosen to maximise the yield.

Plant essences are very chemically complex structures. Using energy obtained from sunlight, the plant combines the chemical elements found in the air, soil and water around it, such as carbon, oxygen and hydrogen, and from these atoms constructs hundreds of different aromatic molecules. These are grouped into eight main categories: acids, alcohols, aldehydes, ketones, esters, phenols, sesquiterpenes and terpenes. Although many of the constituents are found in more than one essence, it is the unique combination of molecules found in each plant that gives it its characteristic perfume and therapeutic properties.

Some of the constituents of plant essences are isolated by pharmacists looking for a single 'active ingredient' to treat a single symptom. The isolated item may be used as it is, or copied (synthesised) in the laboratory, but these single molecules are never as effective, nor as safe used alone as they are when combined naturally as in the plant. The combination of molecules acts synergistically, and also prevents unwanted side effects. Even when an essence contains 80% to 90% of a single type of molecule, there may be a dozen or more other constituents, some present only as traces, and these balance and moderate the effect of the main constituent. This is thought to be the reason why side effects are so rare in aromatherapy, and indeed plant medicine in general.

Essential Oils

Essential oils are the base materials of the aromatherapist. These highly aromatic substances are made in plants by special cells but at this stage the material is not yet an essential oil, but is called an essence. It becomes an essential oil only after it has been extracted by distillation. (See above.)

Although we use the term essential oil loosely to describe all the oils used in aromatherapy, those which are obtained by methods other than distillation should not, strictly speaking, be so called. Those which are extracted by simple pressure (i.e. those from the citrus fruits, Bergamot, Lemon, Orange, etc.) are still the essence when we use them. Others, such as the floral oils of Jasmine, Neroli and Rose, obtained by enfleurage or solvent extraction, are neither essences nor essential oils but are classed as absolutes.

Essential oils are very highly concentrated, and should only rarely be used in their undiluted form. They are very volatile, that is, they evaporate quickly on contact with the air. This is one of the reasons why they are so quickly effective in treatment, but it also indicates the need to keep them in airtight bottles during storage, and to replace the lids as soon as possible when using.

In spite of the fact that they are designated as oils, they are light and non-greasy. Most essential oils are colourless or pale yellow, though there are some notable exceptions to this, such as Blue Camomile. The majority of coloured oils are essences or absolutes, such as Bergamot, which is green, and Jasmine, which is reddish-brown. Ultra violet light damages the oils, so they need to be stored in opaque (dark brown or blue) bottles and kept away from direct sunlight as much as possible. They are also susceptible to damage from extremes of temperature, and the vibrations caused by loud noises.

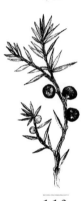

Essential oils dissolve easily in fatty oils, such as olive, soya, sesame, sunflower and other plant oils and also in alcohol. They do not dissolve in water, but can be kept suspended in water for short periods for use as an aromatic skin-wash for example.

Essential oils are highly complex chemically (see **ESSENCES** for more detail), and this very complexity makes them both versatile and safe, since the many constituents act together and balance each other's effects. Newcomers to aromatherapy are often surprised, and sometimes sceptical about the many therapeutic properties which may be attributed to a single oil, but this diversity of properties and actions reflects the complicated chemistry of the oil.

When two or more essential oils are mixed together, they become something more than 'the sum of the parts' as the chemicals making up each oil recombine with each other, and such blends are sometimes more active than any of the oils when used singly. Lavender, in particular, is known to increase the activity of other oils with which it is blended. Much of the art of a trained aromatherapist lies in selecting and blending oils in this way to meet the individual needs of each client.

---

see also the entries for **ESSENCES, QUALITY, CHEMOTYPE,** *and the many entries for individual essential oils throughout the book.*

Esters

Esters are an important category of aromatic molecules that form part of many essential oils. Most esters are antispasmodic, anti-inflammatory, calming and tonic to the nervous system. They are among the gentlest and safest components of essential oils and are harmless on the skin. They include benzyl benzoate, in Benzoin and other resins; geranyl acetate, in Lavender, Eucalyptus, etc.; methyl anthranilate, in Mandarin, Orange and Neroli, and linalyl acetate, the main constituent of Lavender, Bergamot and Clary, also found in Jasmine, Neroli, etc.

Eucalyptus

Eucalyptus globulus, E. radiata and others.

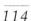

There are about 300 varieties of Eucalyptus. Most essential oil is distilled from the Australians' beloved 'blue-gum', *Eucalyptus globulus*, although there are about 15 out of the hundreds of species that yield a valuable oil. Although *E. globulus* is the most widely used variety, a less well-known species, *Eucalyptus radiata*, is a better choice for use in aromatherapy, as it has all the properties described below, but a pleasanter aroma than the common Eucalyptus, is more easily assimilated and less likely to irritate the skin. One or two other varieties, such as Eucalyptus dives and the lemon-scented *E. citriodora*, have some value particularly in allowing the therapist to vary the oil if it is needed over more than two or three weeks.

The tree was introduced to Europe in the 19th century as an ornamental species, but has developed certain characteristics which do not appear in its native home. In particular, it secretes chemical substances which poison the surrounding soil, inhibiting the growth of other plants in the area.

The leaves of a mature tree are long, pointed and yellowy-green, as opposed to the leaves from younger trees, which are round and a silvery bluish-green. The oil can be distilled from young or old leaves. It is pale yellow in colour, with a penetrating and refreshing smell that is too familiar to need description. The main constituent of *Eucalyptus globulus* is eucalyptol (about 80%), ethyl alcohol, amyl alcohol, various aldehydes, camphene, eudesmol, phellandrene, pinene and the delightfully named aromadendrene. *Eucalyptus radiata* has less eucalyptol (about 70%) with terpineol and other alcohols and some monoterpenes. Its composition is closer to that of the Melaleucas, and like them it is a good immunostimulant, good for people who are tired, run down, prone to frequent colds, etc.

Eucalyptus is best known as a decongestant inhalation for colds and catarrh, but it has many other less known uses. Most important of these is its very powerful bactericidal and antiviral action. A steam inhalation with Eucalyptus is an effective natural treatment for colds, because it not only eases nasal congestion, but inhibits proliferation of the cold virus. Eucalyptus used in **AIRSPRAYS** or any form of vaporisation during epidemics, will give a good measure of protection from 'flu and the infectious illnesses of childhood. In North Africa, groves of Eucalyptus trees have been planted in swampy and unhealthy areas to prevent the spread of malaria. As Eucalyptus is an effective insect repellent, which deters mosquitoes from breeding in the area immediately around the trees, it acts in more than one way towards this end.

Jean Valnet gave precise data on the bactericidal properties of Eucalyptus: a spray containing 2% essential oil of Eucalyptus will kill 70% of staphylococci in the air. Eucalyptus oil used like this has a much greater effect than eucalyptol, its main active principle, which is extracted and used pharmaceutically – indicating once again that essential oils in their natural state are often more effective than the single chemical constituents so beloved of chemists. The effectiveness of oil of Eucalyptus, in this context, appears to be due to the action of aromadendrene and phellandrenes when they come into contact with the oxygen in the air. Their chemical reaction produces ozone, in which bacteria cannot live. The antiviral action of Eucalyptus has not been so well researched, but has been so often observed empirically, that scientific verification must be a formality.

In epidemics and infectious illnesses, then, Eucalyptus serves several purposes at once, as it helps the sufferer but also protects the people coming into contact with him or her. Valnet suggests its use in feverish conditions to lower the temperature and as a measure to prevent the spread of infection in cholera, measles, malaria, scarlet fever and typhoid. In measles and scarlet fever he suggests applying dilute Eucalyptus to the skin of the infected person at frequent intervals, and surrounding their bed with a gauze that can be kept moistened with Eucalyptus solution. For 'flu and bronchitis he combines 4 parts of Eucalyptus with 2 each of Thyme and Pine, and 1 of Lavender in inhalations. A stronger mixture of the same blend (10 grams to a litre of water) can be used to fumigate rooms. I have used Eucalyptus combined with Camomile and Lavender in baths and sprays when my grandchildren had chickenpox. This greatly reduced the fever and itching suffered by the elder child, who became ill first, while her little brother developed only a very mild form of the illness.

Urinary tract infections respond very well to Eucalyptus, too, and here its diuretic action can make it doubly useful.

The antiseptic and healing properties of Eucalyptus have long been known to the Australian aborigines, who bind Eucalyptus leaves around serious wounds. Sophisticated surgeons do not dispute them, and have used a solution of Eucalyptus to wash out operation cavities and Eucalyptus-impregnated gauze as a post-operative dressing. It is valuable for burns, used in the same way, and it helps to form new tissue as the burn heals.

It is useful for septic or congested conditions and combines well with Bergamot for treating cold-sores and genital herpes, caused by the herpes simplex virus, and for the blisters occurring in shingles, which is due to the same virus as chickenpox – herpes zoster. E. radiata is better suited to these uses than E. globulus because it will not irritate the skin or mucous membrane. The acute pain of shingles is due to the fact that sensory nerve tracts are inflamed, and as Eucalyptus is an effective local painkiller it will give some relief. The pain often persists for many weeks, or even months, after the blisters have disappeared, so a Bergamot and Eucalyptus cream can be applied to ease the discomfort.

Eucalyptus can be used in massage to relieve pain in rheumatism, muscular aches and fibrositis. As we have such a wide choice of oils for such applications, I use it only for people who do not mind its powerful odour, or perhaps even find the familiar medicinal smell reassuring. (People unfamiliar with essential oils are sometimes sceptical about the therapeutic properties of some of the more sweet-smelling ones. If you come across this, it is seriously worth considering using the more pungent oils in treatment where appropriate. The psychology of this is 'If it smells so strong, it must be doing me some good.')

I have mentioned that Eucalyptus deters mosquitoes, and in fact insects in general will be inclined to leave you alone if you include a little of this oil in a blend, perhaps with Bergamot, Lavender or any of the other insect-repellent oils. I use a little in room-sprays in the summer, both to keep my home smelling fresh and to keep flies out, and it is another oil which I have used as both a deodorant and flea-deterrent on dogs.

Finally, if you get tar on your clothes or skin on a polluted beach, Eucalyptus oil is an effective and harmless way of removing it.

Evening Primrose Oil

The oil of Evening Primrose *(Oenothera biennis)* is not an essential oil, but is included here because it has proved so valuable in many of the conditions which aromatherapists are often called on to treat, e.g. menstrual and pre-menstrual problems, eczema and psoriasis.

Evening Primrose oil is most often taken in the form of capsules, but it can also be applied to the skin, and in treating allergic skin problems, you could add up to 10% to the carrier oil for massage, and to any creams or lotions.

The action of Evening Primrose oil results from the fact that it contains a high level of gamma linolenic acid (G.L.A.). Please refer to the entry for GAMMA LINOLEIC ACID for more detail.

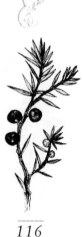

Expression

The essential oils of Lemon, Bergamot, Orange and other citrus fruits are obtained by simple pressure. The essential oil of the citrus fruits is all found in the outer coloured layer of the rind, and the pulp and white pith must be removed before the oil is extracted. This has long been carried out by hand, by one of two methods. The inside of the fruit is either scooped out, leaving a cup-shaped rind, or the peel is taken off in strips, leaving the pulp intact.

The peel is then squeezed to press out the aromatic oil, with a certain amount of juice. This is left to stand until the oil can be separated off from the top of the juice.

Another traditional method was to roll the fruit around in a barrel lined with spikes to puncture the peel so that the oil and juice could be collected and separated.

Various machine methods are now in use, but the best quality citrus oils are still extracted by hand.

By using a new garlic-press (which has never been used for garlic) you can produce very small amounts of Lemon or Orange oil at home, but it is very important that you make sure the fruit has not been sprayed, dyed or coated.

Extraction

Some of the finest flower absolutes are produced by means of solvent extraction. This method was first tried in the 1830s and began to be used on a commercial scale in the 1890s.

Flowers are placed on perforated racks in hermetically sealed containers, which may be connected to each other in a series. At one end is a tank containing liquid solvent, and at the other a vacuum still. The liquid solvent is allowed to flow slowly over the flowers, dissolving the essential oils. The solvent is then distilled off and returned to its tank to be re-used, leaving a semi-solid perfume material known as a 'concrete'. This contains the aromatic material from the plant, together with natural plant waxes. Twenty-five grams of this concrete is equivalent to a kilo of best quality pomade obtained by enfleurage.

Like the pomade, the concrete is then shaken in alcohol to remove the plant waxes, leaving a very high quality absolute.

The solvent originally used in the nineteenth century was petroleum ether, and later benzol was introduced. Modern extraction processes may use liquid butane, or liquid carbon dioxide, which produce very fine oils without damaging the most delicate aromas.

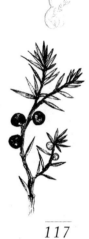

Eyes

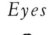

Essential oils must NEVER be used on the eyes, or allowed to come into contact with them even when diluted. If essential oil accidentally comes into contact with the eye, use a pure vegetable oil, such as almond, olive or sunflower to flush it out – do not use water which will make the situation worse. If much oil has got into the eye, or stinging is severe or prolonged, consult a doctor or casualty department.

For eye infections, such as conjunctivitis use a herbal infusion such as camomile, elderflower or eyebright, or distilled rosewater or cornflower water or a homoeopathic preparation of euphrasia. Good quality floral waters can be bought from herbalists and some essential oil suppliers. You can make a herbal infusion just as you would make herb teas. Allow the infusion to cool until it is lukewarm and use it to wash the eyes three for four times a day. Compresses of cottonwool soaked in rosewater, cornflower water or a herbal infusion can be placed over the eyes, especially at night, and if you use camomile tea bags to make an infusion, the cooled teabag will make an effective compress.

Eye infections are often very contagious, and it is very easy to transmit the infection from one eye to the other, or to another person, so great care needs to be taken with hand-washing and the scalding of eye baths or any other utensil used to treat the eyes.

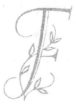

Facials

❧

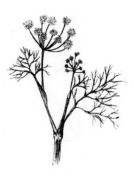

see **SKINCARE**.

Fainting

❧

When we are suddenly frightened, or receive a severe emotional shock, the parasympathetic nervous system diverts a great deal of blood to the abdominal area, and this automatically lowers the blood pressure in the arteries which supply the brain. The decreased blood supply to the brain causes us to lose consciousness, but this is usually very temporary, as falling or lying down brings the head onto the same level as the heart and quickly restores an adequate blood supply to the brain.

Several essential oils are helpful to people feeling faint or in a state of shock, and the most important of these are Peppermint and Neroli. If neither of these oils is immediately available, Lavender and Rosemary are also useful.

Simply hold the opened bottle under the nose of a person who is feeling faint, or put a drop or two on a hankie or tissue for them to inhale; or you may massage a single drop of any of these oils into each temple.

These methods can be used to help somebody who feels faint, and may prevent loss of consciousness, but can equally well be used to help recovery from a faint.

By far the best first-aid, although it is not specifically aromatherapy, is Dr. Bach's Rescue Remedy. I always use this in any emergency, and then follow up with essential oils if needed. Put four drops on the tongue, if the person is still conscious; if not, simply moisten the lips with a few drops. You can give another four drops after they have revived.

Never give alcoholic drinks to a person who feels faint, or who is recovering from fainting. A hot drink with some honey in it is far better, and peppermint tea is probably the best choice.

If anybody faints very frequently, or for no apparent reason, it is important that the cause of fainting is investigated by a doctor, homoeopath or medical herbalist.

Fatigue

A number of essential oils can be helpful in combating fatigue, all of them classed as stimulant, but without any of the dangers associated with such stimulants as coffee, tea, alcohol or drugs. Any of these oils will help the body to recover from fatigue, rather than mask its effects. A massage using Basil, Geranium, Nutmeg, Rosemary, Thyme, Marjoram or Pine, or a blend of two or three of these, will help to restore tone to the body, clear the mind and give renewed energy. Aromatic baths using 6 drops of Geranium, Rosemary, Thyme or Marjoram can be very invigorating, but the two spice oils listed (and all other oils from spices) should be used with caution in the bath, as anything more than 3 drops in an average bath can cause skin irritation. You might like to make a blend of, say, 2 drops of Clove, Nutmeg, etc. with 4 drops of another oil.

Any of these oils will help with physical fatigue, but Rosemary in particular, and Basil to a lesser extent, can be used very effectively to reduce mental fatigue.

Obviously none of these oils should be seen as more than a short term aid to recovery, following a period of intensive work, travel, worry etc. Whether you wish to use them as a self-help technique or as a therapist to help another person, take care not to let the oils become a substitute for getting enough rest, reducing an excessive workload, or whatever other measures may be needed to prevent constant tiredness.

An alternative approach for the aromatherapist may be to use essences which are calming, soothing and enhance sleep, to ensure that the tired-out person gets adequate sleep to replenish his or her energy in a natural way. Lavender and Camomile are the two obvious choices, but you will find many others discussed under the headings of the individual oils.

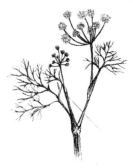

A person who is continually tired, for no apparent reason, may be eating a very inappropriate diet possibly lacking in vitamins and minerals. Junk foods and high sugar consumption also create undue fatigue by causing violent swings of high and low blood sugar levels.

Food allergies may also be an underlying cause, and identification and removal of the guilty food or foods can produce almost magical cures. If you do not feel qualified to give nutritional advice, and your patient is not making progress with the help of aromatherapy, you should seriously consider referring him or her to a nutritionist or clinical ecologist, to determine whether one or other of these aspects of diet could be at the root of the fatigue.

Abnormal fatigue can be a symptom of depression, candida infection, M.E. and of some serious physical illnesses, so do not delay seeking other help for a person who is suffering in this way.

see also **CANDIDA, M.E., STIMULANTS** *and* **SEDATIVES.**

Feet

The feet are a very important area in aromatherapy, partly because of the reflex points on them, which affect every area and organ of the body, and partly because the skin of the feet is particularly good at absorbing essential oils.

In a classic experiment, oil of Garlic was rubbed on the feet of a volunteer. Ten minutes later, the Garlic could be measured in his exhaled breath. Garlic is a very volatile oil, so absorption was rapidly demonstrated, but the same thing will happen with any essential oil, though it may take longer.

Another way of getting oils into the body quickly is by using them in footbaths, and some colleagues have reported that results are further heightened by using a footbath immediately after a reflexology treatment.

Many aromatherapists use reflexology as an adjunct to their treatment with essential oils, sometimes applying the oils very specifically to certain reflex points, but even without studying reflexology it is possible to benefit your client considerably by simply massaging every part of the feet with care.

The feet are one of the few parts of our bodies that we can easily reach, so they offer a simple means of self-treatment if nobody else is available when we need some help.

Massage of the feet can be very important in terms of balancing and energy flow; literally 'grounding' a person who is perhaps living too much in the head. If I have finished a massage with the head – as I most often do – I will usually bring my hands down again to the feet and hold them for a few moments to avoid the possibility of leaving my client feeling rather 'floaty', and to give a sense of harmony throughout the whole body.

see also **FOOTBATHS** *for the method of using them, and* **REFLEXOLOGY.**

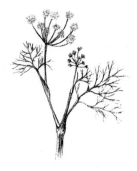

Fennel

Foeniculum vulgare

Fennel takes its name from the Latin word for hay, as it was frequently used in animal fodder. It is a plant of the same family – Umbelliferae – as Aniseed, Caraway and Coriander, and it has a pleasantly aniseedy flavour. However, Aniseed is a fairly toxic oil, and Fennel is safe in use, which gives it greater practical value. The plant grows wild in many parts of Europe, from the Mediterranean, where it originated, through to parts of Russia. It is particularly happy growing near the sea.

The essential oil is distilled from the crushed seeds, and contains anethol, fenchone, estragol, camphene and phellandrene.

Some of the properties attributed to Fennel in the past appear to have more to do with superstition than science. For example, it was thought to give protection from witchcraft, and was hung over cottage doors to keep away the evil eye. Snakes were thought to rub themselves against Fennel plants to improve their eyesight, and it was believed to improve the sight of humans, too. Many old herbals say that Fennel is an antidote to 'all manner venom' (Bankes) such as snake bite, poisonous plants and mushrooms, and we know it now as an important anti-toxic oil. Perhaps one of its most valuable applications in the 20th century is in counterbalancing alcoholic poisoning, and it has played an important part in the treatment and rehabilitation of alcoholics. It also helps in gout, arthritis, etc., to prevent the build-up of toxic wastes in the body which precede the inflammatory condition of the joints.

Like other Umbelliferae, Fennel is a good carminative and digestive remedy, and will quickly give relief from nausea, flatulence, indigestion, colic and hiccoughs. The best way to use Fennel for such problems in is the form of fennel tea. It has a tonic effect on the smooth muscle of the intestine, which is valuable in colitis, and in some cases of constipation, as it strengthens peristalsis (the rhythmic contractions of the intestinal muscle which move the partially-digested food mass through the intestines).

Another application of fennel that connects with digestion, is its reputation for decreasing the appetite. The seeds used to be carried by Roman soldiers on long marches, to chew when they did not have time to stop and cook a meal, and by devout Christians on fast days. This may possibly be the action that Culpeper and other herbalists had in mind when they recommended the use of fennel by 'those that are grown fat'.

It is a good diuretic, which may help some obese people if water retention is part of their problem; but nobody should use diuretics without supervision, or for any length of time, as there is a risk of kidney damage if they are abused. It is also important to remember that fluid retention may be a sign of more serious illness and should be investigated.

As a diuretic and urinary tract antiseptic, Fennel has been used in the past for retention of urine, and urinary tract infections. It may have some value in the prevention of kidney stones.

It is a useful oil for the treatment of cellulitis, when accumulations of toxic wastes and fluid in the subcutaneous fat produce a characteristic wrinkled appearance, often called 'orange peel skin'. Fennel tea should be taken three times a day, combined with a radical reform of eating habits, and a specialised massage to the affected area.

Fennel is one of the plants that has been known for thousands of years for its effects on the female reproductive system. It now seems probable that this is due to a plant hormone – a form of oestrogen – in its structure. It can help to regularise the menstrual cycle, particularly where periods are scanty and painful, with cramping pains. It has been found to reduce the symptoms of pre-menstrual stress, and also the water-retention which many women experience in the few days before menstruation is due. It is useful at the menopause in reducing the unpleasant symptoms caused by wildly fluctuating hormone levels, and it stimulates the production of oestrogen by the adrenal glands after the ovaries have stopped functioning. Oestrogen is needed by everyone, both men and women, to maintain muscle tone, elasticity of the skin and connective tissue, a healthy circulation and strong bones; so maintaining the supply can postpone some of the degenerative effects of ageing. Another hormonal effect of Fennel is to increase the flow of milk in nursing mothers.

Minor uses include that of a gargle or mouthwash for gum infections, and Fennel is often used in toothpaste and commercial mouthwashes.

Fever

Raised temperature is the body response to infection, and all systems of natural medicine see fever as an important healing process. Fever increases most of the body processes, pulse rate and metabolism, and this increased activity helps to strengthen the natural defences against infection. In addition, some invading organisms, particularly viruses, do not thrive in a temperature higher than that of a healthy body. The temperature may rise and stay very high until the fever is resolved by profuse sweating, after which the patient will often sleep deeply for some time, and the temperature will begin to drop towards normal. This is often described as the 'healing crisis'. Allopathic

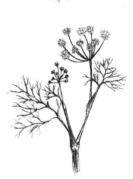

121

CAUTION
Do not use Fennel for young children (under the age of 6) as one of its active principles (melanthine) can be toxic to them, although harmless to adults and older children in normal doses. Fennel must not be used by people with epilepsy.

medicine aims to reduce the temperature artificially, which may bring temporary comfort to the patient, but delays or even suppresses the healing process.

There are two ways in which essential oils can be used in a fever. One is to use those oils which promote sweating (sudorifics) to encourage the resolution of the fever, and the other is to select those oils which will actually help to reduce the temperature. This latter course is wise when the temperature is rising to a dangerous level (say, over 104°F), especially in a young child. Babies and young children may suffer convulsions if their temperature rises and remains very high.

Basil, Camomile, Cypress, Juniper, Lavender, Peppermint, Rosemary and Ti-Tree will all induce sweating if the body needs to sweat. (It is interesting to note that none of these will make you sweat excessively when the body is in a normal state.) If the sick person feels strong enough to get in a bath, put up to 8 drops of one of these oils, or a blend, into a bath which is not too hot, and help the patient into it. Otherwise, give a little gentle massage, perhaps just to the back.

Cooling oils include Bergamot, Eucalyptus, Lavender and Peppermint. As you can see, these last two feature in both lists – this is because their action is mainly normalising. These oils should be used in a fairly low concentration, just a few drops in a bowl of cool water (not cold, as the difference between the water and the body temperature could be too great). Sponge the body with the mixture as often as possible to keep the temperature below a dangerous level.

For details of essential oils and treatment specific to various feverish illnesses, such as Chickenpox, Measles, Scarlet Fever, etc., please also read the entries under these headings.

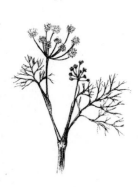

Fibrositis

༄

for oils *and* methods of treatment, *see entry for* **RHEUMATISM.**

Flatulence

༄

Any of the essential oils described as carminative will help to expel gas from the digestive system, and ease the pain that accompanies it. They can be massaged into the abdomen in a carrier oil, always working round the tummy in a clockwise direction. If flatulence is a temporary problem, following a meal containing some particularly gas-inducing food, this is all the treatment that should be necessary, but if this is a constant condition dietary changes will probably be needed, possibly combined with a colon-cleansing programme supervised by a qualified nutritional adviser or a medical herbalist. Excess gas is sometimes experienced after a course of antibiotics, because these kill off millions of the helpful bacteria in the gut, along with the invading organisms for which they are prescribed. This makes digestion inefficient and leads to putrefaction in the colon. A course of lactobacillus tablets or even large amounts of natural live yoghurt will put this right. Using the essential oils as recommended above will ease the intestines until the helpful flora have been re-established. Suitable oils would be Bergamot, Black Pepper, Camomile, Fennel, Lavender or Marjoram.

Floral Oils

❦

see **INFUSED OILS.**

Flower Waters

❦

see **HYDROLATS.**

'Flu

❦

see **INFLUENZA.**

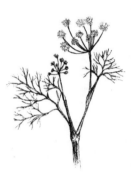

Footbaths

❦

Footbaths have been used by herbalists and healers for hundreds of years. (Maurice Messegué was particularly celebrated for the cures he brought about by this very simple means.) The traditional method of preparation is to make a very strong infusion from the chosen plant, or mixture of plants, and pour this into a bowl of very hot water, but 3 or 4 drops of essential oil in a bowl of hot water is just as effective. The skin on the soles of the feet absorbs essential oils very fast and makes this a good way to get the oils into the body. Some aromatherapists who also practice reflexology have experimented with this method recently, and found it a very good addition to the better known ways of using essential oils. A footbath seems to be even more effective if given after a reflexology treatment, but it can be very good used alone if you are not, or do not know, a reflexologist.

Footbaths are very helpful in situations where a full aromatic bath would not be practical, or is not available, such as when treating elderly or less mobile people who may have difficulty in getting in and out of a bath. I have suggested this form of treatment to people living in flats with a shower but no bath, and have known footbaths to be used very successfully by friends on camping and caravanning holidays.

Frankincense

Boswellia carteri

❦

This beautiful essential oil comes from a small tree native to North Africa and some of the Arab countries. When the bark is damaged the tree exudes a resin in drops or 'tears' and the essential oil is extracted from the resin by steam distillation. In past times the resin was collected from trees in which cracks had appeared naturally, but later cuts were made in the bark systematically to encourage resin production.

123

The oil varies from colourless to very pale yellow, with a clear, fresh, slightly camphorous penetrating odour. Among the chemical constituents which make up this oil are l-pinene, dipentene, phellandrene, camphene, olibanol and various resins.

Frankincense, in the form of the resin, has been burnt on altars and in temples since earliest antiquity. This use probably goes back far further than the earliest written records and is perpetuated in the current practice of many religions. I find it fascinating to reflect on the fact that Frankincense has, among its physical properties, the ability to slow down and deepen the breath, and to breathe more slowly and deeply soon produces feelings of calm, which are very conducive to prayer and meditation. At what stage in the history of the use of Frankincense did our forebears discover this? Almost certainly, the origin of its use as an offering lay in the fact that Frankincense was among the most prized and costly substances in the ancient world. Both the Hebrews and the Egyptians spent vast amounts of money importing Frankincense from the Phoenicians.

Apart from its ceremonial and ritual use, Frankincense was much sought after as a perfume, and used in cosmetics and medicine. The Egyptians also used it in embalming.

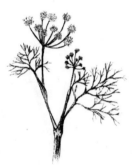

As already suggested, Frankincense is particularly active with regard to the lungs, and is one of the most valuable oils for use in respiratory infections. It is one of the best pulmonary antiseptics, calms coughs, and is indicated particularly where there is bronchial catarrh, for example, in chronic bronchitis. Use it in inhalations, massages and baths. I have found this oil very helpful for people with asthma, because of the way in which it slows and deepens the breathing. Massage is the best form of treatment, concentrating on strokes which open the chest, as this area is often constricted in asthmatics. The heat of steam inhalations may have an adverse effect in asthma, so this method should only be used cautiously.

In skincare, Frankincense is particularly helpful for older skins, and has a definite tonic effect, helping to restore some tone to slack looking facial skin, and slowing down the appearance of wrinkles. It may even reduce the extent of wrinkles that have already formed.

The oil has an affinity for the urino-genital tract, and was used a great deal in earlier times for treating infections in these organs. It is a uterine tonic and may be helpful for abnormally heavy periods, used in baths and gentle massage over the abdomen. It can safely be used during pregnancy.

Frankincense has a calming effect on the emotions, which can be seen as relating both to its use as a meditation aid, and in the treatment of asthma, where anxiety is often a trigger for attacks.

In the past it was burnt to drive out evil spirits. It is also thought to help break links with the past and may be very valuable to people who tend to dwell on past events, to the detriment of their present situation.

An alternative name for Frankincense is Olibanum. This occurs commonly in older texts, and is thought to derive from the Latin *'Olium Libanum'* (Oil from Lebanon). The name Frankincense itself derives from Mediaeval French meaning 'Real Incense'.

Over the past decade it has become increasingly difficult to obtain good Frankincense because drought has caused the desert to spread into the marginal land which is the natural habitat of the Frankincense tree, also because of wars in the producing areas which has made it impossible to collect the raw resin.

Frigidity

The inability to achieve orgasm in women is described thus, and is often bracketed together with impotence, although there are some important distinctions. Frigidity does not affect sexual function, only the enjoyment of it. As with impotence, there is very seldom any physical reason, and the cause may be as simple as an insensitive partner, or as complex as fear, ignorance of the female body and its functions, childhood trauma, upbringing, religious taboos, fear of pregnancy or a multitude of other factors.

Frigid women often have a very negative self-image, sometimes amounting to a real dislike for their own bodies, and careful, nurturing massage with essential oils can go a very long way towards helping such women to appreciate and enjoy their own femininity. Massage may be the first opportunity a woman has had to enjoy touch in a non-sexual context.

Luxurious oils such as Rose, which is particularly connected with female sexuality, and Jasmine, which increases confidence are the ones which are the greatest help. Their very real therapeutic value outweighs the high cost, though in any case only very small amounts of oil are needed for each massage. Neroli is important if there is a lot of anxiety present, and Ylang-Ylang is a very sweet-scented and relaxing alternative. Some women will also enjoy oils such as Clary Sage and Sandalwood that are traditionally regarded as more masculine.

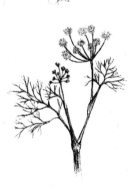

Self-pampering with bath oils, soaps, creams, lotions and body oils perfumed with any of these oils can reinforce a positive self-image and feelings of worth and attractiveness. If the woman's partner is sensitive and concerned about her difficulty, he can be taught to give her some gentle massage with oils of her choice (and if he is not, none of the other suggestions will be of much use).

All of the oils I have mentioned are regarded as aphrodisiacs, though with one exception this action is probably due to the fact that they are all deeply relaxing and so reduce anxiety and fears about sex. The exception is Rose, which is a uterine tonic and cleanser, and generally beneficial to the whole female reproductive system. It seems to have affinities with female sexuality on both physical and emotional levels, and is thought of as the supreme female aphrodisiac.

Some frigid women may feel that they need counselling, Gestalt work or some other form of psychotherapy, but aromatherapy will reinforce any such treatment in a very valuable way.

see also **APHRODISIACS** *and* **IMPOTENCE.**

125

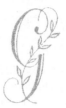

Galbanum
Ferula galbaniflua

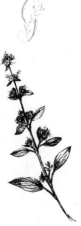

Galbanum is a gum-resin from the stems of a tall plant of the Umbelliferae family which grows mainly in Iran and other parts of the Middle East. The thick juice oozes from natural cracks in old stems, but is collected commercially by making cuts near the base of the stem.

The essential oil is extracted by distillation and is thick, dark yellow, with a hot, strong aromatic odour. The active principles include carvone (50% or more), pinene, limonene, cadinene, myrcene and cadinol. Mrs Grieve says that dry distillation produces an oil with a blue colour similar to that obtained from Camomile *(Matricaria Chamomilla)* but I have never come across this oil.

Galbanum has been used as an incense in various religions for thousands of years, and is mentioned in both the Old Testament and Egyptian papyri. Dioscorides and other early medical writers describe Galbanum as painkilling, antispasmodic, diuretic and emmenagogue.

Although Galbanum is little used in modern aromatherapy, it offers interesting possibilities, especially in chronic conditions such as rheumatism. It will give a lot of relief from persistent pain, particularly when used in hot compresses. It is equally useful for skin infections and inflammations that are slow to heal. (In this it resembles another ancient incense: Myrrh.) Abscesses, boils and slow-healing ulcers respond well to this oil.

Galbanum is used in the perfume industry as a fixative.

Galen

Galen, who was responsible for the first major classification of plant medicines into groups, was born at some time between 129 and 131 A.D. at Pergamum (now Bergama) in Turkey, which was then under Greek rule. His father was an architect, who recognised and encouraged his son's interest in medicine.

Pergamum was the site of a shrine to Aesclepius, the Greek god of healing, and there was a medical school attached to the shrine, where the young Galen studied. Here he met many influential physicians and was able to observe the treatment of a wide range of diseases. He went on to study at Smyrna, in several cities in Greece, and at Alexandria in Egypt. He became physician to the school of gladiators in Alexandria, and it is recorded that, such was his skill, not one gladiator died of wounds during Galen's term of office.

In 161 A.D. he went to Rome, and rapidly gained a reputation for curing people previously given up as incurable by other physicians, and eventually was appointed personal physician to Marcus Aurelius.

His lasting influence on the development of plant medicine, though, was through his eleven books. In these he described a vast number of 'simples' and formulae for combining them in remedies. He divided the plants into specific categories which became the basis of plant medicine for many centuries. The plant categories were called 'galenic' and still exert an influence on herbal medicine.

His books were translated into Arabic in the 9th century and had an important influence on the flowering of Arab medicine. In the 12th century these Arabic versions were translated into Latin, making his knowledge more widely available to mediaeval scholars. In the 15th and 16th centuries, new translations of his books were made, going back to the original Greek texts. Galen was a very important influence during the Middle Ages and Renaissance, his system of description and classification being reflected in many of the great herbals of the period, some of which were, in fact, little more than translations of his work, with commentaries added by later authors.

Not much is known about Galen's later years, but he is thought to have died in 199 A.D.

One of the formulae invented by Galen is the original 'cold cream', the recipe for which you will find elsewhere in this book.

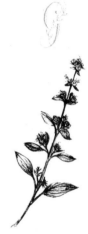

Gallstones

Stones may be formed in the gallbladder due to precipitation of solids from the bile which is stored in this organ. The commonest form of stone is formed of solidified cholesterol.

Treatment is mainly through diet, and surgery may be necessary in severe cases, but massage over the area of the gall-bladder (below the liver in the right-hand side of the diaphragm) can help to reduce pain. Lavender and Rosemary are the two oils that have been found to be the most helpful.

Rosemary is also valuable for inflammation of the gall bladder, the other most common disorder of this organ.

All fats must be excluded from the diet while any inflammation is present, and in the long term kept to a minimum, with vegetable fats preferred to those of animal origin.

Gamma Linoleic Acid

Gamma linoleic acid (G.L.A.) is an essential fatty acid which the body needs to manufacture certain hormones and hormone-like substances called prostaglandins. Prostaglandins are involved in the healthy functioning of many types of body tissue, in areas as different as combating pain and inflammation, controlling blood/cholesterol levels and regulating the menstrual cycle. They appear to have a beneficial effect on the immune system and the brain.

Some people are unable to make sufficient prostaglandins for their body's needs for a variety of reasons, which may include poor nutrition, viral infection, alcohol and hereditary factors. Supplements which provide G.L.A. help to make good any deficiency and relieve the symptoms which a lack of prostaglandins has given rise to.

G.L.A. supplementation helps to maintain the body's own levels of oestrogen and is widely used to help menstrual problems, pre-menstrual tension and menopausal problems such as hot flushes. Ongoing research suggests that oils rich in gamma linoleic acid may be beneficial in Multiple Sclerosis, rheumatoid arthritis, heart diseases, hyperactivity in children and some psychological disturbances, including schizophrenia.

Eczema, psoriasis and other skin conditions often respond well to G.L.A. rich oils. You could include up to 10% of such oils in massage blends or treatment creams.

The best-known plant source of G.L.A. is Evening Primrose *(Oenothera biennis)* probably because the first G.L.A. supplements to be marketed were obtained from that source, but Borage or Starflower *(Borago officinalis)* and Blackcurrant Seed *(Ribes nigra)* and Rosehip Seed *(Rosa rubiginosa)* are also rich sources and provide the basis of some good supplements.

Garlic
Allium sativum

Because of Garlic's reputation for unsavoury smelliness, it surprises many people to find it listed as an aromatherapy oil, for they think of these as being predominantly sweet-scented! However, it is a powerful antiseptic oil and it has many other important actions, particularly in decongesting and detoxifying, and its effect on the blood circulation. Even so, because of the smell this oil is never used externally, but in the form of capsules or 'perles' for internal treatment.

The active principles of Garlic include alliin, allinase, allicin, alithiamin (a form of Vitamin B), antibiotic allistatines, garlicine, nicotinamide (another B vitamin), organic iodine, organic sulphur, Vitamin A and numerous trace elements.

As with many other plants, the history of its use goes back many thousands of years – at least to the Babylonians of 4,000 years ago. It is one of the most widely used plants throughout the world, both for medicinal and culinary purposes. There is a great deal of overlap and those civilisations which have always included a high proportion of garlic in their regular diet, consistently show lower levels of heart disease, high blood pressure and circulatory problems, intestinal disorders and bronchitis. There is evidence that cancers are less common too, but there are still a lot of questions to be asked on this topic, such as whether the life-style in general, or the environment, are factors in addition to the diet.

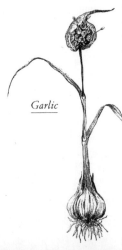

Garlic

From folk medicine, Garlic has found its way into the folklore of many lands – for example any Transylvanian will tell you it keeps the vampires at bay! These beliefs are nothing like as silly as they might appear at first, and modern laboratory testing has vindicated some of the apparently naive methods of use. It is a highly volatile oil – i.e., it releases its properties very easily into the air – and is very quickly and efficiently absorbed through the skin as well as the nose. When we learn that in controlled tests Garlic oil rubbed on the sole of a volunteer's foot was detectable on his breath ten minutes later, then hanging a clove of garlic round a child's neck, nailing slices of garlic to your doorpost or putting them in your shoes, no longer seem so laughable. Garlic's reputation as a protection against the 'evil eye' can be understood too, when we know that it is a preventative measure against many of the minor ailments which were often believed to be brought about by the evil eye. If it kept at bay the coughs and colds, winter ills, stomach upsets, rheumatism and intestinal worms, then Garlic would have appeared to have been doing a very good job of warding off the powers of evil.

In present-day society, Garlic is known as a preventative of high blood-pressure and heart disease, whether eaten fresh as part of the diet or taken in the form of oil in capsules. It is very effective at reducing high cholesterol levels (though we must also make sure that any changes needed in the diet are made).

It is an effective decongestant and antiseptic – of great value in treating catarrh, sinusitis and bronchitis (especially chronic bronchitis) and is probably best known to the lay person in this capacity. Many people take one or more capsules daily throughout the winter as a preventative measure against colds, etc. For acute bronchitis, Garlic should be used in conjunction with other oils to combat the infection, relieve coughing and reduce fever.

Its antiseptic, bactericidal and detoxifying properties make Garlic valuable in treating acne. The (usually young) patient should be encouraged to use Garlic perles daily to help clear the body of toxins. An odourless form of capsule is available, which should give greater confidence to anybody who is worried about what his/her peers will think of smelly breath, though there is a possibility that in removing the odour, some of the properties of the oil are lost.

Garlic has been used for thousands of years to prevent infestation with intestinal worms, both in people and in animals, and it is also effective against certain other parasites. It is used internally as in the treatment of scabies, along with Lavender, Peppermint, and other oils, applied externally.

It is one of the best treatments for gastro-intestinal infections, and can be used as a preventative measure, especially when travelling abroad to areas where stomach upsets are feared; though eating the local food, which is probably rich in garlic, as opposed to that specifically offered to tourists, is perhaps the best safeguard. The widespread use of Garlic in the diet of many peasant communities undoubtedly protects them from infections, in conditions in which rapidly-proliferating bacteria would otherwise be very dangerous. Garlic also increases the individual's resistance to infection.

It was shown in laboratory tests in 1969 that Garlic is highly effective against the E-coli bacteria that cause urinary tract infections. These bacteria of the escherichia genus, inhabit the large intestines and are normally harmless, but if they stray outside the gut they can give rise to bladder and kidney infections. As an antibiotic, Garlic has the advantage of not killing the beneficial flora of the intestine as the synthetic antibiotics do. Well before these facts were established, Garlic was known to be an effective treatment for cystitis, and a good preventative for people who are prone to repeated attacks.

There is little to be said about the method of use, since treatment will nearly always be in the form of capsules: 1 to 3, taken 3 times daily in acute conditions, or once, preferably at night, for chronic conditions or as a preventative. However, there is one other highly effective method of use in certain conditions, and this is to use the capsules as suppositories. One or more capsules should be inserted as high in the rectum as possible, immediately after a bowel movement (disposable plastic gloves can be bought at chemists for this purpose). This method is particularly valuable in treating cystitis, intestinal disorders and worms, and for the very few people who find that Garlic irritates the stomach.

Geranium

Pelargonium graveolens, P.capitatum, P. radens and hybrids of these.

❦

The 'geraniums' of our tubs and window boxes are not, in fact, geraniums but pelargoniums. There are over 200 pelargonium cultivars and some confusion exists as to which of these many varieties provide us with our essential oil. Most of the essential oil currently available comes from a hybrid of *Pelargonium radens* and *P. capitatum*. Even within one variety the oil differs somewhat depending on where the plants were grown, the main producing areas being the island of Reunion, Algeria, Egypt and Morocco. China is exporting Geranium oil, but it is not known from which variety it comes. A product called Bulgarian Geranium oil is not from a pelargonium at all, but a geranium, and is entirely different.

The essential oil is obtained by steam distillation from the leaves. The principal constituents are geraniol and citronellol in varying proportions depending on the variety and the place of origin but usually making up over 50% of the whole with smaller amounts of linalol, limonene, terpineol and various alcohols in different proportions. The oil is a beautiful, pale green in colour, and the odour can also be described as 'green'. It is sometimes described as resembling Rose oil, though a sensitive nose would never confuse the two. It is often used in commercial preparations to 'stretch' the much more expensive oil of Rose.

The plant is another which Culpeper described as being under the influence of Venus, though it is of a less obviously feminine character than Rose. The oil can be described as having a middle position between the sweetness of Rose and the sharpness of Bergamot, and because of this relative neutrality blends well with many other oils, particularly Bergamot and Lavender.

Like virtually all the flower oils, it is antidepressant and antiseptic. It is also a valuable astringent and a haemostatic (it stops bleeding), which makes it very useful in treating injuries. It also promotes speedy healing. It is used in skincare, for its delightful perfume, for its astringent and antiseptic properties and for its action in balancing the production of sebum. This makes it valuable for skins that are excessively dry or oily, or for dry skins with oily patches. It is widely used in commercial skin preparations, soaps, etc. both for its helpful properties and its delightful perfume.

This balancing action arises from the fact that Geranium is an adrenal cortex stimulant. The hormones secreted by the adrenal cortex are primarily regulators, governing the balance of hormones secreted by other organs, including male and female sex hormones; so it is of great assistance in menopausal problems and all conditions where a fluctuating hormone balance is indicated. In particular, Geranium may be used to relieve pre-menstrual tension, and here its diuretic properties also enter into play, helping to relieve the excessive fluid retention which many women experience pre-menstrually.

Geranium also has a stimulating effect on the lymphatic system, and this, combined with the diuretic action, is why I use it in a massage cream for the treatment of cellulitis, fluid retention and oedema of the ankles. The two properties reinforce each other in helping the body to eliminate fluids more efficiently, and in fact Geranium is a valuable aid to elimination in general, having a tonic effect on both the liver and kidneys. It has been used to treat jaundice, kidney stones and various urinary tract infections.

Theoretically it is also a good antiseptic for the mouth and throat, and could be used in mouthwashes and gargles for sore throats, ulcers and gum infections, but in practice many people find the flowery perfume distasteful when it comes to putting it in the mouth, so other oils such as Myrrh and Thyme are more useful, simply because they will be more willingly used.

Some writers describe Geranium as a sedative oil, though Valnet does not, and certainly a number of instances have come to my attention where people were over-excited, restless or unable to sleep quite a few hours after using Geranium, even in quite small amounts. I avoid using it in the latter part of the day, and like to use it in blends with balancing and sedative oils such as Lavender. It is certainly a valuable antidepressant, and some people may prefer its perfume to the sharper scent of Bergamot, though here again I find it better to use the two in combination.

Going back to the window boxes, it may well be that Geraniums originally earned their popularity as windowsill and balcony plants because of their insect repellent properties. The oil is used in a number of commercial insect repellent preparations, often in combination with Bergamot, Lemon or Citronella. Room sprays that include Geranium will help to keep your house free from flying pests in summer, and as it is also a deodorant oil, will also keep it sweet-smelling.

Ancient civilisations regarded Geranium as an exceptionally powerful healer, and credited it with the ability to heal fractures and even eliminate cancers. I do not know of any modern work that has proved or disproved this reputed action. Jean Valnet mentions it, but with caution. I retain an open mind on this question, for our ancestors have been proved right too many times for anybody to dismiss their knowledge too lightly. However, many early references to Geranium actually allude to the wild Geranium (Geranium robertianum) known as Herb Robert or Cranesbill, and not to any of the Pelargoniums. Some of the scented Geraniums do yield essential oils, but they are completely different from Pelargonium oil in smell, chemistry, etc.

Gerard, John

John Gerard, the compiler of one of the most influential herbals of the Tudor era, was born at Nantwich, Cheshire, in 1545, and went to school at Willaston, 2 miles away. At the age of 17 he was apprenticed to Alexander Mason, a successful surgeon. After completing his medical studies, Gerard travelled widely in Scandinavia and Russia – a considerable undertaking at that time – and maybe also in the Mediterranean region, though the records are less clear about this.

In 1595, Gerard was elected to high office in the Barber-Surgeons Company. By this time he had a high reputation as a herbalist, and supervised the gardens of Lord Burghley in the Strand, and at Theobalds in Hertfordshire. Gerard had a garden of his own, too, in Holborn, and in 1596 he published a descriptive list of all the plants in this garden. This was a novel idea at the time, and one which had considerable influence on later writers, in its methodical and scientific approach. A second edition containing both Latin and English names of the plants, was published in 1599.

The book on which Gerard's reputation now stands, his great 'Herball' was published in 1597, with a dedication to Lord Burghley. It consisted to a large degree of translations from classical writers, but to these Gerard added his own observations and comments; for example, descriptions of the habitat and manner of growth of plants, and the regions in Europe and the British Isles where some of the rarer plants could be found.

Gerard eventually became 'herbalist' to James I, and in 1607 he was elected Master of the Barber-Surgeons Company. These two appointments make it clear that at this period no conflict of interest was felt between these two branches of medicine. A marked contrast is seen if we compare this situation with the life and career of Nicholas Culpeper a generation later. John Gerard died at the age of 67, on the 19th February 1612.

Ginger
Zingiber officinalis

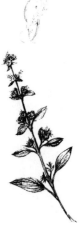

Ginger, like so many of the spices, is a native of Asia, growing originally in India and China. It came to Europe via the 'Spice Route' in the Middle Ages, and was introduced into South America by the Spaniards. It is now grown commercially in all these places as well as the West Indies and Africa. It has been known since ancient times, and its medicinal and cooking uses overlap to a large degree.

The essential oil is produced from the root by steam distillation, and is a pale, slightly greenish-yellow, darkening with age. It smells almost identical to 'green' or fresh root ginger. Its principal constituents are gingerin, gingenol, gingerone and zingiberine.

In traditional Chinese medicine Ginger is used in any condition where the body is not coping effectively with moisture, whether the moisture originates within the body or without. Diarrhoea and catarrh are examples of inability to deal with internal moisture while rheumatism and many of our winter ills are aggravated by external damp, and the fiery properties of Ginger are used to combat this.

Rheumatism, arthritis, muscular pain and fatigue can be eased by hot compresses or massage using Ginger diluted to 1% or 1.5% only since, as you may well imagine, it is a rubefacient and high concentrations will irritate the skin. Alternatively, add a single drop of Ginger to any massage blend.

For colds, 'flu and diarrhoea, stomach cramps (whether of digestive or menstrual origin) use Ginger as an infusion (or 'tea') made from the fresh root. Cut very thin slivers from the Ginger root, and simmer them for about ten minutes, using about six thin slices from a root of average thickness, to each cupful of water. With a little honey this makes a very pleasant drink which is used in traditional Chinese medicine as a preventative against winter ailments. It quells nausea, and can be a great help with both travel sickness and the 'morning sickness' of pregnancy.

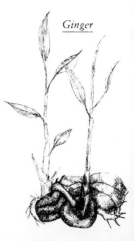

Ginger

The infusion, without honey, can be used as a gargle for sore throats. Alternatively, add 2 drops of Ginger oil to a teaspoon of vodka and dilute this in hot water.

Oil of Ginger, in small proportions, blends well with many others, especially Orange and other citrus oils.

Jean Valnet records that women in Senegal weave belts of pounded Ginger root to revive their husbands' flagging sexual prowess, but this may not be a fashion that European men would take to enthusiastically.

Gingivitis

This is the name given to inflammation of the gums (Latin, gingiva) due to bacterial infection. The gums feel sore, and bleed when brushed or when hard foods are eaten. They may become soft and begin to recede, and because of this, more teeth are lost through gum disease than through tooth decay.

Scrupulous attention to mouth hygiene is important, both in treating and preventing gingivitis, and mouthwashes based on essential oils are a great help.

There are a number of essences which are useful against the bacteria which cause gum infections, the most important of which are Ti-tree and Thyme. (Thymol, a derivative of Thyme oil, is used in the majority of commercial mouthwashes.) Fennel and Mandarin are also valuable in strengthening the gums, and Myrrh is another indispensable ingredient, for its healing and tonic properties.

You will find a formula for a suitable mouthwash in Appendix C, but many variations are possible. You could use Ti-tree in place of the Thyme, or equal quantities (15 drops) of each, or you could replace the Fennel with Mandarin if you prefer the taste.

Keep this mixture in a screw-top bottle and add two teaspoons to a half-tumbler of warm water to swill thoroughly round the mouth at least twice a day.

If the infection is severe, tincture of Myrrh can be applied direct to the inflamed areas of gum. Gentle massage of the gums will improve local circulation and speed up healing. To do this, scrub the hands immaculately clean, and put a drop or two of the mouthwash mixture undiluted on the fingertips. Gently but firmly massage the gums, especially around the base of each tooth. This is specially useful when the gums are so sore that it is painful to brush them.

Vitamin C supplementation will help the infection to clear.

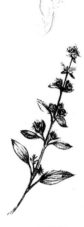

see also **MOUTH ULCERS.**

133

Ginseng

Ginseng (Panax ginseng, or Panax quinquefolium) is sometimes useful in conjunction with aromatherapy treatment, especially if the patient is debilitated.

It has been used in the East, especially China and Korea, for thousands of years, as a tonic and stimulant, and has had so many virtues attributed to it as to have become almost a legend.

It is certainly helpful in times of crisis, and during convalescence, but it is important not to abuse or over-use it. Up to 1200 mgs a day can be taken in capsule form for very short periods only, for example following physical or mental trauma, or when an abnormal amount of effort is required for a short time. The daily intake should not be more than 600 mgs if it is taken for more than a few days, such as during convalescence.

Ginseng is widely regarded as aphrodisiac and although this action stems partly from the feeling of well-being and vigour it produces it does contain a plant hormone equivalent to testosterone.

G.L.A.

❧

see **GAMMA LINOLEIC ACID.**

Gomenol

❧

see **NIAOULI.**

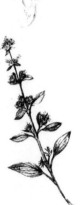

Gout

❧

Gout is a disease caused by a chemical imbalance within the body, which is unable to efficiently process and eliminate uric acid, which then forms into crystals, often around a single joint. The joint most frequently affected, and which has become known as the epitome of the gouty old gentleman, is that at the base of the big toe. Attacks may begin with no warning, and are excruciatingly painful. The joint becomes hot, red and inflamed.

Aromatherapy treatment will include cold compresses, massage and dietary advice, and follows the same lines as those outlined under **ARTHRITIS,** since gout is basically a form of extremely acute localised arthritis.

Grapefruit
Citrus paradisi

❧

The Grapefruit tree is a product of cultivation, being a hybrid between *Citrus maxima* and *C. sinensis*. There are many different varieties grown in different parts of the world especially Israel, Brazil, Florida and California, which produces most of the available essential oil.

The oil is produced by expression from the peel and contains up to 90% of limonene, with citral, geraniol, cadinene and paradisiol. It is yellow to green in colour, with a fresh, citrus aroma closely resembling the fresh fruit.

One of the most important distinctions between Grapefruit oil and the other Citrus oils is that it is not a photosensitiser. It does contain some of the Furocoumarins that have this effect, but it seems that one or more of the other constituents have a neutralising effect. This is a good example of the fact that whole oils are so much safer to use than any part that might be isolated from them. It shares many of the properties of the other citrus oils, and can be thought of as a good alternative to them when the skin is likely to be exposed to the sun after treatment.

Grapefruit is a valuable oil for fluid retention, cellulite and other conditions where toxins are not being eliminated effectively, being a diuretic, detoxifier and a stimulant of the lymphatic system. I use it in lymphatic massage, alone or in a blend with Geranium. If used in a massage after hard exercise, it helps to disperse lactic acid from the muscles, so reducing aches and stiffness. This can be particularly helpful for athletes in training and competition, dancers, and anybody else who needs to keep in peak muscular condition.

It is good for oily skin and acne, and has a tonic effect on the skin and scalp. The delightful smell makes it very welcome in toners, lotions, etc.

It has been suggested that Grapefruit oil can be used to treat obesity. The diuretic effect may help if there is an element of fluid retention involved, but I think this use has more to do with its antidepressant property. Many overweight people are fundamentally unhappy, and helping their emotional state will often lead to weight loss.

In fact, I think that the most important use of Grapefruit is as an antidepressant – one which may have been somewhat overlooked by aromatherapists. It is a 'sunny' oil, non-sedative and mentally enlivening. I use it increasingly for people who are depressed and lethargic, particularly in winter. It does seem to be of great benefit for people with Seasonal Affective Disorder (S.A.D.) but I can hardly think of anybody who would not benefit from having Grapefruit oil around when Spring seems a long way off.

Grief

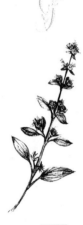

In some books on aromatherapy, you will find certain oils mentioned as helping to allay grief. My belief is that it is the loving care of the therapist, rather than the oil, which is important (i.e. one of these oils in a bath would be far less helpful). However, one or two oils do seem to be exceptionally comforting when used in massage.

Rose is perhaps the best of all. I sometimes use it alone, and sometimes combine it with Benzoin, which has a degree of warmth about it. Marjoram is another very warming oil, and is very good if there is an element of loneliness combined with grief, such as after a bereavement; but this is really an area for sensitive consultation between the therapist and the grieving person, and you might consider the uplifting Bergamot, soothing Camomile, or Lavender or Melissa if any of them feel more appropriate.

The Bach Flower Remedies combine well with aromatherapy in such situations, but you may sometimes feel that other forms of help, such as bereavement counselling, would also be beneficial.

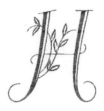

Haemorrhoids

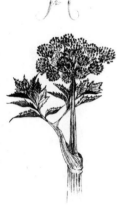

Haemorrhoids, or piles, are varicose veins located in the rectum, just above the opening of the anus. The causes may be various, but a common factor is the restriction of the normal circulation of blood to the rectum. This may occur temporarily during pregnancy, due to pressure from the uterus, or continually due to disease of the liver or chronic constipation. The discomfort of piles encourages constipation, so the two disorders can aggravate each other.

Apart from the discomfort caused by piles, treatment is important because even the small amount of blood that is lost each day from these veins is enough to cause anaemia over a period of time.

Several essential oils can be used for local treatment and to improve the circulation generally. Cypress, Juniper and Frankincense can be used in local applications (suitably diluted) and in baths on a regular basis. Garlic perles and plenty of fresh garlic and onions in the diet will also improve circulation.

If constipation is part of the problem, then dietary changes will probably be necessary in the long run, but Rosemary, Marjoram or Fennel can be used to help in the short term as massaging the abdomen in a clockwise direction with any of these oils in a 3% dilution helps to stimulate natural peristalsis.

Hair

Hair is composed mainly of a protein called keratin, which also forms our nails and the outer layer of skin cells. Keratin is not a living substance, but is produced as the living cells in the hair follicle ('root') die.

Because hair is a dead substance, aromatherapy can do very little to influence its condition. What we are able to do with essential oils is improve the health of the scalp, on which the condition of the hair depends.

Rosemary has been used as a hair tonic, especially for dark hair, for many hundreds of years, and essential oil of Rosemary is used in many commercial hair and scalp products. A few drops can be added to the final rinsing of water after shampooing, or you can make an alcohol-based scalp rub by dissolving 5 mls of essential oil of Rosemary in 100 mls of high-proof vodka.

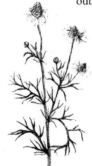

Camomile

Camomile has been used as a rinse for fair hair for centuries, and adds a gold tone, but it can be slightly drying; so if your hair is dry and you want to use Camomile, give the hair a nourishing oil treatment first. Massage jojoba oil into the scalp and leave it on for one or two hours, wrapping the head in cling-film or plastic, covered with warm towels, and then shampoo out. If you have oily fair hair, then you can add a strong infusion of Camomile flowers to the final rinse.

Dandruff can be effectively treated with essential oils. For dry dandruff, dilute Lavender or Ti-tree or a blend of these in a carrier oil to 3% and apply as described above, and repeat once or twice a week. For oily dandruff, Bergamot or Sandalwood would be better, as they help to balance the production of sebum. Using a mild shampoo (many commercial dandruff shampoos are far too harsh on the scalp), pour the amount you need into the palm of your hand and add between 1 and 3 drops of essential oil. Massage the shampoo into the scalp very thoroughly, leave on for up to five minutes and rinse in the usual way two or three times a week.

The health of the hair and scalp depend to a great extent on general health and nutrition, and a diet providing a good balance of minerals and vitamins, or the use of supplements where necessary, is the best way to keep the hair in good condition. Shampoos should be mild, as harsh shampoos strip off the natural coating of sebum, an oily wax produced by glands in the hair follicle. The sebum spreads along the hair shafts and keeps the hair looking smooth and glossy. Without this protective coating, the dead cells which make up the hair for most of its length, will flake and give the hair a dull and lifeless look. External treatments, such as conditioners, help to make the hair look shiny by replacing lost sebum with various other oily substances, but it is simpler and healthier to let the natural sebum do its work.

Hands

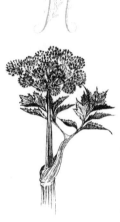

Without hands there could be no aromatherapy! I often think of my hands as the link between the healing oils and the patient.

However, the hands themselves sometimes need help, especially in relation to the skin of the hands, which can so often become dry, rough, cracked or sore from contact with water, detergents and other chemicals handled at work or at home, soil, wind and cold. All the healing and antiseptic essential oils can be useful, but perhaps the most appropriate are Benzoin, Calendula, Lavender and Lemon. All of these are good antiseptics, and Calendula and Lavender are particularly valuable healers for the skin. Benzoin is very effective at healing cracked skin, which may often become a painful condition of the hands in cold weather.

Any of the home-made creams described in **APPENDIX C** will make a good hand cream, the one made with cocoa butter being particularly good for people who work out of doors, as it is thick and rich and provides some protection from soil and other rough materials, and from the weather. To any of the creams you can add a combination of two or three of the oils mentioned above. Lemon is a mild bleach, and will help to remove discolouration of the hands caused by vegetable or fruit preparation, gardening, etc.

Sometimes industrial or household chemicals can give rise to allergic reactions, and the hands are particularly vulnerable to this type of problem, since it is sometimes difficult or impossible to avoid contact with the irritant substance. The two great anti-allergy essential oils are Camomile and Melissa, and either of these may help to relieve eczema or contact dermatitis on the hands. Again, these oils can be incorporated into a cream which will not only treat but protect the hands. Lavender could be included in the cream, too. Obviously, the best remedy is to avoid the substance that is causing the irritation, it if can be identified, but this is not always possible when it is involved in the person's daily work. Gloves should be worn, if possible, to minimise contact if the irritant cannot be avoided altogether.

The hands deserve careful attention when giving a general massage, not only because many people tighten and clench their hands when anxious or stressed, usually without being aware of what they are doing, and massage to release such tension is always valuable; but also because there are a great many reflex points and acupuncture pressure points in the hands. The whole theory of reflexology can be applied to the hands as well as to the feet, but even without studying this, the aromatherapist can do a great deal of good by simply massaging the hands thoroughly and with care.

Hay Fever

Hay fever is a form of allergy affecting the lining of the nose, and often the eyes and throat too. Strictly speaking, as the name implies, it is an allergic response to the pollen of certain grasses, but is used to describe similar reactions to a wide range of pollens and the spores of some fungi. The symptoms are probably too well known to need description; runny nose, sneezing, and streaming eyes when the particular group of pollens to which the person reacts are floating in the air.

Various essential oils help with the symptoms, some people finding one helpful, and some others, just as different sufferers react to various types of pollen in the first place. Any of the oils which relieve the symptoms of the common cold, especially Lavender and Eucalyptus in inhalations, may help to reduce the sneezing and runny nose, but my first line of attack is usually the oils which are helpful for allergies in general, Camomile and Melissa. Of the two, Camomile seems to be effective more often than Melissa, but this is unfortunately a situation in which trial and error seems to be the only way to find out what is most helpful to the person concerned. Also, it sometimes seems that one oil will lose its effectiveness quite soon, and as treatment may be needed throughout the pollen season, you will need to alternate two or more oils to provide some effective relief.

Some people find the heat of a steam inhalation makes them feel worse, so simply give them some oil to put on a hankie or tissue, to sniff whenever they need it during the day. Massage with any of these oils can also be very helpful, as the oil absorbs into the bloodstream, and often decreases the severity of the allergic response.

High levels of Vitamin C supplementation seem to help a lot of hay fever sufferers (at least 3 grams a day), and attention to the diet in general can also be useful. Dairy produce and refined starches, which tend to encourage the production of mucus, should be kept to a minimum, if not cut out altogether, and this does seem to lessen the allergic reaction in quite a lot of people.

For sore, red eyes, cool compresses of rosewater or camomile infusions (NOT the essential oil) are very soothing.

Melissa

Hazardous Oils

❧

Most essential oils are very safe when used in the dilutions and according to the methods described in this book. A few, however, are either too dangerous to use at all, or need to be used with extreme care. These are usually oils which contain large amounts of ketones which may be neurotoxic, cause abortion or provoke epileptic fits, or phenols which are severe skin irritants. A full list of hazardous oils is given in Appendix A. Please consult this before using ANY oil for the first time.

see also the entries for **KETONES** *and* **PHENOLS.**

Headaches

❧

There are many essential oils which can be used to relieve headaches far more safely than the ubiquitous aspirin. Out of the great range of analgesic oils, those which seem to be most effective are Lavender and Peppermint, either separately or in combination. Rosemary is another oil which clears the head and relieves pain, especially if the headache follows a period of mental effort.

Lavender can be rubbed neat on the temples (just a few drops), or made into a cold compress and applied to the temples, forehead or back of the neck. A mixture of Lavender and Peppermint in equal proportions may be even more effective, for Lavender has the ability to enhance the action of other oils when it is used in blends. It is also worth noting that while Lavender is a sedative, Peppermint is a stimulant, and that many commercial headache remedies combine a stimulant (usually caffeine) with one or more analgesics. This is because many of the painkilling drugs have a slightly sedative and sometimes even a depressing effect, and the caffeine is included to counteract this. By using Lavender and Peppermint a similar effect is produced without the dangers inherent in synthetic drugs.

If the headache is caused by catarrh or sinus infection, inhalations with Lavender, Peppermint, Rosemary or Eucalyptus help both to relieve the headache and clear the congestion that is causing it. All these oils are antiseptic, and will combat nasal infection as well as relieving symptoms.

Most headaches can be easily traced to an immediate cause – fatigue, stuffy rooms, eyestrain, tension – but headaches that appear with no apparent reason, and any headache which is persistent or recurrent needs to be given some careful thought. It may be that the sufferer's lifestyle, diet or environment need changing, or less frequently it may be that headaches are a sign of more serious disorders that need proper treatment.

see also **MIGRAINE.**

139

Rosemary

Heart

The heart is a double pump, composed of a special type of muscle which works continuously, day and night, and even when we are unconscious, from well before birth until the moment of death. The right hand side of the heart pumps blood to the lungs, where it collects oxygen, vital to all our body processes, and is cleansed of carbon dioxide and other wastes. The left side of the heart pumps the freshly oxygenated blood round the entire body, taking oxygen and other necessary elements to all the organs and tissues.

A few essential oils act on the heart, Borneol, Garlic, Lavender, Marjoram, Peppermint, Rose and Rosemary are all described as cardiac tonics, i.e. they have a strengthening effect on the actual muscle of the heart. Lavender, Melissa, Neroli and Ylang Ylang are recommended for palpitations, and so on, but my feeling is that all these uses should be approached with great caution, and that we should not attempt to treat any heart condition without a medical training; although the oils mentioned can certainly be used in baths and massages for anybody who is already receiving treatment from a qualified practitioner.

Many of the conditions which we generally refer to as 'heart disease' are, in fact, diseases of the circulatory system, most often due to fatty degeneration of the arteries serving the heart itself. If these become constricted or blocked by fatty deposits inside their walls, the heart muscle is starved of oxygen, and as no muscle can function for more than a few moments without oxygen, it stops working. This is what we describe as a 'heart attack' or 'coronary'. Fortunately, there are a number of essential oils which do have a helpful action on circulatory problems and these are described under the entry for **CIRCULATION**.

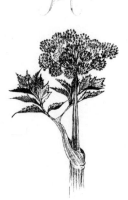

140

Heartburn

see **INDIGESTION.**

Helichrysum

Helichrysum italicum, ssp. Serotinum

Helichrysum oil is distilled from the 'everlasting flowers' popular among flower arrangers. There are many varieties of Helichrysum used in floristry, but only the *H. italicum serotinum,* which has yellow, daisy-like flowers, has the properties described below. You may find the oil described as 'Everlasting' or 'Immortelle' – the French equivalent. Both flowers and oil have a deliciously honey-like aroma. (I used to live near a farm that grew Helichrysums for floristry, and to walk past their fields in summer was a heady experience.)

The oil is usually yellow, occasionally with a reddish tint and its main active constituents are nerol and neryl acetate, together with geraniol, pinene, linalol and some minor additions. It is widely used in perfumery, and in soaps and cosmetics both for its fragrance and its soothing, healing properties.

Helichrysum is one of the oils (like Lavender) that are most active when used synergistically, i.e., in combination with other oils. Fortunate perhaps, as it is expensive and not always easy to come by. It increases the body's own ability to heal, which suggests a possible immunostimulant action.

It is a very safe oil, non toxic, non irritant and tolerated by the most sensitive skins. This makes it a lovely oil to use for babies and children, in their baths, massage, etc., and its rather sweet and 'innocent' fragrance seems well suited to such use. Try blending it with Mandarin – an exquisite combination. Another childhood use is for knocks and tumbles, as Helichrysum contains powerful anti-bruising agents. It is anti-spasmodic and can help calm asthma attacks and the spasmodic coughing (the 'whoop') of whooping cough, which can be so distressing to a child. It is also expectorant, so useful for all kinds of coughs.

Being anti-inflammatory, it is useful in massage for arthritis and rheumatism. A good blend for this would be 95% Eucalyptus (preferably the citriodora variety) with 5% Helichrysum, added to a carrier in oil in the usual 3%.

It is used in general skin care and for many skin problems, including eczema and other allergic conditions, as it is anti-allergenic, anti-inflammatory, antiseptic and healing. Some people have reported using this oil successfully for psoriasis, which is notoriously difficult to treat, whether by aromatherapy or any other means. There is almost always a psychological element in psoriasis, and the non-physical effect of Helichrysum may well be as important as its direct action on the skin.

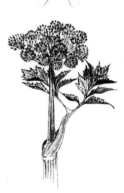

On the mental/emotional plane Helichrysum is comforting and antidepressant – like honey for the psyche. It helps reduce, and possibly even prevent, stress which makes it particularly relevant to all stress-related conditions. Unlike some of the antidepressants, it is a tonic oil and very helpful for people who are exhausted, lethargic or debilitated. I haven't had an opportunity to use Helichrysum for anybody suffering from M.E. but everything about this oil suggests that it would be very valuable.

141

Helichrysum has a variety of other uses, for the digestive and respiratory system, muscular aches, and so forth, but given its cost and relative scarcity, it is probably best reserved for those situations where other oils have been tried without success, or where no alternative is available, at least as far as the treatment of physical conditions is concerned.

Hepatic

Pertaining to the liver. Used in herbal medicine and aromatherapy to describe plants which are tonic to the liver. Essential oils in this group include Camomile, Cypress, Geranium, Lemon, Peppermint, Rosemary and Thyme. In my experience, the last three are the most effective.

Herbal Medicine

The use of plants to help the process of healing is the oldest system of medicine in the world, certainly pre-dating all written history. Early humans probably observed which plants were sought out by sick animals, as well as noticing healing effects of plants which were gathered for food. The example of 'primitive' communities whose lifestyle has survived unchanged into the twentieth century, as well as archaeological evidence, suggests that much of this knowledge was held by a single person in each tribe, who was often also the priest or shaman. The tradition was handed down orally, often within one family, from father to son, or mother to daughter. At a Neanderthal burial site dating from 60,000 years ago, 14 different plant species were found in one grave and of these at least 11 have medicinal properties known to us.

Complex and sophisticated systems of herbal medicine existed in the far East 3,000 years ago, and written records of herbal remedies have been found in Egypt dating from about 1,500 years B.C.

The present day herbalist uses the whole plant, fresh or dried, prepared in a variety of ways, such as infusions and decoctions (teas), tinctures and liquid extracts, tablets, creams and ointments. The use of the whole plant is very important. Unlike a pharmaceutical scientist, the herbalist does not isolate certain active principles from a plant, but uses them in combination with all the other complex chemical structures found in the same plant. This probably accounts for the rarity of side-effects from the use of herbal remedies. The very substances which pharmaceutical laboratories discard as 'impurities' balance and complement the medicinal action.

Herbal medicine and aromatherapy complement each other ideally. Both are based on the use of healing plants, though in different ways, and many plants are used in both systems. Many aromatherapists find it very helpful to be able to refer people to a qualified medical herbalist, particularly if they feel that a herbal remedy would complement the essential oils applied externally by means of baths, massage etc. Conversely, a herbalist may feel that aromatherapy would benefit a patient, especially when stress-related illness is involved.

Herbal Oils

☙

see **INFUSED OILS.**

Herb Teas

☙

Herb 'teas' or infusions can be used to great benefit in combination with essential oil treatments. It is often possible to find a tea, or a dried herb, from the same plant as the essential oil you are using (Camomile, Fennel, Lemon, Verbena, Peppermint, Rosemary, etc.), and taking drinks of these will reinforce the properties and effects of the corresponding oil used in massage, baths, etc. Where this is not possible, you can choose a herb with properties that enhance those of your essential oil, possibly from among the plants used in medicinal herbalism but not in aromatherapy.

The method of preparation is the same as making a pot of tea. Boiling water is poured over the driedor fresh herb and left to infuse for 5 to 10 minutes. The length of time is usually rather more than for a cupof ordinary tea, and will depend partly on which herb you are using. The supplier from whom you buy your herbs shouldbe able to guide you on the right length of time for various plants, or you can find this information in a number of good herbal books.

The most popular herb 'teas' are available in the form of tea-bags, which makes preparation very easy, but these do not usually contain enough of the dried herb to produce a therapeutic dose, so you would either have to use more than one tea-bag per cup, or drink rather a lot of cups to have any real effect. However, even in this somewhat diluted form, these teas provide a healthy alternative to traditional tea and coffee.

Although some writers advise adding a few drops of essential oil to a cup of herb tea, or glass of fruit juice, this is a practice I would strongly discourage. Because essential oils do not dissolve in water, and both teas and juices are largely water, any essential oil taken in this way will remain undiluted. As explained elsewhere in this book, undiluted essential oils can damage the stomach lining. In principle, I feel very strongly that ingesting essential oils is potentially dangerous and best avoided. In the rare instance where a medically trained therapist suggests this, a proper dilutant will be used to avoid the danger.

see also **HERBAL MEDICINE** *above.*

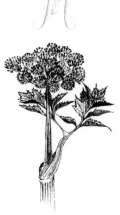

Herpes

Cold sores are caused by the virus herpes simplex I which most of us carry around in our bodies all our lives without symptoms. The blisters may appear when we have another infection, for example, a cold (hence the name 'cold sores') or when we are overtired and run down. In some people the blisters arise in extremely hot or extremely cold weather.

Bergamot, Eucalyptus and Ti-Tree oils are very effective in treating the herpes blisters, particularly if applied immediately at the first sign of an eruption. They are usually applied in an alcohol base. You may be able to obtain isopropyl alcohol at a large chemists; if not, vodka will do very well. Add a total of 6 drops of one oil to 5 mls of alcohol. 6 drops of one oil will do but a blend of two or more is often better. Ti-tree oil can also be used neat. Frequent dabbing at the first onset of trouble will often stop blisters developing, but if they do I use neat Lavender oil in alternation with the alcohol mixture, as this helps to heal the blisters in much the same way as it does with burns.

Genital herpes is said to be caused by herpes simplex II virus, but it is not entirely certain that there are, in fact, two viruses. It is possible that it is the same virus manifesting in different ways. The same oils used for cold sores are helpful, with the emphasis on Bergamot, because of the affinity this oil has with the urino-genital system. Clearly, oils must be greatly diluted. Make an alcohol dilution as above, with 4 drops Bergamot and 2 of Ti-Tree, add to a litre of boiled and cooled water and mix thoroughly before using as a local wash. This is a good preventative treatment. If blisters break out, they can be treated in the same way as cold sores, using a cotton-bud to apply neat Ti-tree or an essential oil/alcohol preparation.

Both forms of herpes seem to erupt more often when the sufferer is under stress so massage and baths with antidepressant and de-stressing essential oils can help.

Herpes zoster is discussed under **ZONA**.

High Blood Pressure

⤫

---

see under **HYPERTENSION.**

Hippocrates

⤫

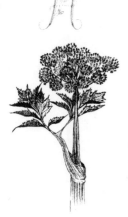

Hippocrates, universally revered as the 'Father of Medicine', was born on the Greek island of Cos in about 460 B.C. He probably came from a family of physicians. References to him written during his lifetime refer to Hippocrates being a member of an Aesclepiad, a term indicating a group of doctors (from the name of Aesclepius, the god of healing). A medical school was commonly referred to as an Aesclepiad, but other references within the same text suggest that in this instance the term referred to a family, particularly as he was known as 'Hippocrates the Great' in his own lifetime, to distinguish him from others of the same name.

Hippocrates' work and writings are of great relevance to aromatherapy on two counts:

1. He used and wrote about a great number of plant medicines.
2. He regarded the body as a whole – not just a collection of parts.

He could with justification be called the 'Father of Holistic Medicine'.

Among the medicinal plants used by Hippocrates and described by him in medical texts were a number of narcotics, such as opium, belladonna, mandrake and henbane, as well as humble fruits like quince, grenadine and rhubarb and many of the plants that are still used in aromatherapy today – aniseed, coriander, cumin and garlic; resins including frankincense, myrrh and styrax; caraway, fennel, thyme and, almost inevitably, roses which played a large part in virtually every early system of medicine.

But perhaps more important was Hippocrates' contribution to medical theory, philosophy and ethics. The 'Hippocratic Oath', still taken by many medical students at the present day, was almost certainly not composed by him, but by his pupils or followers. More important, perhaps, was the importance he placed on the moral qualities needed by anybody involved with the healing of their fellow humans; discernment, self-effacement and devotion, for example. Apart from teaching that the body is a complete organism and must be seen as such when attempting any treatment – surely the first requirement of a holistic approach – he pointed out that it is vital to seek the cause of any disease and eradicate it, rather than treat the symptoms. He taught, too, that an unsuitable diet produced undigested residues and that vapours or 'humours' arising from these residues were a prime cause of disease. Although we no longer subscribe to the theory of 'humours' the importance of diet in all systems of natural medicine is so well established that it seems amazing that it was lost sight of for so long.

Hippocrates travelled widely, teaching and practising wherever he went, and earned the love and respect of all who came into contact with him, not only for his medical skill, but because he lived by the same high moral standards that he taught.

He died at Lirissa in 377 B.C.

Histamine

Histamine is a product of the breakdown of protein. The release of histamine is a normal defence mechanism, and discomfort is only experienced if too much is produced. One of its actions is to cause dilation of the small blood vessels in the immediate area, giving rise to redness and heat. Fluid may seep out of the dilated capillaries into the surrounding tissues, causing swelling and irritation. Other actions of histamine include stimulation of the stomach and intestines, and contraction of the bronchi, leading to asthma attacks.

Histamine may be released in response to a sting from nettles or insects, and as histamine is also present in the poisons manufactured by the plant or insect, an excess of it can very quickly build up in the area immediately surrounding the sting. Inhaling pollens, animal hair and many other irritant substances can also trigger histamine activity, giving rise to the acute discomfort of hay fever and causing asthma attacks. The medical approach is to treat with antihistamine drugs. The antihistamines are chemically similar to histamine, but do not provoke the same responses in the body.

The aromatherapist's response will be to select one of several calming and soothing essential oils, Camomile and Melissa being the most important, and apply them in various ways, which will depend on whether the problem is a skin irritation, or a respiratory disturbance such as asthma or hay fever. For insect stings, direct application of oil of Lavender or oil of Lemon as soon as possible after the sting has happened, will often prevent the local reaction of itching and swelling, suggesting that these oils may have an antihistamine effect.

Inhalations of Camomile, Melissa, Lavender, Hyssop, Benzoin or other oils found to help the individual, can give symptomatic relief to hay fever and asthma sufferers, but in the long term it is important to use massage, baths and possibly dietary advice to try to lessen the individual's response to such stimuli as pollens, animal hair, dust and other irritants.

Nobody fully understands the role of histamine in allergic reactions. In some instances the body produces a flood of histamine in response to a relatively minor threat, and in others it will produce histamine when there is no external threat at all. Without knowing why, we do know that stress plays a major part in these reactions. A person under stress may react to substances that cause no problems when the same person is free from stress. The aromatherapist's approach to allergy involves looking beyond the symptoms and trying to alleviate the underlying stress. All the oils mentioned above have a calming and soothing effect on the mind and emotions, and in many cases will help the allergy sufferer to reach a state of balance where the external irritant no longer provokes an abnormal flood of histamine into the body.

Melissa

see also **ALLERGIES.**

H.I.V.

It is generally thought that the H.I.V. virus (Human Immunodeficiency Virus) is the cause of A.I.D.S. and that everybody diagnosed as being H.I.V. positive will sooner or later develop full-blown A.I.D.S. and die as a result. The longer we live with the A.I.D.S. epidemic, though, the clearer it becomes that this is not necessarily true. Only about 30% of people who are known to be carrying the H.I.V. virus actually develop the full A.I.D.S. syndrome. There are also many more people carrying the virus without knowing it, so the fraction of H.I.V. positive people who eventually develop A.I.D.S. is in fact less than 30%. The longer we live with the A.I.D.S. epidemic, the more people we see who have been H.I.V. positive for a long time – up to 10 years in some instances – without becoming ill. There are also people who have been H.I.V. positive, developed A.I.D.S. and eventually recovered their health, reverting to being H.I.V. positive without symptoms. Some people have developed a condition which, in every other respect, looks like A.I.D.S. without having the H.I.V. virus. So, it is clear that the virus is not the only factor involved.

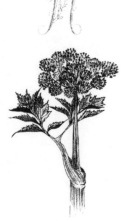

In order to understand why some of these people develop A.I.D.S., while the majority do not, we need to take a look at how the H.I.V. virus operates. Like all viruses, it can only reproduce itself with the help of materials found in living cells. The virus enters a 'host' cell, and once inside the cell begins to multiply, using the cell's biochemical resources to do so. In the case of the H.I.V. virus, the chosen host cells are the T-helper cells of the immune system. The immune system is discussed elsewhere in this book but, briefly, T-helper cells set in motion and accelerate all the processes that combine to make up the immune response, while their opposites, the T-suppressor cells, slow down and stop these processes when there is no threat from infection present. In a healthy body, T-helper cells outnumber T-suppressors, but the H.I.V. virus destroys T-helper cells until eventually there are more T-suppressors than T-helpers.

At this stage, the body is unable to defend itself against invading micro-organisms, and bacteria, other viruses and fungi (such as candida) can wreak havoc. These are known as 'opportunistic' infections, i.e. they seize the opportunity given by the body's lack of defence mechanisms, to proliferate.

The orthodox medical approach is to prescribe drugs that attack the virus, but it is now clear that mutant, drug-resistant forms of the virus can develop within as little as a week of first taking the drug. Most ongoing research is aimed at developing a vaccine against the virus.

The holistic approach is to look at the person involved, rather than at the virus, and to do everything possible to strengthen that person's immune system and general health. Anything that strengthens the immune system and increases its activity, lessens the chances of the full syndrome developing.

There is a body of evidence that people who decide to use natural therapies, improve their nutrition, learn to relax and so forth, are less likely to develop full-blown A.I.D.S. or if they have already done so, have longer periods of remission and a better quality of life.

Aromatherapy can play an important part in such an approach, not only by directly working on the immune system with immunostimulant and tonic oils, but by giving nurture, helping with relaxation and creating a safe space in which people can acknowledge such emotions as fear, anger, etc.

There is a wide range of immunostimulant oils from which to choose, from Thyme, Ti-tree and other Melaleucas, through to less 'medicinal' oils such as Manuka, Ravensara and Rosewood. Any oil which will support your client physically, emotionally or spiritually is appropriate.

An increasing number of aromatherapists are working with people who are H.I.V. positive, often through charities and support groups, and find this a rewarding, though challenging field of work.

Obviously, there is considerable overlap between working with H.I.V. positive people and with those who have developed full-blown A.I.D.S., and you will find much more discussion of the latter in the entry devoted to A.I.D.S.

see also the entry for **IMMUNE SYSTEM.**

Hives

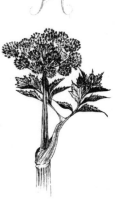

see under **URTICARIA.**

Hoarseness

see under **LARYNGITIS.**

147

Ho-Leaf or Ho-Wood
Cinnamomum camphora, var. *Ho-sho*

Ho-leaf and Ho-wood oils are obtained from a variety of Camphor tree and like all Camphors are hazardous oils and I would strongly advise against home use. Very experienced aromatherapists might wish to use them with caution, but even for them there are safer alternatives available.

I include them here only to dispel the notion that Ho-leaf can be used as a substitute for Rosewood *(Aniba roseodora).* There is no resemblance between the two oils in aroma, properties or uses and where Ho-wood is hazardous, Rosewood oil is a mild, non-toxic, non-irritant oil, safe for virtually any use.

Holistic Medicine

Aromatherapy and other therapies are often referred to as 'holistic' but unfortunately this word is often misused, sometimes simply as a synonym for 'alternative'. This is misleading, for it is not the form of the therapy that makes it 'holistic' but the attitude of the practitioner, whether he or she is a G.P. or hospital doctor, a nurse, masseur, aromatherapist, counsellor or herbalist, or any other caring therapist.

The word 'holistic' is derived from the Greek 'holos' which gives us both 'holy' and 'whole' in modern English (the 'w' got added much later), and also has connections with the Anglo-Saxon word 'hael' from which 'healthy' and 'hale' (as in 'hale and hearty') are descended. The association of the idea of health with wholeness and holiness expresses well the concept of holism. In medicine it means caring for the whole person, often expressed as body, mind and spirit. The whole lifestyle of the person is taken into consideration, including diet, exercise, relationships, relaxation and the interaction between the person and society. In its widest sense, holism implies a relationship between the therapist, the person seeking help and the wider environment.

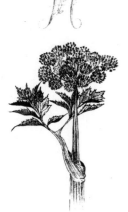

To what extent can aromatherapy be described as a holistic therapy? Once again, this depends more upon the practitioner than the means of treatment chosen. It is possible to apply aromatherapy in a purely mechanistic, symptom-treating manner, but I think it is true to say that most aromatherapists look beyond the treatment of symptoms and seek to help the causes of disease. The very nature of essential oils themselves, and their ability to subtly affect us on many levels – physical, emotional, mental and even spiritual – makes them a very appropriate medium for anybody who is seeking to treat the whole person. During every aromatherapy treatment, the therapist will be breathing in the oils which are being used to treat the client, and will be subtly affected by them. This creates a very special kind of integration between helper and helped, and if we also remember the origin of the oils, in the various plants that the planet provides for our healing, we can see another link between the people involved in the healing process, and the earth itself.

Another aspect of the holistic approach is the willingness of the practitioner to refer a patient to somebody else if some other form of treatment would seem to be helpful, either in addition to or instead of what he or she can offer. Therapists may take a team approach and co-operate closely in the healing process. Aromatherapy lends itself ideally to such an approach, since it can be allied to many other kinds of treatment. Dr. Jean Valnet said, 'Aromatherapy does not claim to be effective, by itself, for every ailment, nor for every patient, nor in every circumstance. It must often be used in conjunction with other medications.' If we bear this in mind, and always keep the health of the whole person as our aim, we can truly claim to be holistic therapists.

Homoeopathy

Homoeopathy is one of the very few systems of natural medicine which may not be entirely compatible with aromatherapy. The reasons for this will be explained a little later.

Formulated in the first half of the 19th century by Samuel Hahnemann, a German physician, homoeopathy means the treatment of like with like. It depends on the fact that infinitely small amounts of a substance will cure the symptoms that are produced by a larger amount of the same substance. Homoeopathic remedies are prepared by making successive dilutions of animal, vegetable or mineral materials and sometimes bacteria and viruses. As each dilution is further diluted, the mixture is vigorously agitated, or succussed, a process which is called potentisation. Conversely to what might be expected, the more a remedy is diluted, the more powerful it becomes. Scientists dismiss homoeopathy because they are unable to measure any trace of the original material in the higher potencies; but yet they are effective, often when more scientifically justifiable treatment has failed.

It seems that homoeopathic remedies work on the level of very subtle vibrational energy and this is why essential oils may be antipathetic to them. Aromatic particles each have their own characteristic rate of vibration, which is involved in the mechanism of smell, but these vibrations are of a less subtle nature than those of homoeopathic remedies, and can negate their action. It has long been known that people taking a homoeopathic medicine should avoid such strong smells as peppermint or eucalyptus and that the remedies must be stored away from all strong smells. However, homoeopaths are by no means unanimous about the relationship between their art and that of the aromatherapist. Opinions vary from a total ban on the use of essential oils, to a feeling that no harm can be done provided that Eucalyptus, Peppermint and a few other strong-smelling oils are avoided. Other suggestions include separating aromatherapy treatment from taking a remedy by at least half an hour, restricting it to some of the gentler oils, such as Camomile and Rose, and that while low potencies are probably not antidoted by essential oils the higher potencies almost certainly are.

The only practical course of action is to make sure that the homoeopath is consulted before using essential oils for anybody who is currently taking a homoeopathic remedy. This would, in any case, be correct professional etiquette. If necessary, massage can be given with a carrier oil alone until the course of homoeopathic treatment is finished.

Having said that, I have to follow it by saying that I know people who combine homoeopathic remedies quite happily with aromatherapy, with no apparent detriment to either treatment!

Homoeopathic remedies need to be stored quite separately from essential oils or any other highly perfumed materials. Keep them in a separate room if possible, or if not, at least in a separate cupboard. One homoeopath with whom I have discussed this question suggests that if you use essential oils all the time, any homoeopathic remedies you may have should be replaced at fairly frequent intervals if not used up. Throw them away and replace at least every six months would seem to be a sensible guideline, or buy and use only as needed.

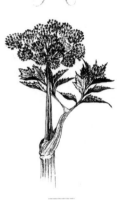

149

Honey

The healing properties of honey have been known for many centuries, and it is a substance that works well in association with essential oils, especially in the treatment of skin conditions. Small amounts of honey can be incorporated into ointments (along with the closely-related beeswax) both for general skin care, and to help with more serious conditions such as eczema.

Hormones

The name hormones is given to a number of chemicals produced in the body which are secreted into the bloodstream and affect the functioning of many body systems and organs. The word hormone is taken from a Greek root meaning to excite, since the action of the hormone is often to stimulate activity in an organ. A characteristic of hormones is that they influence bodily functions at a distance from the point of origin of the hormone. For this reason they are often referred to as 'chemical messengers'.

The group of glands which produces hormones is known as the endocrine system, and is responsible for regulating growth, metabolism, reproduction, our response to stress and the levels of various vital nutrients in the bloodstream. None of these glands works in isolation from the others; there are very complex and finely-balanced relationships between them, and the whole is regulated by the pituitary gland. This is situated just below the brain, which is itself influenced by the hypothalamus, which acts as an interface between the brain, the nervous system and the endocrine system.

As well as regulating the activity of the other glands, the pituitary governs growth. The thyroid gland is involved with growth and metabolism. The parathyroids regulate the levels of calcium in the blood. The adrenal glands are involved in a variety of body functions, including the metabolism of starches, our response to stress and the functioning of the testes and ovaries. The Islets of Langerhans (specialised cells in the pancreas) produce the hormone insulin, which is involved in the maintenance of levels of sugar in the blood. The ovaries and testes produce the male and female hormones, oestrogen, progesterone, testosterone and others, and regulate the reproductive cycle, lactation and secondary sexual characteristics (facial hair, breast development, etc.).

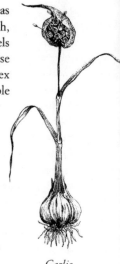

Garlic

Many essential oils have an effect on the endocrine system, and they may do so in one of two ways: some oils contain plant hormones, known as phytohormones, which are similar in action to our own, and act in the body in a similar manner, reinforcing the action of the corresponding human hormones. Phytohormones can be used in a similar way to some of the synthetic or animal-derived hormones used in orthodox medicine, but without the dangers and moral objections associated with them.

Other essential oils act as a trigger or balancer of hormone production from various glands. For example, Garlic and Onion help to balance thyroid secretion, and are useful when the thyroid gland is under-active. Basil, Geranium and Rosemary stimulate the adrenal cortex, though Geranium is also a balancer of hormone production in general. Eucalyptus and Juniper help to reduce excessive blood-sugar levels, and here again Geranium acts as a balancer.

A number of oils (mostly from the Umbelliferae family) contain anethol, which has oestrogen-like properties and are very valuable in disturbances of the menstrual cycle and menopausal problems. These include Fennel, Star Anise and Tarragon. Sclareol, found in Clary Sage, is another oestrogen-like substance. Cypress has a similar action: the active substance responsible has not yet been identified but is thought to be a di-terpenic molecule.

Oestrogens always need to be balanced with the use of progesterones, but no essential oils contain progesterone-like molecules, so we need to turn to medicinal herbs such as Vitex agnus castus or Ladies Mantle (*Alchemilla mollis*) which can be used in the form of tinctures or tablets.

The influence of essential oils on the endocrine system is one of the most important ways in which they act on the human body, and there is still a lot that is not known about plant hormones. It is very probable that many more essential oils which influence the body do so through subtle hormonal effects that are not yet understood.

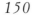

Hungary Water

Hungary Water, or 'The Queen of Hungary's Water' is an aromatic compound reputed to have had such a powerful rejuvenating effect on an aged 14th century queen, that she was restored to youthful good looks and courted by the King of Poland. As the queen was over 70, semi-paralysed and suffering from gout, the effect must indeed have been remarkable!

Most tall stories have a foundation in truth and this one is no exception. The essential oil of Rosemary does help with gout, and has for many centuries had the reputation of curing paralysis (though obviously not paralysis caused by damage to the spinal cord). Rosewater and orange-flower water are good skin tonics, so some of the supposed rejuvenating effect would have arisen from an improvement in the queen's general appearance.

Modern versions of Hungary Water are used mainly as a refreshing summer perfume or an astringent. Ingredients vary a lot but all include Rosemary and rosewater. You can make your own quite easily using the following formula:

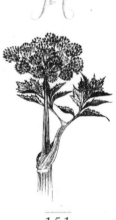

> 4 drops of oil of Rosemary
> 6 drops of oil of Lemon
> 2 drops of oil of Orange
> 5 mls triple-strength orange-flower water
> 5 mls triple strength rosewater
> 40 mls 90% alcohol (vodka) or ethyl alcohol if you can obtain it.

Blend the essential oils, and then stir them into the alcohol, finally add the rosewater and the orange-flower water and shake thoroughly. Put the mixture away to mature, but shake it every few days at first, and then once a week for at least two months, or longer if you can bear to wait. It makes a very refreshing toilet water, skin tonic or mild deodorant, but please don't be too disappointed if you don't look fifty years younger after using it!

151

Hydrolat or Hydrosol

A hydrolat or hydrosol (both names are commonly used) is the water that is collected when plants are distilled to make essential oil. In some cases the amount of oil that can be produced by distillation is so small that the process is carried out specifically to obtain the hydrolat, and the essential oil is regarded as a by-product – though a valuable one. For example, a very small amount of distilled Rose oil is collected during the production of rosewater.

Hydrolats are valuable therapeutic materials in their own right and can be used alongside essential oils or in place of them especially in cosmetic applications and for treating skin disorders. They can be applied to the skin direct, without further dilution and are particularly useful where a non-oily or water-soluble treatment medium is needed, for example in some forms of eczema where oils or oily creams seem to make the condition worse. Melissa or Camomile hydrolats would be particularly appropriate here. It is also possible to use them as bath additives and in inhalations and sprays.

The best-known hydrolats are the flower-waters which have been used in skin-care and perfumery for centuries: lavender water, orange-flower water and rosewater, but hydrolats of Camomile, Clary Sage, Eucalyptus, Linden Blossom, Melissa, Rosemary, Thyme, etc. are also obtainable. Cornflower hydrolat makes a good eye-bath for tired eyes or minor eye infections.

Hydrolats usually contain a tiny proportion of essential oil along with many water-soluble extracts from the plant that do not occur in the oil. The water passes through the plant material many times during distillation so a high level of these water-soluble elements is obtained. Their properties, therefore, are not identical to that of the corresponding essential oil, but do closely resemble them. You can safely take what you know about an oil as a guide to the use of its hydrolat.

Because of their gentleness, in comparison with the equivalent essential oil, hydrolats are particularly well suited to use for children, the elderly and people who are very debilitated by illness.

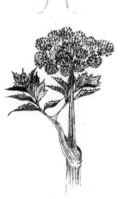

Hypertension (High Blood Pressure)

It is perfectly normal for the systolic blood pressure (the pressure of the blood as it is being pumped out of the heart) to increase during exertion or emotional stress, but in a healthy body it will return to normal quite quickly.

A continual state of raised blood pressure is potentially dangerous, even if no symptoms are felt, because of the strain that it imposes on the heart, blood vessels and kidneys. There is a delicate relationship between the kidneys and blood pressure, in that high blood pressure can damage the kidneys. Conversely, kidney disease which interferes with the flow of blood through the kidneys and the secretion of a hormone (renin) which helps to maintain blood pressure at a normal level, can lead to high blood pressure. The latter stages of kidney disease leading to high blood pressure, is virtually indistinguishable from high blood pressure leading to disease of the kidneys. It is therefore extremely important for any aromatherapist treating raised blood pressure to ensure that the sufferer has been examined and diagnosed by a person with adequate medical training.

Continued high blood pressure places strain on the heart. Initially, the heart muscle will enlarge to deal with the added workload, but may later be unable to keep up an adequate circulation (heart failure). One of the major risks involved in continued high blood pressure is that it increases the likelihood of the individual suffering a stroke or coronary thrombosis. It is often associated with atheroma (the forming of fatty deposits in the lining of the arteries) and arteriosclerosis (the thickening and hardening of the arterial walls).

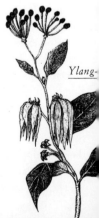

Ylang-

Aromatherapy can help to lower blood pressure, although it is important to make sure that changes in diet and lifestyle are also made. Massage with one or more of the essential oils known to decrease blood pressure is the most important aspect of treatment, and it is significant that all these oils are also calming, soothing and deeply relaxing, for the person with high blood pressure is often somebody who finds it hard to relax, who drives him or herself relentlessly, or is unduly stressed. An interesting parallel is found here between the words we use to describe the physical state 'pressure' and 'hyper (i.e. excessive) tension', and the mental/emotional state that is often involved. Long-term studies in a London teaching hospital have shown that massage effectively reduces high blood pressure, and that this effect persists for a long time. The benefits are cumulative and when massage is given regularly blood pressure may be lowered for several days after a massage.

The most important oils are Lavender, Marjoram and Ylang-Ylang. Ylang-Ylang is valuable if there is shortness of breath or over-rapid breathing or heartbeat, which often accompany high blood pressure. All these oils are pleasing and enjoyable to use for massage and in the bath between treatments.

It is essential to direct aromatherapy treatment at a long-term change in the attitude of the sufferer towards his or her lifestyle and goals, rather than the mere removal of symptoms, and a pleasurable and de-stressing massage at regular intervals is a positive step in this direction. I will often back up and vary the oils which directly act on high blood pressure by selecting other sedative, antidepressant and uplifting oils according to the individual's needs at a particular time. Camomile, Bergamot, Neroli, Rose and Frankincense are some of those I have used in this way.

I also use cleansing, detoxifying oils such as Fennel, Juniper and Lemon combined with changes in diet to help maintain blood pressure at a healthy level; Garlic is important in this respect and should be taken as capsules or included in the diet as fresh garlic if acceptable. A reduction in animal fats is one of the most important changes to be made, as they are a major factor in atheroma. Salt intake should be considerably reduced, and stimulants such as tea, coffee and alcohol cut to a minimum. If they can be cut out altogether for a short period, and maybe re-introduced into the diet in small amounts in the long term, it will certainly help recovery.

Gentle exercise is one of the best ways to keep the circulation in good health, so I am always pleased if I can persuade a person with high blood pressure to investigate a yoga class, since this will combine safe and gentle exercise with relaxation and possibly a period of meditation. Any of the systems of meditation can be a valuable way of learning to slow down and maintain a degree of calm in daily life.

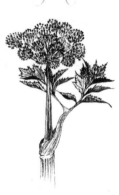

153

see also entry under **BLOOD PRESSURE.**

Hypotension (Low Blood Pressure)

Blood pressure which is lower than the normal limits is less common than a level higher than normal, and the long term implications for health are less serious. However, people whose blood pressure is consistently lower than normal may be prone to dizziness and fainting, as the supply of blood to the brain may be interrupted momentarily if the pressure falls below that necessary to maintain the flow to the head. They tend also to feel cold and tire easily.

Rosemary oil has been used to raise blood pressure to a more normal level. It is tonic and stimulating and responds in many ways to the needs of people with low blood pressure. Other stimulant oils such as Black Pepper and Peppermint are helpful, particularly if fainting is a frequent problem, but they should not be used to excess. Hyssop and Sage are other possibilities, but both present some risks of toxicity, so I would advise against their use except by very experienced therapists.

Massage, perhaps of a brisker and more vigorous nature than we usually use in aromatherapy, is once again the best form of therapy, and I would always combine this with recommendations to take regular exercise, gentle at first, as a means of improving the general efficiency of the circulatory system.

see also entry under **BLOOD PRESSURE.**

Hyssop
Hyssopus officinalis

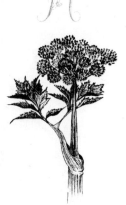

Essential oil of Hyssop should only be used with great caution and there are many circumstances in which it should not be used at all (see **APPENDIX A**). However, it does have some therapeutic applications, so with these cautions in mind it may be considered in some situations.

Hyssop

The earliest medical writers praise Hyssop and many of the renaissance herbalists list a multitude of uses, but we must remember that they are referring to the plant itself, and not to the essential oil in which all the chemical compounds are so highly concentrated.

Hyssop was regarded by both the Greeks and the Hebrews as a sacred herb, and is mentioned several times in the Old Testament. It was used to clean out temples and sacred places, quite literally by using bundles of the herb as a broom. Later, it was a popular strewing herb, and these two uses might lead us to consider burning or vaporising a little Hyssop to disinfect rooms and protect from infection. It is still used in perfumery and cooking, and is an ingredient of Chartreuse liqueur.

The plant is a member of the Labiatae family, and a native of the Mediterranean which grows to two or three feet in height, with spikes of flowers that may be blue, mauve, white or pink. The flowering tops are used to distil the essential oil, which is yellowish in colour, with a spicy aromatic scent a little like Thyme or Basil. The active constituents include a high proportion of pinocamphene (a ketone) with pinene and traces of geraniol, borneol, thujone (another ketone) and phellandrene. It is the high ketone content which makes this a 'borderline' oil in terms of toxicity.

Among the possible applications of Hyssop is in chest infections where there is thick mucus. Hyssop helps to fluidify the phlegm so that it can be expelled more easily. However, there are other oils with these properties and I would always use them in preference to Hyssop. It is a cephalic oil and also has a tonic and stimulant effect on the respiratory system and the heart.

Another use is for bruises: it can be applied in a cold compress as soon as possible after the bruising has occurred. Hot compresses, on the other hand are helpful for rheumatism.

Hysteria

Various essential oils have been used to treat hysteria at different times and places. These include Camomile, Clary Sage, Lavender, Marjoram, Melissa, Neroli, Peppermint, Rosemary and Ylang-Ylang, but my own experience suggests that the majority of these are more valuable in helping to prevent hysterical crises than in dealing with them if they arise. Hysteria is an extreme example of violent swings of mood, and any of these oils can help to create a calmer emotional state in which a hysterical outburst is less likely to occur. The reasons which lie below a tendency to hysteria need to be sought, and a responsible aromatherapist may well suggest that the client seeks some form of counselling or psychotherapy. As far as aromatherapy itself is concerned, the choice of oils depends very much on the immediate circumstances and emotional state of the person needing help. In the long term approach, massage is the most important form of treatment, though baths, room sprays or essential oils burnt in the room and used as a personal perfume are all useful back-ups.

In an immediate crisis, the essential oils which may be helpful are those which are used for shock (hysteria is often a response to shock). These are Melissa and Neroli, the former being the one I have found to be the greatest comfort if an element of grief is also involved, such as when the shock is caused by the news of an unexpected death.

The oils may be inhaled though it may be that the hysterical person is not in a state even to co-operate by inhaling from a bottle, in which case you could spray the oil around them, maybe even on them. I would also give Dr. Bach's Rescue Remedy as soon as possible.

The traditional idea of a hot, sweet drink is a good one, and as soon as you can get the sufferer calm enough to sit down and drink, a calming herb tea such as camomile, lemon balm (Melissa) or valerian sweetened with honey will be useful. Honey is, in itself, a mild sedative. On no account give alcohol.

If you can possibly offer a massage as soon as possible after the crisis, this is probably the best way to restore calm and balance. A blend of Rose and Benzoin is one which I have used in such circumstances for their gentle, calming, almost insulating properties, but Lavender, Neroli, Melissa, Clary or Ylang-Ylang might be more appropriate for different people. More massage, aromatic baths and caring support over the next few days are really important, for hysteria is often followed by deep depression.

Finally – and I am not being in the least facetious in making this suggestion – I would suggest that anybody who has had to cope with somebody hysterical could benefit from taking a dose of Rescue Remedy, or inhaling one of the oils mentioned for shock, themselves.

CAUTION
This oil must never be used for anybody who suffers from epilepsy, as it may trigger an attack. It should also be avoided in pregnancy and by people with high blood pressure.

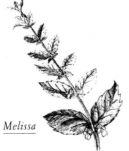

Melissa

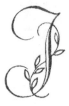

Immune System

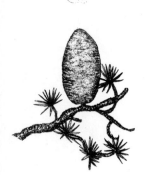

The way in which the human body protects itself from infection is extremely complex, involving several different organs and systems.

Infection arises when the body is invaded by bacteria, viruses or fungi: collectively called micro-organisms, but many such organisms enter the body continuously, and some live permanently in it without causing harm. Infection is only said to be present when an invading organism begins to reproduce and multiply within the body to the extent where it causes problems.

The first line of defence is the skin, and the mucous membrane which lines the mouth, nose, lungs, etc. Bacteria cannot penetrate the skin unless it is broken, and both sweat and sebum are mildly antiseptic. The mucous membranes are a somewhat less effective barrier, being able to exclude certain bacteria but not others.

Once any threatening micro-organisms enter the body, a chain of events is set in motion, involving various specialised cells in the blood, lymphatic system, spleen, thymus and tissue fluids. This is known as the immune response. Although the cells most actively involved in this response are collectively known as white blood cells, they are found in large numbers in the lymph nodes, tissue fluids, etc., and it is possible that their major activity takes place outside the bloodstream which merely serves to transport them to where they are most needed.

Phagocytes, formed in the bone marrow, are large white cells which literally wrap themselves round foreign particles, including bacteria, and kill them, although often the cell itself dies in the process. The pus which gathers at an infected wound, for example, contains vast numbers of these cells together with the dead bacteria. Phagocytes are often referred to as 'scavenger' cells.

Lymphocytes, which are formed both in the bone marrow, and in lymph tissue (lymph nodes, spleen and thymus) have a different function: they are able to manufacture antibodies which are produced in response to threat from a specific micro-organism. When the same organism is encountered in future, the antibodies already present in the blood help to suppress its growth and activity. When sufficient antibodies to any organism are present to prevent disease symptoms arising, we are said to have immunity to that particular organism.

Co-ordinating the activity of these cells are the T-cells. T-helper cells stimulate the production and activity of phagocytes and lymphocytes, while T-suppressor cells initiate the 'winding-down' process when danger from the infection has passed. When the immune system is functioning normally, T-helper cells outnumber T-suppressor cells by about 2 to 1, but if the system is damaged or depleted the number of T-helper cells declines.

The lymphatic system plays an important role in the immune response. Large numbers of lymphocytes are formed in the lymph-nodes in response to infection. A larger than usual number of bacteria circulating in the lymph causes production of lymphocytes to increase dramatically. Also in the lymph nodes are large 'scavenger' cells called macrophages, which filter and engulf bacteria and other unwanted particles. During infection, all activities of the lymph nodes are heightened and the accumulation of active and dead cells and bacteria may cause the nodes to become enlarged. This can often be felt and seen in the neck, armpits and groin, and this swelling is characteristic of some illnesses, such as glandular fever.

The adrenal glands also play a part in the immune response, secreting hormones that trigger some of the processes. Stress lowers the body's resistance to infection partly because periods of stress exhaust the adrenals.

Although an orthodox definition of the immune system does not include the colon, it is now thought that a healthy colon is an important part of the protective mechanism. Millions of 'friendly' bacteria in the gut (the intestinal flora) help to control and suppress micro-organisms that could otherwise endanger the body.

Essential oils can support and strengthen the immune response in two ways: by directly opposing the threatening micro-organisms or by increasing the activity of the organs and cells that fight them. A number of essential oils combine both these actions, for example Bergamot, Eucalyptus, Lavender, Manuka, Ravensara and Ti-tree all act against a wide variety of bacteria and viruses, while at the same time increasing the immune response. Rosemary and Geranium support the adrenal glands in their action and are also stimulants of the lymphatic system. Black Pepper and Lavender strengthen the spleen. The use of these oils, as well as those mentioned above, therefore assist the body very effectively in resisting and combating infection. This action is especially marked if the oils are used at the first onset of symptoms.

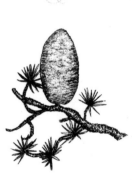

However, virtually every essential oil in therapeutic use is active against one or more bacteria, and almost all of them stimulate production of white blood cells, though Lavender, Bergamot and Ti-tree do this most markedly. People who use essential oils all the time, as part of their daily bathing, skincare and household routines, mostly have a high level of resistance to illness, 'catching' fewer colds, etc., than average and recovering quickly if they do.

Where infection is recurrent or prolonged, and the immune system is depleted, treatment with a variety of essential oils should be continued for at least a month, so that not only are micro-organisms in the body brought under control, but the immune system repaired and strengthened to resist further attack.

Nutrition is also important, because a variety of essential nutrients are needed for the manufacture of the white blood cells. A diet with adequate protein and a high proportion of raw, fresh fruits and vegetable, seeds and grains with a little unsaturated vegetable oil, will usually provide all that is needed, but if the system is very depleted, supplementation is vital until a healthy balance has been restored.

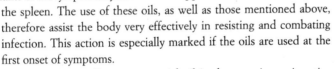

Lavender

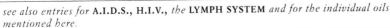

see also entries for **A.I.D.S., H.I.V.,** *the* **LYMPH SYSTEM** *and for the individual oils mentioned here.*

Impotence

Impotence is, obviously, a terribly distressing situation both for the person who is suffering, and for his sexual partner. There is seldom any physical reason for the inability to achieve an erection, and the causes are nearly always mental and emotional. Anxiety about a specific sexual encounter, or about a man's sexuality in general, will often be enough to bring about a failure, and this in turn gives rise to further anxiety, creating a vicious circle. External stress and anxieties about other areas of life, such as finance, health, work or redundancy can have the same depressing effect.

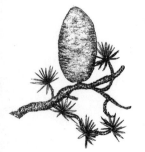

Jasmine

The vicious circle can often be broken by the judicious use of aphrodisiac essential oils, and by those which work on stress in general. If at all possible, massage by a trained therapist is the very best treatment, for it provides the opportunity to enjoy touch in a completely non-sexual situation, as well as being generally relaxing and de-stressing. Aromatic baths just before going to bed offer a simple means of using the oils at the time when they are most likely to be beneficial, and some of them could even be used as a perfume or aftershave, as they have aromas that are quite often used in masculine toiletries, Sandalwood being the best example. If the man's partner can learn to give him some simple massage at home, this may be the best therapy of all, though it is vital that it is understood from the beginning that the massage is not intended to lead to lovemaking and intercourse. If it does, so well and good, but if it does not the session must not be regarded as unsuccessful.

I have already mentioned Sandalwood, which is a powerful aphrodisiac, and an odour which is liked by most men. Jasmine, the most luxurious of all essential oils, often called the 'King of Oils' is another, and helps to restore or increase confidence. Neroli is particularly appropriate if anxiety is the main problem. Clary Sage is deeply relaxing, and sometimes described as 'euphoric'. Although I know few people who have experienced anything like the 'high' sensations sometimes attributed to Clary, it is a very good aphrodisiac because it is so relaxing, and again it has a delicious nutty fragrance that many men enjoy. Clary Sage should never be used if any alcohol has been taken, or is likely to be within a few hours, but I think everybody is aware that alcohol is one of the greatest enemies of virility.

All the oils I have mentioned so far depend for their aphrodisiac effect on their ability to relax the mind and emotions, though there may be other factors involved that are not completely understood, such as a possible hormonal effect with some of them, especially Jasmine and Sandalwood. Some oils classified as aphrodisiac are stimulants, and about these I feel much more doubtful. They might be helpful temporarily in situations where a man is generally fatigued and debilitated, but they should be used with caution, like all stimulants. One or two of them can irritate the kidneys if over-used. Excellent nutrition, vitamin and mineral supplements and a short course of ginseng capsules are probably safer in such circumstances.

see also **APHRODISIACS** *and* **FRIGIDITY.**

Indigestion

❧

Indigestion can be helped by gentle massage over the stomach with a soothing and comforting oil, such as Camomile, Lavender or Marjoram or a hot compress with one of these oils can be put over the stomach and renewed as often as needed.

Drinking Camomile, Fennel or Peppermint herbal infusions will speed up relief.

Infectious Illnesses

❧

Essential oils are very valuable in dealing with infectious illnesses, on three counts:

1. Increasing the body's ability to combat infection from bacteria or viruses.
2. Attacking the bacteria or viruses themselves.
3. Preventing the spread of infection.

All essential oils which are described as antiviral or bactericidal have the ability to attack bacteria or viruses, either killing the invading organisms, or slowing down the rate at which they multiply in the body. These oils are much too numerous to list here, since virtually every essential oil is active against certain infecting organisms. Some oils, though, are active against a very wide range of bacteria and viruses, and these include Bergamot, Eucalyptus, Juniper, Lavender, Manuka, Rosemary and Ti-tree. Most of these also increase the body's ability to fight off the infection – Manuka and Ti-tree most notably so.

You should never massage anybody who has a high temperature (they probably won't feel like being massaged, anyway) so gently sponging the body with essential oils diluted in tepid water is a good method. If the sick person feels well enough to get into a warm bath with some oils added, this is even better.

If the illness affects the respiratory passages (nose, throat, lungs) inhaling essential oils with steam is an effective treatment, and oils can be vaporised in the bedroom with a purpose-designed fragrancer or other apparatus, or on a light bulb or any other heat source, such as a radiator.

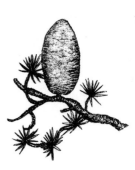

159

see also entries under the names of individual illnesses, and under **INHALATIONS** and **EPIDEMICS.**

Inflammation

❧

An inflammation is one of the body's ways of responding to damage or threat. It may be provoked by bacteria, injury, or contact with irritants, and is an indication that the defence mechanisms are being mobilised. To this extent, inflammation can be seen as a useful process, as the increased blood supply and locally raised temperature both serve to neutralise infections and speed healing.

However, inflammation often continues beyond the point where it is helping the healing process and gives rise to considerable pain or itching and then it is helpful to be able to reduce it. Camomile is the anti-inflammatory oil par excellence with its cooling, soothing, pain killing actions. Lavender comes a close second, and Myrrh is another to be borne in mind, particularly if the inflammation is associated with a wound that is slow to heal. An example might be a deeply embedded splinter or a cut that has become infected.

Where painful swellings are associated with the inflammation, hot compresses are valuable but where there is surface inflammation, such as is seen in contact dermatitis, bathing with a cool solution of one of these oils is better. Add a few drops of Camomile to some boiled water cooled to a little below blood heat and gently swab the inflamed areas as often as wished.

Inflammation may be internal, as in arthritis, cystitis, etc. and helpful methods are described in the entries for these conditions.

Influenza

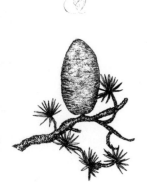

Severe colds and various unidentified virus infections are often referred to as ''flu', and some authorities would argue that this is incorrect, and that true influenza is a much more severe infection, appearing in widespread epidemics, often at intervals of approximately ten years. However, I shall take the first, and most usual definition since such infections are so widespread, and since this is an area where rapid self-help with essential oils is really effective.

The first thing to remember is that treatment is most effective if started at the very first sign of infection. At this stage, a moderately hot bath with a few drops of anti-viral essential oil added will usually provoke profuse sweating, followed by a deep, restful sleep. I hardly need point out that the sick person should go straight to bed after bathing. Very often, this will be enough to avert a full-blown attack of 'flu completely, though it is a good idea to repeat the bathing for the next two or three days. The most spectacularly effective oils for this purpose are Ravensara and Ti-tree. If you do not have either of these to hand, try a 'cocktail' of Lavender and Eucalyptus, using 3 drops of each.

I would like to make it clear that this approach is not suppressive, i.e. we are not trying to mask the symptoms of illness. To understand this, it may help to know how the infection progresses. Between the time when the virus enters the body and the time when the person infected begins to feel ill, the virus reproduces itself rapidly. (Viruses can only reproduce in the body of a host.) No reaction is experienced until the number of viruses in the body reaches a certain level. If the immune system is working at maximum efficiency, the invading virus may be neutralised before it can reproduce sufficiently to make its host feel ill. The person is then said to have good resistance to infection, and this explains why some people 'catch' colds or 'flu in an epidemic and others do not.

At the point where the first symptoms of illness are felt, all the defence mechanisms of the body will be working at full tilt, and an antiviral essential oil will reinforce that effort. Eucalyptus, Lavender, Ravensara and Ti-tree act in two ways, by both attacking the virus itself, and stimulating the immune response. This can be enough to prevent any further proliferation of the virus in the body, so the bout of illness progresses no further.

The effect of an essential oil bath can be increased by taking a steam inhalation, or

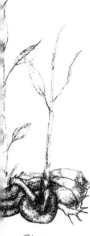

this can be used if bathing is not practical, or if the person feels too ill to take a bath. Use any of the oils suggested for the bath.

If this sort of intervention does not stop a 'flu attack from developing, it will almost certainly reduce its length and severity. In this case, bath with the oils daily, if not feeling too ill, and take an inhalation at least three times a day. This will also help to prevent secondary infections of the respiratory tract by bacteria.

Bacterial side infections are the greatest risk of 'true' influenza, and were responsible for thousands of deaths in past epidemics. The use of antibiotics has dramatically reduced such deaths, although the very young and the elderly are still at risk and a really severe infection of this kind may be one of the situations in which the use of antibiotics is sensible. In this case, do not stop the treatment with essential oils – it can only be beneficial and will not conflict with the more orthodox drug treatment.

Ginger

Burning or diffusing essential oils in the sick person's room is a good additional measure. Again, Ti-tree or Eucalyptus are good choices, possibly with some Bergamot added. Another anti-infectious oil to vaporise is Clove, which has been used in epidemics for hundreds of years. Remember, though, that this is a skin irritant, and do not use for bathing.

Recovery from influenza is often slow, and the convalescent may feel very weak and lacking in vitality. Bergamot can be very helpful at this stage, used in massages if possible, but if not, in baths. Rosemary is a tonic and stimulant oil, valuable in helping the convalescent to get back on his feet. A course of Floradix or ginseng can be beneficial.

Infused Oils

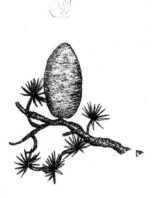

161

An infused oil differs from an essential oil both in its qualities and in the method by which it is made.

Whereas an essential oil is extracted directly from the plant by one or other of the techniques described in this book and nothing else is added to it, an infused oil is made by placing the plant material – usually leaves or petals, but sometimes stalks are included – in a container of vegetable oil. This is kept in a warm place for two or three weeks, or until the base oil has absorbed all the perfume from the plant material. The petals or leaves are removed as they turn brown, and replaced by fresh batches until the base oil has attained the required strength.

This method has been in use for many thousands of years, long pre-dating the making of essential oils. In oriental and mediterranean civilisations, the pots were simply stood in the sun until the process was complete, but in the British Isles, unless we have an exceptionally hot summer, some other source of warmth needs to be provided, such as an airing cupboard or a shelf above a boiler or other fairly consistent source of heat. Some people stand the jar in a tray of water and heat the water, but this does not give such a good oil as the slower and more traditional method.

Because of its simplicity, and the fact that no expensive equipment is needed, this method provides anybody who has access to a supply of fresh herbs or flowers with the opportunity to make excellent massage oils at very little cost.

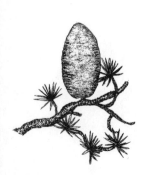

Juniper

If you would like to experiment with making your own infused oils, take a large clean jar, preferably wide-mouthed, and fill it about one-third full with petals or leaves. Fill the jar almost to the top with almond oil, grape-seed, sesame, sunflower-seed or other good quality bland oil, then cover the top of the jar as tightly as you can to exclude the air which can quickly turn the oil rancid. Put the jar in an airing cupboard, on a shelf above your central-heating boiler, or an Aga – or put it in the sun if we have a really hot spell. In this case, bring the jar indoors at night and put it out again when the sun is sufficiently hot the following day. When the petals begin to turn brown, remove them and put in a fresh batch, and repeat this two or three times until your oil is strong enough. Then strain out any little bits of plant debris and bottle the oil, capping it tightly. It will last a few months if stored away from light and air.

Infused oils are quite complex substances, and should not be looked on merely as a 'poor relation' of essential oils. Although it is quite safe to take your knowledge of the corresponding essential oil as a guide to the properties of an infused oil they will not be identical to those of an essential oil from the same plant, but similar and complementary. There is not a hundred-per-cent correlation as an infused oil will not have every property of the essential oil, but on the other hand, it will have absorbed other substances from the plant which are not present in the essential oil.

It is also possible to make infused oils from plants that do not yield an essential oil, or do so only in minute amounts, thus extending the range of plants that we can work with in aromatherapy. Devil's Claw, used for rheumatism and arthritis, Meadowsweet, an excellent analgesic, Comfrey and Echinacea are all useful additions to our repertoire. They can be used in massage blends, singly or in combinations, adding between 3% and 10% to your carrier oil. If you wish you could also add some essential oil, but in very small amounts as the infused oil is already rich in active principles.

Infused oils are sometimes referred to as Floral Oils, if the plant material used is all petals, or Herbal Oils. A more technical name, which you may sometimes come across, is Phytols.

Inhalations

Inhalations have been traditionally used for many centuries to ease problems in the respiratory tract – colds, catarrh, sinusitis, sore throats, coughs, etc. The most usual method is to put some appropriate plant material in a bowl of near-boiling water, lean over the bowl with a large towel enveloping both the bowl and one's head, and inhale the steam for five or more minutes. Literally hundreds of different herbs and plants have been used for this purpose at different times and in various countries.

Essential oils give us a very simple and effective way of making an inhalation, by adding three or four drops of a suitable oil to a bowl of steaming water, and inhaling it as described above. There are also several forms of electrical apparatus for generating steam for inhaling, the simplest and most readily available being sold under the name of a 'facial sauna'. It can, as its name implies, be used for skin treatments, but is also a very neat and convenient way of making a steam inhalation. If using this, or any similar apparatus, you will need to put in only one drop of essential oil as only a very small amount of water is used to produce the steam.

Inhalations should be very carefully monitored if the person using them is known to suffer from asthma, hay fever or any other allergy. If this is so, they should use the inhalation for only 30 seconds on the first occasion. If this provokes no adverse reaction, this time can be increased to 1 minute for the next inhalation a few hours later, and gradually increased to 3 to 5 minutes.

Children need close supervision the entire time they are taking an inhalation to ensure that they do not risk scalding themselves.

For suggestions about which essential oils to use, look at the entries under CATARRH, COLDS, SINUSITIS, etc.

Injuries

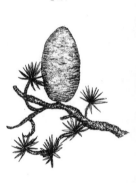

Aromatherapy can be very useful in treating minor injuries, or as a first aid until medical help is available for more serious ones, both where the skin is broken, as in cuts, burns, etc. and in sprains, strains and pulled muscles.

Essential oils can be applied in a variety of ways, according to the nature of the injury, and these are discussed in detail under the entries for BURNS, SPRAINS, WOUNDS and so forth. Also please see under SHOCK.

If an injury is more serious than would normally be dealt with by a non-medically qualified person, do not move the patient in case of causing worse damage, as can be done with fractures, for example.

Shock often follows an injury, even a relatively minor one, such as a fall that causes nothing worse than some bruising, so it is also helpful to use essential oils and Bach Rescue Remedy to minimalise this.

163

Insomnia

Insomnia, whether temporary or of long standing, can be dramatically helped by aromatherapy. There are many essential oils which help to induce sleep safely and naturally, without any of the possible side-effects of sleeping tablets, and the simplest methods of use, such as aromatic baths, or a few drops of essential oil on the pillow, are usually very effective.

Lavender, Camomile and Neroli are the essential oils which I have found to be the most effective in helping insomnia, and it is worth notice that each of them has a profound effect on the mind and emotions; calming, soothing, balancing and relieving anxiety. Any of the oils classified as sedative can be helpful, and indeed it is important to vary the oils used, especially if help with sleeping is needed over a period of more than a week or two.

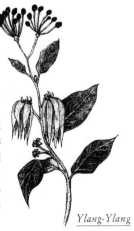

Ylang-Ylang

The sedative oils include Benzoin – very helpful where external worries are at the root of sleeplessness, Bergamot – a good choice where insomnia is linked with depression, Clary Sage – a very profound relaxant which should never be combined with alcohol, as the two together can induce nightmares or very strong dreams, Marjoram – very warming and comforting, Sandalwood, Juniper, Ylang-Ylang, and others. This list is not exhaustive but includes the oils I have found most useful. Almost any of these can be mixed together in blends, so experiment until you find those you consider most pleasing and most effective.

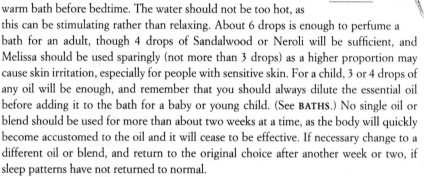

Camomile

Any of these oils or blends can be put into a comfortably warm bath before bedtime. The water should not be too hot, as this can be stimulating rather than relaxing. About 6 drops is enough to perfume a bath for an adult, though 4 drops of Sandalwood or Neroli will be sufficient, and Melissa should be used sparingly (not more than 3 drops) as a higher proportion may cause skin irritation, especially for people with sensitive skin. For a child, 3 or 4 drops of any oil will be enough, and remember that you should always dilute the essential oil before adding it to the bath for a baby or young child. (See **BATHS**.) No single oil or blend should be used for more than about two weeks at a time, as the body will quickly become accustomed to the oil and it will cease to be effective. If necessary change to a different oil or blend, and return to the original choice after another week or two, if sleep patterns have not returned to normal.

These simple uses of essential oil are safe, enjoyable and very effective in helping anybody who is unable to sleep for a few nights; but if insomnia is a long-term problem, simply relying on baths and other uses of essential oils night after night, is little better than taking prescribed pills. The underlying causes should be sought and remedied.

Very often, relatively simple physical reasons can be found for insomnia, such as a sedentary lifestyle, unsuitable diet, stimulating drinks such as tea or coffee late in the evening, an uncomfortable bed or some other physical discomfort; and more exercise, lighter suppers, a change of mattress and so forth may be all that is needed to put matters right.

However, insomnia is increasingly caused by the anxieties and stresses of modern living so some form of structured relaxation may be helpful. Yoga, meditation and breathing techniques can all be very helpful, but perhaps the best approach is regular aromatherapy massage. The combination of gentle, therapeutic touch and deeply relaxing essential oils will work on both the mind and the body to reduce the level of stress, and sleep will follow quite naturally. Most people feel very relaxed, and possibly drowsy, after such a massage, and an evening massage given at home is obviously the very best therapy. But even if it is necessary to visit a salon or clinic earlier in the day, the benefits of increased relaxation will last for many hours, or even days, and combine ideally with aromatic baths. A single massage session can break the vicious circle of sleeplessness, though a course of treatment is obviously better if insomnia has persisted for a long time. The benefits of massage are cumulative, with really significant reduction in stress being experienced after several sessions.

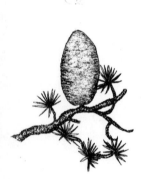

Internal Medication

The question of whether essential oils should be taken internally at all, and if so, how and in what amounts, is probably one of the most vexed in the whole of aromatherapy. I believe very strongly that essential oils should not be taken by mouth, but it is interesting to look at the context within which the two opposing views have arisen.

One school of thought, largely following the tradition of Marguerite Maury, holds that aromatherapy consists of external treatments only. This means massage, baths and inhalations as major methods of treatment, with some secondary use of essential oils in creams, lotions and other skin preparations. The effectiveness of these forms of treatment has been proved empirically over thousands of years, but in recent decades controlled experiments have demonstrated just how much and how quickly essential oils get into the bloodstream when applied to the skin. In addition, some oil will be inhaled, whatever the method of application, and inhaled oils also reach the bloodstream along with the oxygen and other gasses passing through the lungs. These two routes of entry both by-pass the digestive system, where the greatest potential damage from swallowing essential oils is likely. They also offer a faster way of getting essential oils into the bloodstream, the digestive route being much slower.

The other tradition, which advocates the internal use of essential oils, arose in France, where virtually all aromatherapists are qualified medical doctors, and this is an important factor to bear in mind. These therapists have a thorough knowledge of both the pharmacological aspects of essential oils and of human physiology. They also have access to a body of pharmacists trained in the dispensing of essential oil in a suitable dilutant. (By way of comparison, we may consider the garlic capsules or 'perles' which are available at most chemists and health-food stores: these are made from essential oil of garlic diluted in a vegetable oil, usually soya or sunflower. Garlic oil alone, without the vegetable oil and the surrounding capsule would be far to potent to ingest.)

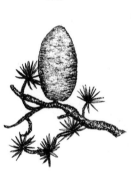

In Great Britain, America and other countries where only the tiniest minority of aromatherapists have a medical training, the situation is very different. If we suggest internal use of essential oils to our clients, without the years of training followed by our French counterparts, we risk serious harm to our clients, and in many countries will also be breaking the law. The general body of opinion now inclines to external use only, and even therapists who were using oils internally a few years ago are discontinuing this practice in the light of evidence about the risks. The International Federation of Aromatherapists specifically requires its members to use essential oils externally only.

The question of self-medication by lay people is even more worrying. There are a number of popular books available which suggest taking essential oils on sugar or honey, usually 3 drops at a time, but sometimes much more. As essential oils dissolve only in alcohol or other oils, the sugar does not dissolve the oil, but merely makes it palatable enough to swallow. (Perhaps we should let the fact that an undiluted essential oil is virtually impossible to swallow, act as a warning that they are not meant to be used in this way?) Evidence collected by Robert Masson in France shows that undiluted essential oil can cause serious irritation, and even damage to the stomach lining. A further risk is that many people, particularly if they are not fully aware of the great degree of concentration of essential oils,

Garlic

think that if a little is good for them, a bit more will be even better! 3 drops may appear too little to people accustomed to taking medication by the teaspoonful, and there is a dangerous fallacy that if a substance is natural, it is safe. If too much essential oil is taken, a great burden is placed on the organs of elimination, the kidneys and liver, as they try to remove them from the body. In several cases where people have died as a result of essential oil overdoses, the cause of death has been massive destruction of the cells of the liver.

Adding essential oils to fruit juice, herb teas, etc., is equally dangerous, and the oil will not dissolve in these water based liquids, and the same risks to the stomach lining exist.

In short: my advice regarding taking essential oils by mouth is – DON'T.

Inula
Inula graveolens or I. odora

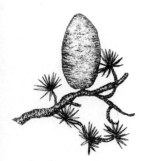

The oil generally known as Inula comes from a variety of Elecampane but is so rarely known by its English name in aromatherapy that I will refer to it as Inula to avoid confusion.

The plant is a very tall perennial, up to six feet in height, with very large oval leaves and yellow, daisy-like flowers. It originated in Asia but is now cultivated throughout the world as a medicinal and ornamental plant. The essential oil is extracted by steam distillation from the roots and rhizomes and sometimes from the flowering tops and contains bornyl acetate, 1.6 cineol, linalol, borneol, etc. It is unusual in that it is a beautiful deep green in colour and it has a very pleasant, honey-like aroma.

Inula has only been known to aromatherapists for the past ten years or so, and even now is not widely used, partly because it is relatively expensive (comparable in price with Neroli, for example) and supplies are limited. In spite of this it is an important addition to our repertoire because it is one of the most powerfully mucolytic oils known: in other words it breaks down mucus so that the body can get rid of it more easily. This is of great benefit in any condition where there is an accumulation of mucus, such as colds, sinusitis, catarrh, earache (when this is a complication of catarrh) and coughs, especially when somebody is coughing a lot without actually bringing up phlegm. Experience in France suggests that Inula is particularly valuable in treating chronic conditions that have not responded to other treatments so it would be well worth introducing where Myrrh and other mucolytic oils have not resolved a problem. It is particularly valuable for chronic bronchitis, where mucus is trapped deep in the smallest structures of the lungs and acts as a 'breeding ground' for bacteria. As Inula is also antibacterial and expectorant it works in several ways to combat the infection.

Inula has a variety of other uses, but they all duplicate the action of cheaper, more easily obtainable oils. My inclination would be to keep it for difficult conditions that have not responded to treatment with other oils.

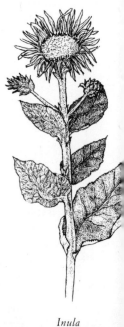

Inula

166

CAUTION
Do not confuse *Inula graveolens* with *I. helenium*. The latter is a very severe skin sensitiser and should never be used on the skin. The best precaution is not to use Inula oil on the skin at all unless you are absolutely certain that it is *Inula graveolens*.

Itching

Itching is something of a mystery – we all know that we may itch in response to some external irritant, such as an insect bite, nettle sting or any substance to which we might, as individuals, be allergic. What nobody has yet understood is how this happens. There are no nerve-endings which can be identified as 'itch' receptors, though it seems likely that very mild stimulus of the nerves which are pain-receptors gives rise to the sensation of itching, and this is why scratching gives some relief, as the mild pain of the scratch is a more powerful stimulus than the original itch. What is still a complete mystery is how we can itch simply through thinking about itching, for example, when somebody talks about head-lice and you immediately have an urgent need to scratch your head. The fact that many people with allergies and other itchy skin disorders suffer more when under stress may be linked to the same response.

Camomile, more than any other essential oil, has the ability to relieve itching, though Lavender and very dilute Melissa are all good alternatives. I have found that Camomile and Lavender combined are more effective than either of them alone, and that Blue Camomile is the best of the various Camomiles. Depending on the location and the extent of the itching, you can use these oils in the bath – especially if a large area of the body is affected as in some allergic conditions – in a cream or lotion, or even, for a very small itchy area, one or two drops of the neat oil rubbed directly onto the skin.

see also **PRURITUS.**

167

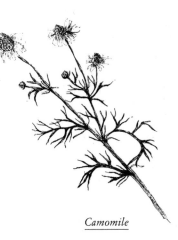

Camomile

Jasmine

Jasmineum officinale and *J. grandiflorum*

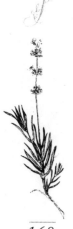

Where rose is often considered the 'Queen of Oils', Jasmine is regarded as the 'King'. This may at first seem rather surprising, given the delicate appearance of the Jasmine flowers, which give an impression of femininity. But the oil extracted from them has a far more 'masculine' nature. It is dark in colour, viscous, and has a heavy, almost animal quality to the aroma, which is very long-lasting. Like Rose, Jasmine oil is very costly, because of the enormous quantity of flowers needed to produce a relatively small amount, and because it is extracted by the labour-intensive method of enfleurage. In the case of Jasmine, the labour costs are further increased by the need to gather the flowers at night, for the odour of Jasmine is more powerful after dark, due to changes in the plant's internal chemistry. The flowers continue to release essential oil for several days after being picked, so are left on the cotton cloths soaked in olive oil until all possible oil has been extracted. The olive oil is afterwards extracted with spirits, leaving the true Jasmine essence. A cheaper grade of Jasmine oil is made by extraction directly from the petals with petroleum spirits. This does not produce the quality or intensity of odour, and the spirit kills the flower instantly, so that the maximum amount of essential oil is not extracted. This grade of Jasmine oil is of little use in aromatherapy, and 'bargains' in Jasmine oil will be avoided by caring therapists. As in the case of Rose oil, the initial cost is offset by the fact that the essence is so concentrated that very little is needed in treatment.

Also in common with Rose, the odour of Jasmine has never been satisfactorily synthesised. Synthetic Jasmine has a sickly sweetness that is nothing like true Jasmine oil, and can only be described as 'cheap' – which of course it is. It is interesting though, that it does smell very like oil of Jasmine which has been left too long after mixing with a carrier oil and 'gone off' (i.e. been spoilt by the oxidisation of the carrier oil).

Two varieties of Jasmine used in making the essential oil are grown in great quantity around Grasse and excellent Jasmine oils are also being produced in Egypt and India. The chemical constituents of the oil include methyl anthranilate, indol, benzyl alcohol, benzyl acetate, linalol and linalyl acetate.

The properties of Jasmine overlap in some respects with those of Rose, being a valuable uterine tonic. It is valuable for menstrual pain and cramps (though less costly oils, such as Marjoram, can be used just as effectively) and is very helpful in childbirth. If it is used as a massage oil on the

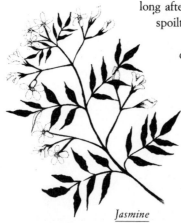

Jasmine

abdomen and lower back in the early stages of labour, Jasmine will both relieve pain and strengthen contractions, and it helps with the expulsion of the placenta after delivery and aids post-natal recovery. Being also an antidepressant, it is a good oil to help relieve post-natal depression.

Conversely, it is equally valuable in certain male disorders, such as enlargement of the prostate gland, and is said to strengthen the male sexual organs. It has had a reputation as an aphrodisiac since antiquity, and is one of the best means at our disposal to help with sexual problems. An important fact to remember is that Jasmine, like all essential oils, acts on the mental and emotional levels as well as the physical. Since the majority of sexual problems arise from tension, anxiety, depression or fear, rather than from any physical cause, a relaxing antidepressant oil such as Jasmine can be a real aid in relieving them, and it is doubtless in this way that Jasmine has earned its aphrodisiac title.

As well as relaxing, Jasmine is often said to be 'warming'. This can be confusing, for it is not a rubefacient like many of the warming oils (that is, it does not make the skin red by dilating the surface capillaries when used in massage) but it does have a gentle and deeply penetrating effect which makes it an ideal massage oil. Culpeper described it as being 'good for hard and contracted limbs'.

On the emotional plane, we find once again that the actions of this oil parallel its physical effects, for it is relaxing and emotionally 'warming'. It is a powerful antidepressant of a stimulating nature, which makes it one of the best oils to help where depression has given rise to a certain lethargy. Jasmine is a good oil to choose for massage or baths for any person who lacks confidence, either in their own worth as a person, or their ability to overcome immediate problems.

Jasmine is described as being a good remedy for coughs (particularly catarrhal coughs), chest infections in general, and loss of voice; but I have to say that I have never used it for any of these purposes, because it is so costly, and there is a wide choice of other oils that are very effective for pulmonary problems.

Jasmine is a beautiful oil to use in skincare, and enjoyed by almost anybody using it for the delicious perfume, though it is particularly good for skin that is hot, dry and sensitive. It needs to be used in tiny amounts, as too much can have an opposite effect to what is needed. However, the very strength of Jasmine's perfuming power is usually enough to ensure that too much is not used.

169

Jaundice

A small number of essential oils have been found to be helpful in treating jaundice, but I would emphasise that this is a serious illness, and the patient must be under the care of a doctor. Aromatherapy treatment can be given at the same time, and may be used to relieve discomfort and strengthen the body's powers of recovery.

The oils which are most likely to help are Camomile and Peppermint, to relieve nausea in the early stages, Lemon, Rosemary and Thyme to strengthen the liver. Jean Valnet also mentions Geranium, but I have no experience of using this oil for jaundice.

Massage very gently over the whole area of the liver, stomach and abdomen. If the liver is too distended for massage to be comfortable, use cold compresses of Camomile, Rosemary or Thyme. Once the patient feels strong enough to take a bath, put 6 to 8 drops of Camomile or Rosemary in each bath to strengthen the liver. If you want to use Lemon, Peppermint or Thyme in the bath, restrict them to a maximum of 3 drops, as they are all potential skin irritants in larger amounts, making up the rest with Camomile or Rosemary.

The recovery period from jaundice is often very long indeed, with general debility and digestive difficulties lasting for many months, and in some cases even longer. During this time, aromatherapy baths and massage to tone and stimulate the entire body, as well as the liver and digestive systems are needed, and very often the convalescent may become quite depressed, so inclusion of any of the antidepressant oils would be welcome. Bergamot is the one which seems to be the most valuable during convalescence.

see **LIVER** *and* **HEPATIC.**

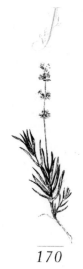

Jealousy

Certain essential oils are sometimes attributed with the ability to dispel jealousy, among them being Rose, Benzoin and Camomile.

While not for one moment denying the profound effect of essential oils on the mind, I am not sure whether it is wise or possible to be as specific as this. Perhaps it would be wiser to say that these oils, and indeed any of those listed as sedative, have a generally calming and soothing effect, and will combine with the gentle and caring attitude of the therapist to enable a jealous person to confront their own situation in a more constructive manner.

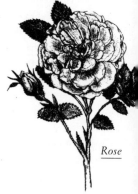

Rose

Jealousy, like any other emotion, can take many forms, and a jealous person might be roaring with rage, or very withdrawn and depressed. Obviously the choice of essential oil or oils, and the way in which they might best be used, needs to be very carefully matched to the needs of the individual at a particular moment, and the therapist must use all his or her skill and intuition.

Juniper
Juniperus communis

Juniper is a small tree of the cupressus family, with needle-like leaves, and berries which are at first blue, but turn black after two years, when they are considered ripe. The best essential oil is obtained by steam distillation from these berries and its active principles include alpha pinene, cadinene, camphene, terpineol, borneol and camphor of juniper. An oil is also distilled from berries and twigs together but the oil from berries alone has greater therapeutic value, so make sure you buy oil described as Juniperberry and not simply Juniper. The essential oil is very fluid, and may vary from colourless to yellowy or a pale green. The odour is reminiscent of turpentine (to me, it smells like very high quality artist's oil paints), but is surprisingly pleasing when diluted and especially in blends, to which it gives a characteristic smoky note. This works well with citrus oils.

Juniper has been known since antiquity as an antiseptic and diuretic, and these two properties are important ones in aromatherapy; but I would always consider the most important action of Juniper to be detoxification. It is one of the most valuable oils in all situations where the body needs to throw off toxic wastes. Very often, the diuretic action of Juniper will be useful in such situations, too.

Juniper has a special affinity with the urino-genital tract, being tonic, purifying, antiseptic and stimulant. It is one is the best oils to choose for treating cystitis, pyelitis and urinary stones – though it is vital to ensure that a doctor or medically qualified homoeopath is consulted in any kidney infections. Cystitis often responds very well to aromatherapy treatments, but if there is blood or pus in the urine, or fever, do not delay in getting medical help. The same remarks apply to all cases of pyelitis, though you can usefully continue with aromatic baths and massage at the same time.

Juniper

Juniper will dramatically reduce retention of urine, which often occurs in men when the prostate is enlarged. Again, it is obviously important to ensure that treatment for the prostate condition is undertaken. Larger amounts of Juniper oil can actually cause retention of urine – another example of the principle discovered by Samuel Hahnneman, the 'father' of homoeopathy: that a symptom which can be produced by a large amount of a certain substance will be relieved by very small amounts of the same substance. While in aromatherapy we are not talking about the infinitely tiny quantities used in homoeopathy, the same principle applies in many instances.

Juniper is sometimes used to treat leucorrhoea, but again I would emphasise that no discharge should be treated without investigating the cause. Scanty or missing periods can be treated with Juniper in baths or in a massage oil used over the abdomen. It is as effective as Sage, with none of the side-effects associated with that oil.

It is a very good astringent, and is used (sometimes combined with Frankincense) in the external treatment of haemorrhoids (piles) either in the bath or as a local wash.

The astringent, antiseptic and detoxifying properties all combine to make this a good treatment for acne. I have found Juniper particularly useful when treating adolescent boys with acne, as they will happily accept the woody smell, and use creams or lotions made up with Juniper regularly, where they might reject some of the sweeter-smelling oils as too feminine.

Juniper is another of the many aromatics which has been used for hundreds, if not thousands, of years to protect from infection. It is known for this in lands as distant, geographically and culturally, as France and Tibet, and sprigs of Juniper were burnt with Rosemary in French hospital wards until relatively recently for this purpose. The essential oil makes a very good household disinfectant – simply use a few drops in water for washing paintwork, floors, etc. – and can be used in sprays, on a light bulb or in one of the various types of essential oil burners, particularly during epidemics.

Juniper has been traditionally used in France as a tonic, especially in convalescence, and where a generally sluggish condition is due to poor elimination. It stimulates appetite – hence the use of gin and tonic as an aperitive. Poor elimination is one of the root causes of rheumatism, gout and arthritis, and Juniper should be considered as a means of improving elimination. It is a very helpful treatment for cellulitis, because here accumulated toxins are associated with fluid retention, so the detoxifying and diuretic actions of Juniper work hand in hand.

It can be a valuable oil in several skin conditions, such as eczema (particularly if it is weepy), dermatitis and possibly psoriasis. Juniper should be considered if any skin condition is very slow to heal, but you should bear in mind that, because it will stimulate the body into throwing off toxic residues, the skin may first appear to get much worse before it begins to improve. This is a classic example of a 'healing crisis' – a phenomenon which is common to many forms of natural medicine.

Juniper has several veterinary uses, including the treatment of canker in the ears of dogs and cats, mange in dogs and the removal and prevention of fleas and tics. I have used Juniper to treat a dog with dermatitis, as well as to keep animals free from fleas.

The cleansing properties of Juniper work on the mental/emotional plane as well as the physical. It is a psychically purifying oil, especially for individuals who are exposed to contact with a large number of people in the course of their work, or with few, but emotionally draining people. I have used this oil for myself and my colleagues when we felt depleted and confused after talking to huge numbers of people at public events; for myself after giving treatment to seriously disturbed patients; for the mother of a large family when she felt exhausted by the constant demands of her own and other people's children. A bath containing a little Juniper oil is probably the most effective treatment (it combines beautifully with Grapefruit if you don't like the smell very much on its own) but in a crisis, putting one or two drops of Juniper on your hands and stroking them over your arms, or even just inhaling the oil, will help enormously. Juniper seems to clear 'waste' from the mind just as it does from the body.

Keratin

Keratin, which is the main constituent of hair, nails and the tough outer layer of the skin (the epidermis) is a protein. The skin, hair and nails are all dead tissue, formed from cells pushed up from the living layers beneath, and consequently no form of treatment, whether aromatherapy or other, can influence them in any way. What aromatherapy can do is to increase the health and vitality of the growing (germinative) layer of the skin, the follicles from which individual hairs grow, and the nail base. Regular massage of the hands, scalp and entire skin surface will improve the circulation and therefore the vitality of these growing areas. Essential oils of Lavender and Neroli in particular are valuable as they stimulate the growth of healthy new cells, but many other oils are helpful and are described under SKIN, HAIR, etc.

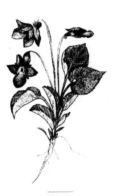

Ketones

These organic molecules are the most potentially toxic compounds in essential oils. They exert a very powerful action on body systems and essential oils with any significant proportion of ketones are generally too hazardous for use in aromatherapy. They may be toxic to the central nervous system, abortifacient and/or epilepsy-provoking. In VERY small amounts they have valuable properties: immunostimulant, antifungal, etc. but safer alternatives can usually be found.

Examples: thujone (perhaps the most dangerous of all the ketones), found in Mugwort, Sage, Thuja, etc. – abortifacient, neurotoxic; borneone, in Camphor, Cinnamon, Mugwort, Spike Lavender; carvone, in Caraway, Peppermint and many other oils; pulegone, in Pennyroyal, causes abortion; pinocamphone, in Hyssop, provokes epileptic fits.

If you see any of these high in the list of active constituents of an oil, you should assume that the oil is very hazardous.

Kidneys

The kidneys are involved in several vital body processes including cleansing and filtering toxic wastes out of the blood and excreting them from the body in urine, controlling the balance of potassium and sodium in the blood, and regulating the amount of fluid in the body. If any of these functions break down the build-up of poisons in the body can become life-threatening. The kidneys also help to regulate blood pressure, by means of the amount of water extracted from the bloodstream, and are helpful in the production of red blood cells. They are twin, bean-shaped organs located towards the back of the body on either side of spine, protected by the lower ribs. They connect with the urinary bladder by means of two tubes called the ureters, which carry the urine produced in the kidneys to the bladder.

Essential oils have a profound effect on the kidneys, because the oils circulate in the bloodstream, and all the blood in the body passes through the kidneys twice in each hour. The dangerous practice of taking essential oils by mouth and even the use of excessive amounts on the skin (through which the oil is quite soon absorbed into the bloodstream) can overload the kidneys and cause damage to them.

Oils which are beneficial to the kidneys reach them in the same way, but obviously we need to be careful about the amounts used, keeping to the proportions, methods and quantities described throughout this book. Camomile, Cedarwood and Juniper have an affinity with the kidneys, and are valuable for their tonic effect on these organs, and for kidney infections such as pyelitis and nephritis. However, I cannot state too strongly that nobody should ever attempt to treat such infections by means of aromatherapy alone. All kidney ailments need prompt medical attention, proper diagnosis and supervision. By all means use the essential oils as first-aid until a doctor can be called, and continue with them parallel to any medical treatment, to strengthen the kidneys and help their recovery.

Diuretic essential oils increase the flow of urine, and can be helpful where there is retention of fluid or when the body needs to get rid of a lot of toxic waste, but they should be used with care, and never for a long period. Over-dependence on diuretics can not only mask serious conditions of the kidney which should be urgently treated, but is dangerous also because artificially increasing the amount of urine produced can disturb the mechanisms which control fluid balance, potassium/sodium balance, etc. The diuretic oils include the three already mentioned, and Cypress, Eucalyptus, Fennel, Frankincense, Geranium and Rosemary.

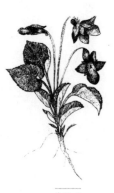

174

see also entries for **CYSTITIS** *and* **URINARY TRACT.**

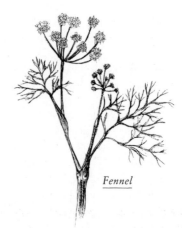

Fennel

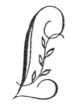

Laryngitis

Laryngitis can indicate any acute inflammation of the larynx, whether this is caused by infection – often following a cold, cough or sore throat – or by mechanical irritation caused by shouting, smoking or inhaling irritant particles. Dry air causes further irritation, and some kinds of central heating and air conditioning will therefore aggravate the condition. Because the vocal cords lie in the larynx, hoarseness or complete loss of voice is one of the complications. Laryngitis following a cold may be aggravated by the fact that air is inhaled through the mouth because the nose is blocked, and so is not warmed, moistened and filtered before it reaches the larynx.

The accepted medical treatment includes steam inhalations, since the vapour eases the breathing and soothes the inflammation. This can be made doubly effective by adding essential oils to the inhalation. The traditional choice is Benzoin, which has been used to treat laryngitis, in the form of Friar's Balsam; but Lavender, Sandalwood or Thyme are also effective.

Laryngitis seldom lasts for more than a few days, so any symptoms of hoarseness which persist for longer than this may be due to other, more serious causes and should be properly investigated.

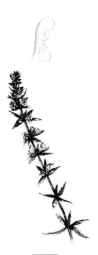

Lavandin
Lavandula hybrida

Lavandin is a hybrid Lavender which grows wild in areas where true Lavender is cultivated or grows wild. There are several varieties, originally created by natural cross-pollination by bees who fertilised Spike Lavender (*Lavandula spica*) flowers with pollen from the true Lavender, but now it is increasingly cultivated. The most widespread varieties in cultivation are Abrial, Grosso, Reydovan and Super. Of these, Abrial has the finest aroma and is more often used as a substitute for Lavender in perfumery, etc. Super contains a high proportion of esters, and is the most antispasmodic while Reydovan is high in linalol and the most bactericidal. If you can be certain which variety you are using, you can make informed choices about its best use in aromatherapy.

The bushes have larger, darker blue flowers than Lavender, and are extremely fragrant. They give a much higher yield of essential oil than true Lavender, and for that reason the oil is cheaper. It is sometimes sold as Lavender and widely used to 'stretch' true Lavender. However, if we are going to use Lavandin it should be as an oil in its own right and not confused with Lavender.

The essential oil is a darkish yellow, with a refreshing, slightly camphorous smell. It contains about 30% of linalyl acetate, linalol, cineol, camphene and other minor constituents.

The properties of the oil reflect its hybrid parentage, having something in common with both true Lavender and Spike Lavender. Most notably, it is far less sedative than Lavender. It is very effective as an inhalation for colds, catarrh, sinusitis and other respiratory problems and a good alternative to Lavender for these uses, especially during daytime when Lavender's sedative property might be a slight problem.

I have found Lavandin good for muscular pain and stiffness, being both analgesic and rubefacient. It is very refreshing in the bath, and excellent for clearing headaches.

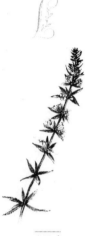

Lavender

Lavandula vera, L. officinalis, L. angustifolia and others.

Of all the essential oils, that of Lavender is undoubtedly the most versatile, with a spread of properties ranging from analgesic, via antidepressant, antiseptic, bactericidal and decongestant, to hypotensive, insect repellent, sedative and vermifuge. The properties can, however, be best summed up as calming, soothing and, above all, balancing. Perhaps the most important property of Lavender oil is its ability to restore unbalanced states – whether of mind or body – to that state of balance in which healing can take place.

The versatility of the plant mirrors its complex chemical structure. The active constituents of the oil include the ethers of linalyl and geranyl, geraniol, linalol, cineol, d-borneol, limonene, l-pinene, caryophyllene, the esters of butyric acid and valerianic acid, and coumarin. The proportion of the various constituents will vary from place to place, according to the soil and conditions in which the plants were grown, and from year to year according to the weather conditions. For example, after a dry and hot summer, the oil will have a higher proportion of esters than after a dull one, and Alpine Lavender is always higher in esters than plants grown at lower altitudes.

Lavender has been used continuously for thousands of years, either in the form of the essential oil, or as the fresh or dried flowers. Where some of the medicinal plants known to ancient civilisations fell out of use, only to be 'rediscovered' in recent years, Lavender has never lost its popularity. It is one of a small handful of essential oils which is still listed in the British Pharmacopoeia.

The name of the plant derives from the Latin 'lavare' – to wash, probably from its use in cleansing wounds, although it was also widely used for personal bathing and washing linen (the word laundry comes from the same source, there being no distinction between 'v' and 'u' in Latin).

Lavender is a native of the Mediterranean. It flourishes all over Europe, since the Romans introduced it to Britain and other Northern European lands, but the best Lavender is still that grown in its original home, around the Mediterranean. The finest quality grows at altitudes between 700 and 1,400 metres.

There are several varieties of Lavender in cultivation which are of use medicinally, and confusion sometimes arises over the names of the various species. The 'common' Lavender, or *Lavandula officinalis,* which is the most important *Lavende* medicinally, can also be called *Lavandula angustifolia,* or *Lavandula vera,* meaning 'true Lavender'. This is the most delicately scented Lavender, and the one we associate with lavender water, and the bags used to perfume clothes and linen, and keep moths at bay. It is also probably the best-loved and most widely used oil in the whole of aromatherapy.

Very few people show any allergic reaction to true Lavender *(Lavandula vera),* and in my experience they are often asthma or hay fever sufferers, or have a family history of allergies (hay fever, asthma, eczema or other skin reactions). Fortunately, these people often seem to have their own 'early warning system' and will express a strong dislike for the smell of Lavender, which is in most instances one of the best-loved perfumes of all. Always heed an expression of dislike for the smell of ANY oil – it will often indicate that it is not to be used for that person.

It was René-Maurice Gattefossé's observation of the dramatic healing effect of Lavender oil when he burnt his hand in a laboratory accident, that led him to research essential oils in greater depth, and eventually to coin the word 'aromathérapie'. Dr. Jean Valnet used Lavender oil to treat serious burns and war injuries when he was a French army surgeon. Lavender is both antiseptic and analgesic, which makes it an ideal choice for treating burns and all kinds of injuries. It also promotes rapid healing, and helps to prevent scarring.

The analgesic, antiseptic and antibiotic properties of Lavender oil also make it a valuable treatment for colds, coughs, catarrh and sinusitis, as well as 'flu, the most effective form of treatment being a steam inhalation (q.v.). Steam alone – as hot as you can bear it without risking scalding your throat – is an effective antiviral agent, and with oil of Lavender added, it can soothe, decongest and attack the bacteria which cause secondary infections, leading to catarrh and sinusitis following colds or 'flu. Lavender is also an effective sedative, so such an inhalation, used last thing at night, will aid sleep, and this in itself helps recovery. A little oil of Lavender (neat) can be massaged into the throat to relieve a tickly cough. The sedative action of Lavender calms the tickle, and the warmth of the body releases some of the volatile oil to be breathed in, and this works on the cause of the cough – the infection in the respiratory tract. A drop or two can be massaged in the same way along the bony ridges of the eyebrows and on either side of the nostrils to help catarrh. In doing this, you will be working on some important acupressure points for catarrh, as well as using the decongestant and antibacterial action of the Lavender.

Massaged into the temples, Lavender will relieve many forms of headache. If this alone does not help, a cold compress of Lavender can be placed on the forehead or back of the neck.

One of the most important uses of Lavender is for the relief of muscular pain, whatever the cause. It is best used in a massage oil, either alone or preferably blended with another oil, such as Marjoram, Rosemary, etc.; for Lavender is not only enhanced in its action by being mixed with other essential oils, but also heightens the action of any oil with which it is mixed. If there is nobody available who can give massage, an aromatic bath with Lavender will also give relief to muscular pain following exercise, or arising from tension, etc. Low back pain can be helped in this way, providing it is first established that the pain is muscular in origin, and does not arise from any spinal irregularity (it is as well to have this checked by an osteopath or chiropractor before undertaking treatment).

The same methods can be used to relieve the pain of rheumatism, sciatica, arthritis, etc., because of the multiple action of Lavender oil in reducing pain locally, lowering

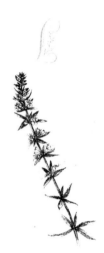

177

the reaction to pain of the central nervous system, reducing inflammation and toning the system generally.

Lavender is also valuable in reducing menstrual pain or scanty menstruation, either massaged gently into the lower abdomen, or made into a hot compress. During labour, Lavender will both reduce pain and strengthen contractions, thus speeding labour, if it is massaged into the lower back (a useful job for the expectant father). It can also be used as a compress or massaged gently into the abdomen to help with the expulsion of the afterbirth.

Lavender can help with many of the minor upsets of infancy, too – colic, irritability and childhood infections – provided it is borne in mind that the essential oil should always be very well diluted. A single drop of Lavender oil in a baby's bath will help a fretful infant to sleep. Dilute the oil first, either in a little almond oil or a few teaspoons of vodka, for, as oil and water do not mix, the essential oil will float in a fine film on top of the water. With young babies, there is a danger that if they get a little undiluted oil on their fingers, they may rub it in their eyes, causing irritation and possible permanent damage to the cornea.

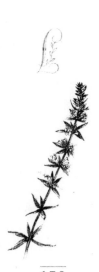

The action of Lavender on the muscle of the heart is both tonic and sedative, making it valuable for the treatment of palpitations, etc., and it also helps to reduce high blood-pressure, though it is obviously necessary to look at the diet, life-style, etc. of the sufferer, too. Massage or aromatic baths (not too hot) are the most suitable mode of use.

The soothing, antiseptic and anti-inflammatory properties of Lavender make it valuable for many skin conditions, and its delicate and well-loved aroma lends itself well to blending in creams, lotions, skin-tonics, etc., in concentration of 1% to 2%. Lavender is one of the most valuable oils for the treatment of acne. It inhibits the bacteria which cause the skin infection, while soothing the skin, helping to balance the over-secretion of sebum, which the bacteria thrive on, and helping to reduce scarring. Lavender is one of the three essential oils which most powerfully stimulate the growth of healthy new cells – Neroli and Ti-tree are the others, although all essential oils share this property to some extent. Lavender will also help many cases of eczema, although Camomile or Melissa may be the first choice oil in some cases. All three of these oils share the qualities of being calming, soothing and antidepressant, so they act on the emotional factors which so often underlie the physical manifestations of eczema.

The insect repellent and insecticidal properties of Lavender have been used for many centuries to protect clothes and household linens from moths and other small pests, and to delicately perfume the linens at the same time. It has long been used to freshen rooms, both in pot pourris, and as bowls of dried flowers. Lavender oil (perhaps mixed with Grapefruit or Eucalyptus) applied to the skin will help you avoid being bitten by mosquitoes, midges and other insects, but if you should get bitten or stung, a little of the neat oil, applied as soon as possible to the skin, will take the pain out of the sting and help to stop the irritation spreading and infection entering at the puncture point. The oil can also be used to help keep animals free from fleas, and to treat infestations of head-lice. It is also used in treating scabies – once found only in rural areas (where the miniscule parasite is harboured by sheep in their wool) but now occurring increasingly in towns. Lavender is fungicidal, too, and valuable in treating such infections as athlete's foot and ringworm (see also **MYRRH** and **TI-TREE**).

On the psychological plane the actions of Lavender can be seen to 'mirror' many of its physical effects. Because of its primarily balancing nature, it is of great value in helping people who are in an unbalanced emotional state – hysteria, manic depression or widely fluctuating moods. Massage of either side of the spine with Lavender can help profoundly in such situations, and here the physical touch of the therapist is also a very important part of the healing process. Lavender baths are also very useful – both between treatments and as a very valuable and effective form of self-help. People who are depressed and/or anxious will benefit from using Lavender in the bath, particularly at night. Insomnia is one of the states for which Lavender is the supreme choice of essential oil, whether the causes are physical discomfort or mental stress, anxiety or an overactive brain at night. While an aromatic bath is probably the very best method of use, a few drops of the oil on a hankie, or on the pillow case can also be very effective. One or two drops on a nightie or pyjamas will often soothe a sleepless child.

Lavender

From the aesthetic point of view, Lavender blends well with many other oils, particularly some of the other flower oils, such as Geranium, and with citrus oils such as Bergamot; also with some of the other members of its own plant family – the Labiatae – such as Marjoram and Rosemary. It blends less well with the more exotic oils, such as Sandalwood, Jasmine, etc.

The very versatility of Lavender oil arouses suspicion in some people, particularly if they are accustomed to the allopathic idea of specific drugs for individual diseases or symptoms, so it is worth mentioning again that its great variety of uses is, to a certain extent, related to the chemically complex structure of the oil and its numerous active constituents. The other, and perhaps more important, point to remember, is that the action of Lavender is primarily balancing and normalising, and this is why it can be used in so many different contexts.

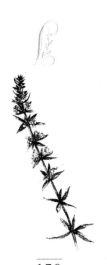

179

Lavender, Stoechas
Lavandula stoechas

Lavender stoechas contains large amounts of ketones which makes it a potentially toxic oil, unlike the other Lavenders. Simply inhaling it for two to three minutes would make you very dizzy. It is a very powerful mucolytic, useful in chronic conditions, but I would leave its use to those aromatherapists who are also medically qualified.

Lemon
Citrus limonum

The Lemon tree is thought to have originated in India, and to have been introduced into Italy towards the end of the 5th century. From Italy, cultivation spread throughout the Mediterranean basin, and particularly to Spain and Portugal, though California now rivals the traditional growing areas in commercial terms.

The essential oil is pressed from the outer rind of the lemons (it takes as many as 3,000 of them to produce a kilo of essential oil). The oil is a pale greeny-yellow in colour, and has the unmistakable smell of fresh lemons. Its active constituents include pinene, limonene, phellandrene, camphene, linalol, acetates of linalol and geranyl, citral and citronellal.

Lemon oil has a number of very important properties, of which one of the most important is its ability to stimulate the white corpuscles that defend the body against infection. This is of great value, both in the treatment of external wounds and in infectious illnesses. Dr. Jean Valnet mentions tuberculosis, typhoid, malaria, syphilis and gonorrhoea, but it is very important to remember that he is speaking from the standpoint of a fully qualified doctor of medicine. The aromatherapist without such qualifications should never be tempted to treat such conditions, except as a back-up to treatment by a doctor or naturopath. In less serious conditions, though, such as bronchitis, 'flu and gastric infections, Lemon also has the property of reducing temperature. For this purpose, slices of lemon in water, or the fresh juice squeezed into water with a little honey, can be given as often as the sick person feels like drinking.

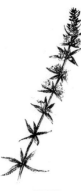

The ability to stimulate the body's own defence, in the action of the white corpuscles, is also a very good reason for using Lemon for all kinds of cuts and wounds; and, in addition, Lemon is also haemostatic, i.e. it helps to stop bleeding. I have used this for minor and not so minor injuries, as well as to arrest bleeding after tooth extraction, and for nosebleeds. If the gum is bleeding after a tooth has been extracted, take some fresh Lemon juice and hold it in the mouth for as long as possible. Don't swill it about, as the movement will prevent the clotting which is needed to stop the bleeding. A mouthwash of Lemon juice is also a good gum tonic, a treatment for gingivitis and for mouth ulcers. For nosebleeds, soak a small pad of cotton wool in Lemon juice and insert it into the nostril.

Lemon is a powerful bactericide, which is yet another excellent reason for using it in treating cuts. Dr. Valnet cites research which has shown that the essential oil will kill diphtheria bacilli in 20 minutes, and even when diluted to 0.2% it will make tuberculosis bacilli completely inactive. The juice of one lemon can be added to each litre if you are ever doubtful about the source of drinking water. Lemon oil mixed into an air spray, or vaporised in a burner or diffuser gives some protection against the spread of infection at the same time as delicately scenting the home.

Another very important property of Lemon is its ability to counteract acidity in the body. This may at first appear surprising, in view of the obviously acid nature of lemons, but the citric acid is neutralised during digestion, giving rise to carbonates and bicarbonates of potassium and calcium, and these help to maintain the alkalinity of the system. This has useful applications in all conditions where the acid/alkaline balance of the body is unbalanced in the direction of excessive acidity, the example that first springs to mind being gastric acidity, leading to pain and ulcers. Lemon is also a good general tonic to the digestive system, including the liver and the pancreas.

Other situations in which too much acidity in the body gives rise to painful symptoms, include rheumatism, gout and arthritis, when the body does not rid itself effectively of uric acid, and this forms crystals which cause pain and inflammation of the joints.

Lemon has a tonic effect on the circulatory system, and is especially appropriate in treating varicose veins. It is helpful in cases of high blood pressure too, and can be used in preventative regimes against arteriosclerosis.

Among the minor uses of Lemon are a number of applications in skincare – it is a mild bleach, and is useful in brightening dull and discoloured skin, especially on the neck, and it might have some effect on freckles, if applied every day over a period of time. It is astringent, and will therefore help greasy skin, and the same antiseptic properties which make it helpful for cuts, etc., are equally valuable in treating spots and boils.

Oil of Lemon can be used as an alternative to chemical treatments to remove corns, warts and verrucae. I have always used oil of Lemon undiluted for this purpose, though some sources suggest 2 drops of Lemon oil in 10 drops of cider vinegar. Whichever you choose, apply it daily to the verruca, corn or wart, taking care to avoid the healthy surrounding skin. Cover the area with a plaster in the daytime, but leave it open at night. Repeat this every day for as long as needed. If wished, mix or alternate with Ti-tree.

There is some suggestion that Lemon has an anti-ageing effect. I am sorry to have to say that I haven't enough evidence to support this, but the tonic, anti-acid and other beneficial effects could certainly help to prolong vigour.

Lemon oil can cause skin irritation unless used in very low dilutions, so I do not exceed 1% in massage oils, making the blend up to 3% with other oils. In the bath, not more than 3 drops should be used, or even 2 drops for people with sensitive skins.

Lemongrass
Cymbopogon citratus

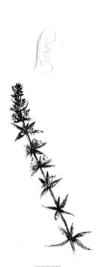

This is one of the more important members of a family of scented grasses native to India, which are also cultivated in other tropical areas, particularly Brazil, Sri Lanka and parts of central Africa. The grass grows to three feet or more in height, and two or more crops may be cut each year. After harvesting the grass is finely chopped to facilitate the extraction of the essential oil by steam distillation.

The main constituent of Lemongrass oil is citral, which accounts for between 70% and 85% of its volume. The remaining 15% to 30% varies in composition depending on the freshness of the leaves at the time of distillation, and also according to which of several varieties of the grass is used, but all varieties include geraniol, farnesol, nerol, citronellol and myrcene, with a number of aldehydes and other traces. The oil ranges from yellow to a reddish-brown and has a very strong lemony perfume.

Lemongrass has a very long history of use in traditional Indian medicine, particularly against infectious illnesses and fevers. It has a tonic and stimulating effect on the whole organism and is a very powerful antiseptic and bactericide. A large number of laboratory trials have given scientific confirmation of its traditional uses.

Lemongrass has been found to have a soothing effect on headaches, but unlike Lavender, should be diluted in a carrier oil before gently massaging the temples and forehead, as the neat oil would be damaging to the skin.

As a bath oil, Lemongrass is refreshing, antiseptic and deodorant but again needs to be used with care because of

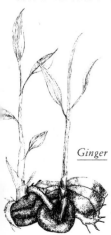

Ginger

possible skin irritation. Do not use more than 3 drops at a time, and dilute before adding to the water. Another possible way of using the oil is in footbaths – very refreshing for tired feet, and helpful for excessive sweating.

Like all the lemon-scented oils, this is a good insect-repellent. It can be used alone or in any number of possible blends with other insect-repellent oils, and has been used extensively to protect animals from fleas and tics. I have used it in a blend with Lavender to sponge my son's dog in summer when fleas become a real problem: the blend also kept doggy odours to a minimum. I often use Lemongrass in a burner in summertime, too, to keep the flies and other insects away from my kitchen, and sometimes add a drop or two to the water for washing the tiled floor.

The essential oil is sometimes used to adulterate more expensive oils, and occasionally turns up labelled as 'Verbena' which is similarly lemon-scented. Here is another example of why it is so important to insist on knowing the botanical name for all oils you buy.

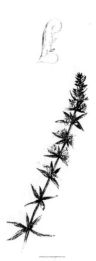

Leucorrhoea

A white or colourless discharge from the vagina, which may be no more than a slight increase of normal secretions, or may be the symptom of infection or irritation. Thrush (candida albicans) is often responsible.

No vaginal discharge should ever be neglected, and the cause must be investigated to rule out any more serious illness. However, douches incorporating Bergamot, Lavender, Myrrh or Ti-tree are a good local treatment which can be used while fuller investigation is carried out, and often concurrently with any other treatment that may be necessary. Use 0.5% to 1% of the essential oil in boiled water cooled to blood heat. Douching should not be carried out excessively or over a long period, as it can disturb the normal vaginal secretions. An alternative treatment is to use Ti-tree pessaries, which can be bought in some health food stores, or make pessaries from essential oil and cocoa butter, using 2 drops of essential oil to each 5 grams of cocoa butter.

see also **THRUSH.**

182

Lice

Head lice have always been a major problem in schools, and other places where people congregate together, and this has now been complicated by the fact that lice have become resistant to most of the chemicals commonly used to control them.

Fortunately, a number of essential oils are effective in removing and preventing head lice: Bergamot, Eucalyptus, Geranium and Lavender being the most effective. A 'cocktail' of three or four of these oils seems to act better than any one of them alone.

Mix the blend of oils in a fairly high proportion (5% to 10%), in a carrier oil, such as sunflower or safflower oil, and massage very thoroughly into the hair and scalp. Cover the head and leave on for several hours – overnight if possible, before washing out with a mild shampoo. Comb through the hair with a fine-toothed comb sold by chemists to remove lice and eggs loosened by the shampooing. This procedure will need to be repeated at 48 hour intervals to deal with the eggs as they hatch out. The eggs or 'nits' are stuck to individual hairs with a kind of cement by the female louse and are difficult to detach, but the treatment with oils and shampoo, followed by careful combing will help to dislodge them. Three or four treatments at 48 hour intervals will usually get rid of an infestation.

To prevent re-infestation, it is important to remember that lice and eggs can lurk in coat collars and hoods, hats, scarves and bedding. Wash anything that can be washed, and thoroughly sponge mattresses, pillows, coat collars, etc., with an alcoholic blend containing 10% of any one, or more, of the above oils. I usually include Camphor in the mixture for such use, but not in that to be used directly on the head. Even surgical spirit will do for the sponging mixture, though I have on occasions used commercial lavender water with essential oils added. This is probably the best choice, since it is not possible to buy pure alcohol without a licence, surgical spirit is evil-smelling, and vodka is expensive.

Contrary to general supposition, lice actually prefer clean hair and heads, so there is no stigma involved in becoming a host to them. Very few children get through their schooldays without picking up some lice at least once, and they will often infest the whole family before the first child becomes uncomfortably aware of the parasites. Adding some essential oil to the final rinse after shampooing might help to prevent a fresh infestation. Any of the oils listed above would do, but obviously the sweeter-smelling ones, such as Bergamot or Lavender, will be more welcome.

Ling, Per Henrick

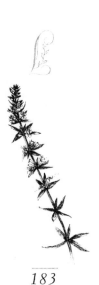

Per Henrick Ling is widely known in the world of alternative therapies as the originator of Swedish massage, but this is a somewhat limiting view of a man with wide-ranging interests in the human body, and indeed the soul.

As a young man Ling (who was born in 1776) seemed to be destined for a literary career, and wrote romantic poetry and novels. But while travelling abroad, he became interested in gymnastics, and when he returned to Sweden after a few years, in 1804, he obtained a post as fencing master at the University of Lund in southern Sweden. He was fascinated by the human body in movement, and began to make a detailed study of the limb movements of his fencing students. From this, he developed a system of exercises to be used in schools and the Swedish armed forces. Older readers may remember 'Swedish Drill' from their schooldays, and this method is still in use in some places. He also became very involved with the 'Lar dig Folkdans' folk dance revival movement, his interest here being as much in the human body in movement as in the scholarly preservation of old dances.

In 1813 he received Royal permission to open in Stockholm the 'Central Institute for Gymnastics' (still in existence) for the education of future professionals in 'Sjukgymnastik'; that is, naturopathy and what Ling termed 'movement cure'. This was the name he gave to his system of massage designed to create movement within the body – the different systems, muscles and joints.

This form of massage is still known in Sweden as 'Lingism' and is still taught in the Institute that he founded. It was only when it began to be known in other countries that the term 'Swedish Massage' was used to designate Ling's original method. Unfortunately, in the process, the sensitive and serious approach which Ling advocated was discarded, and much of what is now known as Swedish Massage is far from what was envisaged by this poet-masseur.

The movement towards more sensitive forms of massage which originated in California during the 1960s, and which gave rise to Esalen and Intuitive massage, did much to restore to massage an element which, after Ling's death in 1839, had been in danger of being lost.

Litsea Cubeba or May Chang

Litsea cubeba (syn *Litsea citrata*)

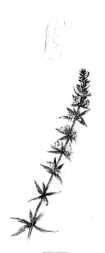

Litsea cubeba is a small tree related to the Laurel and Cinnamon. It is native to China and other parts of E. Asia, and has lemon-scented leaves and flowers and small berries resembling peppers.

Most of the essential oil comes from China and is extracted from the fruits by steam distillation and is very rich in citral (up to 85% of the total) with some linalol. It is a light yellow, with a very strong, pleasant 'citrus'-type aroma – somewhere between orange and lemon.

The main uses of Litsea cubeba are in skin care, and it is used in many commercial preparations. It is non-irritant, very antiseptic and very effective in treating oily skin, acne, and spots in general. I have found it a good alternative to Bergamot, especially for facial application as there is no risk of photosensitivity. It reduces excessive perspiration and is a very good deodorant. It makes a very refreshing bath oil.

It is one of my favourite oils for spraying or vaporising in the house. Being antiseptic and deodorising it is very suitable for the bathroom but it is another oil that is good to use during epidemics. I use it a lot in winter when there is 'flu about, and when the weather makes it impossible to have windows open for long, though I confess I use it as much because I love the smell as for any other reason. Nothing has been written about the mental/emotional effect of this oil, but my own observation is that it is a very good antidepressant, always welcome during the grey days of winter.

The Liver

The liver is the largest organ in the body (apart from the skin) and one of the most complex in its actions. It lies on the right side of the body, protected by the lower ribs, and on average weighs about 3lbs (1.5 kilos) though there can be a lot of variation. The liver has at least four functions which are vital to life: manufacturing, metabolising, storage and detoxification. In addition, because of the continued chemical activity involved in these processes, the liver provides most of the body's heat.

Substances manufactured in the liver include bile, which is needed for the digestion of fats; heparin which helps to prevent the blood from clotting, and most of the proteins found in the blood plasma. Vitamin A can be synthesised in the liver from carotene if needed.

A large part of the liver's activity is concerned with metabolism: i.e. the breaking down of elements from food and converting these into forms in which they can be utilised by the body. Glucose, from sugars and starches, is converted into glycogen which is the fuel used for all muscular activity. Fats cannot be used by the body in the form in which we eat them. In the liver they are oxidised and broken down into simpler forms which can either be used or stored in the liver until needed. Amino acids, which are the 'building blocks' of protein foods, are vital for health, but the body can use or store only limited amounts at any given time, so if too much protein is eaten the liver breaks down the excess by a process called de-amination. Both amino acid residues and fatty acids can also be converted into glycogen and stored. The storage of glycogen and other nutrients in the liver means that they can be released into the bloodstream in regulated amounts as the body needs them. Fat soluble vitamins A and D are also stored in the liver, and so is iron.

The fourth very important function of the liver is detoxification. In this organ substances that could damage other body tissues, such as alcohol, drugs and poisons are broken down into forms in which they can be excreted via the faeces or urine. As well as toxic substances taken into the body, the liver also breaks down and prepares for excretion substances produced naturally in the body which could cause self-poisoning if they were not removed once their purpose had been served. These include dead red blood cells and hormones. The haemoglobin from red blood cells is converted into pigments that colour the bile, and eventually leave the body in the faeces. When this process goes wrong, the pigments cannot be excreted as fast as they are formed, and they accumulate in the blood and other cells and give the skin a yellow colour – the condition we call jaundice.

A number of essential oils, referred to as hepatic, have a tonic and beneficial action on the liver and strengthen its various actions. By far the most important of these is Rosemary, which stimulates the production and flow of bile, helps in cases of jaundice and is a general liver tonic. Other helpful oils are Camomile and Peppermint, which benefit the liver and the digestive system as a whole, Cypress, Lemon and Thyme which are useful when the liver is congested, and Juniper as an aid to detoxification.

General body massage or baths with these oils will enable them to enter the bloodstream and reach the liver quite quickly, but relief from discomfort in the liver area is best achieved by means of warm (not too hot) compresses over the liver. In cases of jaundice and congestion, alternating hot and cold compresses, finishing with a cold one, will stimulate the liver and improve its function.

Essential oils which are described as toxic (see **APPENDIX A**) are nearly all capable of damaging the liver to the extent where very serious illness or even death would follow.

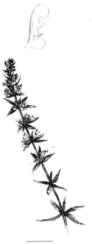

Camomile

Loss of Appetite

Several essential oils are of value in stimulating appetite, where this has been lost, particularly in convalescence, and sometimes in depressive states. The best known and probably most effective of these is Bergamot, though many of the oils derived from culinary herbs and spices have a similar action. Among these the most often used are Caraway, Lemon and Coriander.

The use of small amounts of these oils in baths and massage is the best method, for these will help to stimulate the entire organism. Ginger and Fennel are also mentioned by some authorities, although others say that Fennel decreases appetite. It is probable that the action of Fennel is neither stimulant nor depressive of appetite, but that it has a regulating effect. Both Fennel and Ginger can be used effectively and pleasantly as teas or infusions, and Earl Grey Tea is flavoured with Bergamot.

If the loss of appetite is the result of emotional stress of any kind, it is important to treat this rather than symptomatically try to stimulate the appetite. Massage with a wide range of essential oils is probably the best choice of treatment, because of the human contact involved, and the comforting effect of touch.

see also **ANOREXIA NERVOSA.**

Lotions

Lotions are prepared by blending an oily and a watery ingredient, with an emulsifier such as lecithin or various waxes to keep the oil particles in suspension in the water. A typical combination might be almond oil, rosewater and wax, but the resulting lotion will be of a lighter and more fluid consistency than a cream made from the same ingredients, and the proportion of rosewater much greater. Essential oils are added both for their perfuming ability and as a treatment for a variety of skin problems. I find lotions better tolerated than creams when treating eczema, and in skincare they are best for dry and sensitive skins.

Lotions are much more difficult to make without professional equipment than creams, and few aromatherapists attempt to make their own, though they are better suited to the treatment of certain skin problems than the more easily made creams. Some essential oil suppliers offer an unperfumed base to which you can add your own essential oils or you can find some good lotions made from pure plant ingredients, and lightly perfumed or unperfumed, which can be bought commercially, usually in healthfood stores.

Low Blood Pressure

see under **HYPOTENSION.**

Lungs

The lungs and the skin are both vital to the practice of aromatherapy, as these are the two routes by which essential oils enter the body.

Essential oils evaporate on contact with the air, so when breathed in they are carried with the inhaled air through the nose and into the lungs. The two primary bronchi, which first bring the air into the lungs, divide into smaller passages, which in turn divide and subdivide into tubes of ever decreasing size, the smallest being called bronchioli. This is sometimes called the 'bronchial tree' and that indeed is a very graphic description. If you imagine an upside-down tree, with the trachea forming the trunk, the primary bronchi the two main branches, and a network of branches, smaller branches and twigs, you will have a fairly clear picture of how air is distributed within the lungs.

The smallest of these air passages, the bronchioli, lead into even smaller ones, called alveolar ducts, and each of these ends in a group of structures resembling miniscule balloons. If seen in magnification, they look like bunches of grapes. These are the alveoli, and this is where the vital process by which oxygen is supplied to the blood and waste matters removed takes place. The process is sometimes called the 'exchange of gases'.

The walls of the alveoli are made of the thinnest tissue in the body, and through this fine membrane fluids can pass. The surface of the membrane is always moist, so that oxygen and other soluble particles dissolve before passing through it. Around each cluster of alveoli is a network of miniscule blood-vessels (capillaries) which are also moist, and which also have very, very thin walls. Through these permeate the oxygen and other dissolved substances, and the carbon dioxide and other wastes on the return journey.

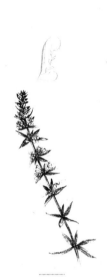

The importance of this process in understanding aromatherapy, is that particles of essential oils that have been breathed in can pass through these thin-walled structures, and that is how they enter the bloodstream for circulation to other parts of the body.

Disorders of the lungs, including **ASTHMA**, **BRONCHITIS**, **COUGHS** and **PNEUMONIA** are discussed under their individual headings.

187

Lymph/Lymphatic System

Lymph is a colourless fluid similar in composition to intercellular fluid (tissue fluid). As part of the continual process of circulation, some of the tissue fluid is absorbed into the bloodstream via the capillaries, and the remainder, containing the greater part of the proteins found in tissue fluid, is absorbed into the smallest lymphatic vessels. These form part of a system which parallels the blood circulation, but with the important difference that it has no central pump (i.e., the heart) to help it circulate. Instead, the movement of lymph depends on pressure from the normal activity of the surrounding muscles. A sedentary lifestyle may, therefore, lead to inefficient circulation of lymph.

Lymph is involved in the absorption of fats from the intestines, in the drainage and removal of toxic wastes from all parts of the body, and in the body's response to infection. (This is discussed elsewhere, under the heading of **IMMUNE SYSTEM**.)

Rosemary

The other main function of the lymphatic system is the drainage of fluids and poor circulation of lymph may lead to localised or general retention of fluid. This can be seen in people whose work involves long periods of standing, and who may have swollen ankles at the end of the working day. Cellulite, involving the retention of toxic waste and fluids, particularly in the region of the thighs, hips and buttocks, is also related to sluggish lymph function.

Specialised forms of massage are very effective in reducing swelling and encouraging a more efficient drainage of lymph, especially when combined with such essential oils as Geranium, Juniper and Rosemary. When treatment is continued over a long period, Black Pepper can be used in place of Rosemary and some therapists include Birch or Patchouli. The massage is directed from the extremities towards the area of the clavicle (collarbone) where the lymph drains into the subclavian veins. There are several different systems of lymph massage, but most aromatherapists are trained in one or other of them. Because this form of massage increases the amount of lymph entering the bloodstream, the amount of water extracted from the blood as it passes through the kidneys is also raised. As a result, increased urination is usually experienced after lymph drainage massage, and this is heightened by that fact that several of the oils used with this massage are also diuretic.

The benefits of such massage can be increased by bathing with a selection of the same oils, and by gentle exercise and skin brushing. This is done with a dry brush, and follows the same direction as the massage strokes (from the extremities towards the collarbone). A cleansing diet may also be necessary.

In rare cases, fluid retention will not respond to lymphatic drainage massage, or reoccurs very quickly after treatment, and medical help must be obtained urgently, as this could indicate serious illness.

Pre-menstrual fluid retention can be greatly reduced by lymphatic massage carried out one or two days before swelling is usually experienced.

Apart from such easily visible disorders as oedema and cellulite, a less than efficient lymph system can contribute to many conditions where poor elimination of toxins is involved. Catarrh is a typical example, also some skin disorders, headaches, migraine etc.

People who have very poor resistance to infection, can also benefit from regular lymphatic massage, and it may be of help during convalescence. This is related to the role played by lymphoid tissue in fighting infection and is more fully described elsewhere in this book.

A very important contra-indication for lymphatic massage is cancer. The lymphatic system is a route by which malignant cells can move from one part of the body to another (metastasis) and give rise to secondary cancers, and treatments involving this system are generally advised against.

see also entries for **CELLULITIS, PRE-MENSTRUAL TENSION** *and especially for* **IMMUNE SYSTEM,** *which discusses the other functions of the* **LYMPHATIC SYSTEM.**

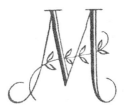

Maceration

A method of preparing herbs by prolonged soaking in water. The term is sometimes used to describe the process whereby flowers or herbs are infused in a bland oil.

see **INFUSED OILS.**

Mandarin

Citrus nobilis or *C. madurensis* or *C. reticulata*

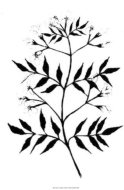

The Mandarin probably originated in China, and has certainly been known in that country since antiquity. It takes its name from the fact that, in the past, the fruit was traditionally offered as gifts to the mandarins. The names Mandarin and Tangerine are both used to describe the same oil, with a tendency to use the name Mandarin in Europe and Tangerine in America.

The essential oil has a very delicate aroma, true to the scent of the fruit, and is golden-yellow in colour, with a slight blue-violet fluorescent tint visible in bright light. The major constituents are limonene, methyl anthranilate and smaller amounts of geraniol, citral and citronellal.

A major application of Mandarin is in treating digestive problems, as it has a tonic and stimulant effect on both the stomach and liver. Its effect on the intestines is calming (in common with both Neroli and Orange) and it has been found to be even more effective when used in a synergistic combination with other citrus oils.

Because of its gentle action, Mandarin is often regarded in France as 'the children's remedy' and is often chosen to help with the tummy upsets of childhood, including 'burps' and hiccoughs. A 2% dilution in almond oil can be gently massaged into the tummy, always in a clockwise direction. I would extend this to say that it could be a wise choice of oil for anybody who is a little fragile, particularly the elderly.

Mandarin is one of the oils which is safe to use during pregnancy, as it will not harm either the mother or the developing child. It is an excellent component of massage oils for the prevention of stretch-marks: 1 drop each of Lavender, Mandarin and Neroli to 10 mls of almond oil and 2 mls of wheatgerm oil is a good blend. It must be used daily, preferably twice daily, from about the fifth month of pregnancy to be really effective.

Manuka
Leptospermum scoparium

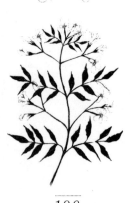

This oil from New Zealand is a fairly recent addition to the European aromatherapist's repertoire of oils but promises to be a very valuable one. It has a long history of use by the Maori people, particularly for bronchitis, rheumatism and similar conditions. You may see it described as 'New Zealand Ti-tree' which is very misleading in one sense, as it is only very distantly related botanically to Ti-tree. (Ti-tree is, of course, one of the Melaleuca family, and the Melaleucas are a sub-group of the larger Myrtaceae family that includes Clove, Myrtle and the Leptospermums.) On the other hand, it does give you a fairly good idea of the properties and uses of this oil, though Manuka also has properties that Ti-tree does not.

The shrubs grow in the bush and are harvested from the wild. The best Manuka oil comes from plants growing at high altitudes, and has been found to be more antibacterial than that from lower altitudes. The essential oil is extracted by steam distillation from the leaves and is virtually colourless. The main constituents are caryophyllene, geraniol, pinene, linalol and humulene and there is also an unusual constituent, Leptospermone which is very insecticidal. The smell is quite elusive – very sweet and gentle.

As you may expect from the comparison with Ti-tree, Manuka oil is antiviral, anti-fungal and highly bactericidal across a wide spectrum. It can be used for all respiratory tract infections: colds, catarrh, sinusitis, bronchitis, etc. and the fact that it is also decongestant is a bonus. I have tried it in the bath for colds, as a gargle for sore throats and dabbed neat on to incipient cold-sores, against all of which it proved highly effective. Because of the pleasant aroma, it is a very agreeable oil to use in vaporisers during an epidemic.

It is an excellent antiseptic for use on the skin, and can be applied to cuts, spots, boils, ulcers, etc., being particularly indicated where healing has been slow. Manuka can be used neat on the skin when needed, but it does have a drying effect, particularly if used repeatedly. This can be useful in treating acne and oily conditions of the skin but for general use it should be used well diluted to avoid the drying effect. Between 1.5% and 2% is a suitable dilution for massage, and it is a good idea to use a rich carrier oil, such as avocado or jojoba for people with dry or sensitive skin.

Manuka has an antihistamine action and is anti-allergic generally. It is good for insect bites and stings, and would be worth trying for allergic rashes: possibly for asthma and hayfever. (I say 'possibly' here because I have not yet had an opportunity to try it for such conditions.) It is good local analgesic, helpful for muscular pain and rheumatism – as illustrated by the Maori's use.

It is an effective insecticide and the pleasant scent makes it particularly suitable for use in air sprays or burners. One friend is currently using Manuka, diluted in water with a dispersant, to keep her cat free from fleas. Here again, the gentle aroma makes it very acceptable, as many cats, with their acute sense of smell, will not tolerate the stronger-smelling oils.

The delicate scent means that you can blend Manuka with virtually any other oil that would be therapeutically appropriate. It can be used in situations where the stronger and more medicinal smelling oils might not be welcome.

Manuka oil gives us a good alternative to Ti-tree as an anti-infectious oil, which is welcome especially when long-term treatment is needed, though it may not have the same immunostimulant properties. It does, as you can see, have other valuable properties which merit a place in our essential oil repertoire.

Marigold
Calendula officinalis

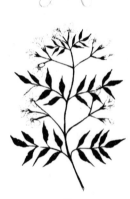

The true Marigold is occasionally used to produce small amounts of absolute, but this is very rarely available commercially and most oil of Calendula is produced by infusing the petals and sometimes leaves, in a bland oil. This infused oil is very valuable in aromatherapy for its powerful skin-healing properties. Although appearing green in the bottle, it gives a beautiful golden tint to any cream to which it is added, and this is its main mode of use. I often put Calendula oil into creams for badly cracked skin, especially for people whose hands are damaged by rough work, cold, exposure to water, etc. It is also very useful in creams for the minor skin problems of children, nappy rashes and grazes. Nursing mothers have used this cream to heal cracked nipples which would not respond to other treatments: it is totally non-toxic to the baby, which is a very important consideration, though the mother may need to wash her nipples before breastfeeding if the baby dislikes the taste. If preferred, the infused oil can be used on its own instead of in a cream.

Regular daily application of Calendula oil, or a cream made with it, can help to reduce old scars and it will also help varicose veins and chronic ulcers.

The old herbalists ascribe a host of useful properties to the Marigold flower, ranging from strengthening the eyesight to drawing evil humours out of the head. Virtually all the early writers state that Marigold 'comforts the heart' and it would seem that this is meant both physically and metaphorically, for such phrases as 'comforteth the heart and spirits' recur as often as 'strengthens and succours the heart in fevers'. Fresh or dried Marigold petals were added to broths, both for the flavour and their beneficial properties, and are a delightful addition to salads. From such uses the flower acquired the name of Pot Marigold.

Calendula

It is important to distinguish between the true Marigold (Calendula) and the African Marigold (Tagetes). Although the oils are unrelated to each other in terms of properties or botanical families, some suppliers and therapists confuse them, and indeed I have even seen an oil listed as Calendula/Taget! If you want to use Calendula, be quite certain that this is, in fact, what you are buying. Tagetes is a very hazardous oil, due to its high level of ketones.

191

Marjoram
Origanum majorana

ॐ

The Latin name for Marjoram, *Origanum majorana,* is derived from 'major', meaning greater; not because the plant has a smaller relative, but because it was thought, in ancient times, to confer longevity, hence a greater lifespan. The plants thrive on sunny hillsides, and are indigenous to the Mediterranean, Yugoslavia and parts of Hungary and Iran, though like most of the great labiatae family it grows in gardens almost everywhere. It was certainly well known in English country gardens, and even as an escapee along the edges of fields, by the early 17th century, for Culpeper says that 'It is so well known, being an inhabitant in every garden, that it is needless to write a description thereof.'

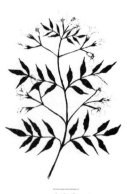

The essential oil, which is produced by steam distillation from the flowering tops, is yellowish, darkening towards brown as it ages, and its active constituents include borneol, camphor, origanol, pinene and sabinene. The aroma is warm, penetrating and slightly peppery, and indeed the outstanding property of Marjoram is its warming action, both on the mind and the body.

Culpeper says, 'It helpeth all diseases of the chest which hinder the freeness of breathing' and it is one of the best oils to use in treating asthma, bronchitis and colds. Used as a steam inhalation it will clear the chest and ease respiratory difficulties very quickly. A hot bath containing 6 drops of Marjoram will often prevent some of the secondary miseries arising from the common cold. It can be massaged into the throat and chest to soothe tickly coughs, for it is warming, analgesic and sedative.

The sedative properties of Marjoram must not be abused, for it can dull the senses and cause drowsiness, and in large amounts is stupefying. Obviously no responsible aromatherapist will use Marjoram (or, indeed, any other oil) in the amounts that could entail such risks.

As you might expect from this, Marjoram is a very good remedy for insomnia, especially when used, together with Lavender, in a warm bath before bedtime. Its warm, nutty perfume is rather more masculine than many of the oils that can help with sleeplessness, and this makes it more acceptable to men who are unable to sleep, than some of the sweeter perfumes.

It is used in treating high blood pressure and heart conditions, as it dilates the arteries, thereby reducing strain on the heart. The same action on the tiny capillaries just beneath the skin produces a feeling of local warmth when Marjoram is used in a massage oil, and this is one of the reasons why it is so valuable in massaging tired, tight and painful muscles, especially after heavy physical exertion. The increase in the local circulation

Marjoram

helps to carry away the toxic wastes left in the muscle after heavy exercise, and this in turn reduces the pain and stiffness. It is in massage blends that I make the most use of Marjoram, not only for muscular stiffness, but to reduce the pain of rheumatism and arthritis. Here again, the warming effect is very valuable and it will often permit a joint that is normally too stiff and painful to be moved to regain some mobility.

Marjoram, as we might expect from its ages-old use in cooking, has several helpful actions on the digestion. It reduces colicky intestinal cramps and strengthens peristalsis (the wavelike movements of the gut that propel the partly digested food along). The antispasmodic effect is also very much welcomed for its action on the uterine muscle, and a hot compress of Marjoram over the abdomen will ease menstrual cramps more effectively than anything else I know.

Marjoram is used for its warming effect on the mental and emotional level, too, and can be very comforting for people who are lonely or suffering grief. It should not be abused, though, as over use can have a deadening effect on the emotions. While this may be welcome for a short time, prolonged use of this or any other essential oil is never a good idea.

By its action in lessening both emotional response and physical sensation, Marjoram has the effect of being anti-aphrodisiac, and has been used in the past, particularly in religious institutions, for this reason. It may sometimes be useful to know about this effect when seeking to help a person who has chosen to be celibate or who finds him/herself in a situation of enforced celibacy, such as bereavement or after the breakdown of a relationship.

There is one Marjoram chemotype: *Origanum majorana,* Vivace, when grown in the north of France, becomes an annual plant instead of a perennial, as in its Mediterranean habitat. This annual Marjoram has quite a different chemistry, with a preponderance of thujanol, and is comparable with the thujanol-rich chemotype of Thyme.

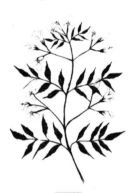

Massage

❧

Massage with essential oils is by far the most important application of aromatherapy, allying as it does the therapeutic power of touch with the properties of the individual essential oils chosen for a particular person at a specific time.

Massage itself – with or without essential oils – can be described as a formalisation of a very primitive instinct. If a child falls over, his mother will 'rub better' his bumped knee: if you or I trip and bruise ourselves, our unthinking first reaction will be to rub the painful area: if we find a friend in a state of distress, we offer a reassuring hug. All these are forms of healing, whether on a physical or an emotional level. The simple action of rubbing a painful part of the body encourages an increased flow of blood in the tiny capillaries just below the skin, and this in itself helps to ease the pain. A hug is a non-verbal way of communicating to our friend the sympathy and love that we may not be able to put into words in a crisis.

Both of these kinds of healing enter into massage. The masseur learns a variety of movements, or strokes, which are designed to relieve pain, ease tense and tight muscles, increase circulation, or benefit the physical body in other ways. These strokes are applied to the superficial muscles – that is, those muscles which are visible below the skin – but the effects also benefit the deeper layers of muscle and possibly the underlying organs.

Some forms of massage aim only to benefit the physical body in this way, but even so, a general feeling of mental wellbeing will usually result, and the most important effect is the degree of relaxation experienced after a massage. Often renewed energy and vigour will follow this deep relaxation. The benefit of massage is cumulative: although the client will almost always feel good following a massage and for some hours afterwards, regular massage will prolong the feeling of wellbeing for ever increasing periods after each treatment.

As well as releasing tight muscles during the treatment, massage can act as a form of re-education, helping us to become aware of the fact that we are tensing certain muscles unnecessarily, and to feel the difference between a tight, or contracted, muscle and a relaxed one. Very often we do not recognise the fact that we are tightening certain groups of muscles until we experience those muscles in a relaxed state during and after a massage. Although it is a perfectly normal reaction to tense muscles when we feel mentally tense, it is important to be able to let go of this physical tension before the tight muscles themselves convey a sense of discomfort and unease to the mind, thus setting up a vicious circle of tension. This is one of the ways in which mental stress can lead to real physical symptoms, but massage can break this chain of events, especially when we work with essential oils that have a calming, soothing or uplifting effect on the mind as well as the body.

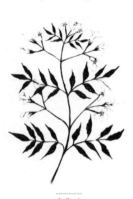

Some systems of massage, such as Esalen massage, and the various kinds of intuitive massage that have been developed in the past thirty years or so, take this link between mind and body further, and aim to work mainly on the connection between the mental and physical states of the person receiving the massage. The letting-go of physical tensions can often lead to a release of emotion. This may relate to the present situation of the person involved, or to something that has been 'stored' in the body for a very long time. Clearly, a relationship of great trust and sympathy between the masseur and the client must be built up before such a catharsis can take place, and this may need to be built up over a number of treatments. One of the ideas inherent in Esalen massage is that by very gently working on the physical surface tensions, deeper tensions will be enabled to come to the surface and eventually be released.

Different aromatherapists have quite different ways of giving massage, depending partly on their training and background, and partly on their personal outlook and preference. The variety of techniques used is enormous, and it would be pointless to try to describe all of them here, particularly as I believe that it does not matter too much which method is used, provided the therapist has been thoroughly trained in his or her chosen system, and uses it with care and a nurturing attitude towards the person who needs help. I have certainly received treatments from masseurs trained in widely diverging systems (both with and without essential oils) and benefited just as much from one approach as another. Far more important than this or that method is to ensure that the massage physically encompasses the whole body, and that the therapist takes into consideration the whole person – body, mind and spirit.

From the purely physical point of view, massage is vital to aromatherapy because it provides us with the most effective way of introducing essential oils to the body. The skin absorbs these oils very readily, and when the whole body is massaged a useful amount of essential oil can be taken into the bloodstream in a fairly short time. (The oils are always added to a carrier oil, usually in a dilution of 3%.) If it is not possible, for any reason, to carry out a full massage, then a back massage offers the next best possibility of getting sufficient essential oil into the body to have a therapeutic effect, since the back presents the single largest expanse of skin of any body area. In an emergency it is possible to massage the back repeatedly at intervals of as little as half an hour, to get the maximum possible amount of essential oil circulating in the body. (I should emphasise that this is a technique to be used only by very experienced therapists, and preferably only those who also have medical qualifications. I mention it here only as an illustration of the ability of the back to absorb essential oils during massage.)

M.E.

M.E. (short for myalgic encephalitis) is also known as chronic fatigue syndrome, post viral fatigue syndrome, chronic fatigue and immune deficiency syndrome (C.F.I.D.S.), Epstein-Barr syndrome or, insultingly, as Yuppie 'flu. The very diversity of names indicates the bafflement of doctors and lay people alike when trying to understand this debilitating and often long-drawn-out condition. The fact that it may take different forms in different people adds to the confusion and there is disagreement as to whether a viral or other infection is responsible.

Some recent research has found candida albicans proliferation in a very high percentage of people with M.E. but whether that is a cause or a result of the wider syndrome it is impossible to tell. Some doctors have simply refused to acknowledge that such a condition existed, and implied that the patient was either neurotic or malingering, though fortunately such an attitude has become rarer as more and more cases have come to their attention.

I think the truth is probably that there is no one single cause of M.E. Stress, environmental pollution, infection, may all be involved and I have seen people who first experienced this syndrome after an accident or emotional shock.

As aromatherapists, we do not need to involve ourselves in such academic arguments, and can do most to help by considering every M.E. sufferer individually, in the light of their physical symptoms, emotional needs, lifestyle and so forth – in other words, in the way a holistic therapist always works.

The one thing that is common to everyone with M.E. is an almost unbearable weariness. Some have acute muscular pain all or some of the time, others become so weak that they are confined to wheelchairs. Loss of co-ordination, giddiness, headaches and digestive problems are also possible and – not surprisingly – most victims are very depressed.

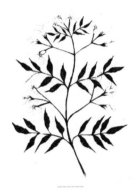

195

This means that we may need to consider a very wide range of oils to help with different problems and at different times, though I think the core of any treatment must be aimed at strengthening the immune system. Ti-tree and other immunostimulant oils need to be used in alternation, as treatment is inevitably long-term. Analgesic oils are needed for the ongoing pain. Tonic oils such as Rosemary and Thyme have been very valuable in every case of M.E. I have encountered, and Bergamot, Orange, Petitgrain and other citrus oils seem to be enjoyed more than some of the other anti-depressant oils though, as I have already said, we need to be very sensitive to individual tastes and needs.

People who are very weak and exhausted may not be able to tolerate full-body massage, but massage is such an important part of their therapy that as much as is enjoyed should be given as often as possible. Remember that M.E. sufferers often have periods of remission followed by relapse (especially if they try to do too much when they are feeling a bit better) and somebody who enjoyed a full massage last week may only be able to tolerate having their hands and feet massaged at the next appointment.

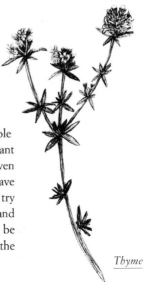

Thyme

Some advice on nutrition is often needed, as high levels of vitamin and mineral supplementation often help, especially in increasing energy levels. I mentioned above that the majority of people with M.E. have been found to have a problem with candida albicans. This seems to me to be a 'chicken and egg' situation: has the weak immune system which it seems is part of M.E. allowed the candida to proliferate, or has the candida caused the symptoms of exhaustion, pain etc., as it certainly can? Either way, using dietary measures to reduce the candida problem often seems to help, and if you are using Ti-tree and similar oils as part of the overall treatment, this will also help. A good strategy is to give some pre-diluted Ti-tree to the client to be rubbed into the abdomen every morning. This is something even the weakest person can do, and it is psychologically helpful to be able to do something towards one's own recovery.

These are only general guidelines, and many other oils and methods of treatment will suggest themselves as appropriate according to the needs of each individual.

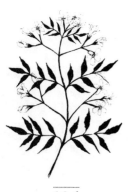

Meadowsweet
Spirea ulmaria (or Fillipendula ulmaria)

☙

Meadowsweet is one of the plants that contain salicylic acid – Nature's own 'aspirin' and in fact the name aspirin was originally derived from spirea. It comes as no surprise, then, to know that the infused oil of Meadowsweet is analgesic, anti-inflammatory and mildly sedative. It can be used on its own or with a little essential oil added (1% to 2%) in massage for joint pains, tendinitis, rheumatism and arthritis.

Measles

☙

Measles is caused by a virus which is not in itself particularly dangerous, but during an attack the child is weakened and much more vulnerable than usual to bacterial infections. These side infections, especially of the chest and ears, are the main danger associated with measles, and careful use of essential oils can reduce this danger.

The best and simplest method is to keep up a continuous vaporisation in the sick child's room of Ti-tree or Eucalyptus, using a burner or other type of diffuser. Failing any specialised equipment, the essential oil can be put in a humidifier attached to a radiator, or even on wet cloths hung over a radiator or it can be mixed in a spray which will need to be repeated at frequent intervals. These methods will not only help to protect the sick child from secondary infections, but may be useful in reducing the risk of measles spreading to other members of the family. Dr. Jean Valnet recommends surrounding the patient with a veil which is repeatedly sprayed with Eucalyptus oil. Vaporisations of this kind can be safely used for even the youngest children.

If the sick child is old enough to be safely treated directly with essential oils (from about 4 years upwards) gently sponging with tepid water and a febrifuge oil, such as German Camomile or Bergamot

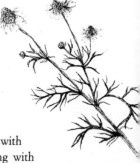

Camomile

will help to reduce fever. Put 2 drops of Bergamot and 2 of German Camomile into a pint of lukewarm water and gently sponge the child's body every few hours.

Steam inhalations can be used to ease the sore throat that accompanies measles, again, if the child is old enough to safely manage this. If not, vaporising oils in the child's room would be an alternative.

Major outbreaks of measles occur every two or three years. Spraying or vaporising Ti-tree and Eucalyptus oils in the home can give children a degree of protection, and older children can take baths with 2-3 drops of either of these oils. It may not be possible to avoid infection, but such measures will often ensure that the attack is a mild and uncomplicated one.

It goes without saying that a doctor should always be called: it would be totally irresponsible to attempt to treat acute childhood illness with essential oils alone. Do, however, continue the measures described above with whatever treatment is suggested by your doctor.

Meditation

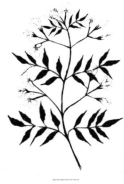

In various places in this book you will find references to meditation as an aid to relaxation and a generally more harmonious lifestyle. Many people who consult aromatherapists do so because they are stressed, anxious, depressed or suffering from physical symptoms which result from these mental states; and although aromatherapy massage, aromatic baths, etc., can be very effective in reducing the level of stress, it is important in the long run that the patient should take some active steps towards helping him or herself.

Some aromatherapists teach clients a simple form of meditation, while others may suggest a class or centre where one or other type of meditation can be learnt. People sometimes have fears and misconceptions about meditation, such as that they may 'lose control' or 'float away'; or that it is very difficult and great efforts of concentration must be made to master the technique. Another objection may be that meditation is some kind of odd religious practice, but although meditation does form a central part of some of the great world religions, it is perfectly possible to practice it outside any religious context. If I pick up any such hesitation or fear on the part of a client who I feel would benefit from meditating regularly, I may not even mention the word, but simply say, 'I am going to teach you a little breathing exercise to help you relax.'

Awareness of the breath is one of the most basic and widely practised forms of meditation, the two other major forms being repetition (aloud or silently) of a word or phrase, or visualisation of an object or (in the religious context) a deity. Different people will find these different approaches more or less appropriate to their own needs, and may need to try several before hitting on the form with which they feel at ease.

Many therapists, both in aromatherapy and other disciplines, use meditation as a preparation for giving treatment, and sometimes, if the patient/client is a person who will feel at ease with such a suggestion, include a short period of meditating together at the beginning or end of a treatment.

Melissa
Melissa officinalis

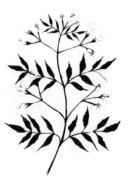

Melissa officinalis is the botanical name of the Lemon Balm found in so many cottage gardens. It was introduced to this country at a very early date, possibly by the Romans. The name derives from the Latin name for honey, and it is a plant much loved by bees. The word 'officinalis' in its name is a clear indication that its medicinal properties have been known for hundreds of years.

All parts of the plant yield essential oil, which has a very pronounced scent of lemon. It has at least three active principles in common with oil of Lemon (citral, citronellal and linalol) and should be treated with respect, as far as use on the skin is concerned, as it is capable of causing irritation. Use very diluted, both in massage oils – not above 1% – and in baths, where 3 or 4 drops to an average bath is the safe limit. Dilute the oil before adding to the water. I have seen weals (similar to burning) caused by only 5 drops of Melissa in a bath. In spite of these warnings, Melissa in very low concentration is a very valuable oil indeed in treating eczema and other skin problems.

Melissa is frequently adulterated: Lemon grass, Lemon or Lemon Verbena being mixed with, or substituted for the genuine oil. True Melissa is rare and costly. I am often asked why this is so, given that the plant is as prolific as a weed. The answer is that the plant has an unusually high proportion of water in its make-up with only a very small amount of the oily essence. So, like other costly oils, it takes a huge amount of plant material to produce a very, very small amount of essential oil.

The overriding property of Melissa is that it is soothing, both to the body and the mind. It is one of the two oils most often used to treat allergies, whether these manifest as skin problems or respiratory difficulty. The other one, of course, is Camomile, but where a particular individual has not responded to Camomile, Melissa has sometimes produced almost dramatic improvement. I never use Melissa in concentrations of more than 1% for fear of aggravating the very conditions I am seeking to help, and in many cases there will be a slight worsening of symptoms before healing begins. This 'healing crisis' is of course common to many systems of natural healing.

Asthma and coughs are often relieved by inhalations of Melissa, although asthmatics should avoid steam inhalations.

It has a calming and regulating effect on the menstrual cycle, and helps to regularise the pattern of ovulation where this is erratic. It may in this way be helpful to couples who wish to use natural methods of birth control, and also to those who have difficulty in conceiving because the time of ovulation is uncertain.

Melissa will also help to lower high blood pressure, and has a calming effect on over-rapid breathing and heartbeat, which makes it a good remedy for shock.

The mental and emotional actions of Melissa mirror those of its effects on the physical body, as is so often found with essential oils. It is soothing and calming, but also uplifting in a similar manner to Bergamot. Gerarde says that 'It maketh the heart merry and joyful and strengtheneth the vitall spirits.' A Swiss manuscript by an unknown author says that Melissa 'chasse les idees noirs', (chases away black thoughts) and with this in mind,

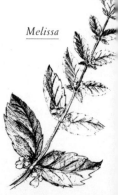

Melissa

I have used Melissa to help bereaved and shocked people who have lost somebody close in an accident or through sudden, unexpected illness. Of course, it is necessary to grieve, but the subtle energy of Melissa, together with Dr. Bach's Rescue Remedy, can help people through the first terrible hours of shock and distress.

Minor uses of Melissa include room perfuming and as an insect repellent but given the cost of true Melissa it is probably better to use Lemon, Citronella, etc., as all the lemon-scented oils have this property.

Memory

All the essential oils described as cephalic are thought to aid the memory, especially Rosemary which has enjoyed this reputation for many hundreds of years, hence 'Rosemary for remembrance'.

The area of the brain which registers smell is very closely connected to the area which is involved with memory, and both are situated in the oldest part of our brain: the part which was already well developed in our most primitive ancestors. This would seem to suggest an explanation of why perfumes and smells of all kinds can so powerfully and mysteriously trigger complete recall of past events and emotions.

see also the entry for the **MIND.**

Menopause

Strictly speaking, the term menopause refers to the point in a woman's life when ovulation – and therefore menstruation – has completely ceased. However, most people use the term to describe the time leading up to that point, which may last for several months or a year or two from the time when the normal pattern of menstruation first changes.

Many women stop menstruating at some point during their 40s or 50s with little or no discomfort or disturbance of their lives, while others experience depression, irregular menstruation, excessively heavy periods amounting almost to haemorrhage, hot flushes, insomnia and other symptoms for long periods of time, sometimes several years. The progress of menopause does not seem to relate in any predictable way to previous menstrual history, childbearing, marriage or celibacy. It has been suggested that women with a career, or other sources of personal satisfaction are less likely to suffer depression and physical symptoms, while those who have devoted themselves to childrearing and housework are more likely to be affected as the physical changes often coincide with the time when children are leaving home. However I have seen many cases which make nonsense of this theory.

Every woman's experience is different, and the aromatherapist needs to take this into account when considering treatment. Many of the essential oils which help with menstrual irregularities earlier in life can be used to minimise the physical problems. In particular, Geranium which is a hormonal balancer and Rose, which tones and cleanses the uterus and helps to regulate the menstrual cycle. Camomile is another oil which is often found helpful, being gently calming, soothing and antidepressant. All the antidepressant oils, such as Bergamot, Clary Sage, Jasmine, Lavender, Neroli, Sandalwood and Ylang-Ylang can be helpful.

In the earlier stages of menopause, the regime described in the following section (**MENSTRUATION**) can be used to stabilise an irregular cycle and reduce heavy bleeding. Cypress is particularly indicated for heavy bleeding, but this should always be discussed with a doctor or gynaecologist, as it may be a symptom of fibroids or other problems that require treatment. Fibroids are not caused by the changes of menopause, but often cause trouble at this time, simply because they grow so slowly that a fibroid which has been forming for 20 years will only reach a size where it gives rise to pain or bleeding when a woman is in her 40s.

It is difficult to discuss menopause without raising the question of hormone replacement therapy (H.R.T.). The drop in oestrogen levels that occurs when a woman stops ovulating underlies most of the problems

Clary Sage

that can be experienced during menopause and after, from hot flushes to osteoporosis and heart disease. However, many women are reluctant to take replacement hormones, because they cannot tolerate the short-term side effects, worry about the long-term side effects or have ethical objections to products produced from the urine of pregnant mares. Fortunately, aromatherapy and herbal medicine offer a number of natural alternatives. Oestrogenic oils, such as Clary Sage, Fennel, Star Anise and Tarragon, hormone-balancing oils such as Geranium or herbal remedies like Agnus Castus, False Unicorn Root, Ladies' Mantle, etc., all help to maintain hormone levels in the body. Supplements of Evening Primrose oil (or equivalent) are important, because they provide gamma linoleic acid which the body needs to make oestrogen.

A reasonable amount of exercise and excellent nutrition are good preventive measures against heart disease and osteoporosis so older women should make sure that their diet includes the whole spectrum of vitamins as well as minerals and trace elements which become even more important at this stage in life. Calcium supplementation is advisable to protect against osteoporosis.

Many menopausal and post-menopausal women feel that their femininity is fading, and Rose, again, can help them to feel feminine, nurtured and desirable. This isn't just a 'feel-good factor' – Rose genuinely helps many menopausal problems, as well as being antidepressant, aphrodisiac, an excellent oil for older skins, etc., all of which boosts morale.

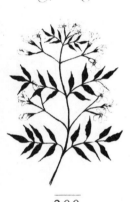

Menstruation

Although the idea of menstruation as a malady is now outmoded, a sizeable number of women experience some difficulty, either long-term or temporarily and aromatherapy is ideally suited to alleviating their problems.

Probably the most commonly experienced problem is period pain, or menstrual cramps, caused by spasm or contraction of the uterine muscles. Very gentle massage over the abdomen with an antispasmodic oil will almost always disperse the pain. Some women find a hot compress over the abdomen even more comforting, renewed as often as necessary. The most effective of the antispasmodic oils are Marjoram, Lavender and Camomile – in that order according to my observations. Some women may get more relief from massage or compresses over the lower back, and for others both lower back and abdomen will need to be included to get maximum relief.

Several antispasmodic oils are also emmenagogues, i.e., they will bring on a period or increase scanty menstruation. Women whose menstrual flow is normal or heavy need to avoid these when choosing an oil for period pain, as their use may cause the period to become very heavy. The oils most likely to have such an effect are Clary Sage, Myrrh and Sage in my experience, though Basil, Juniper, Fennel and Rosemary might also do so. It is safer to restrict the use of these oils to the first half of the menstrual cycle.

Obviously, all the oils classified as emmenagogues can help women whose periods are scanty or delayed, but these oils must be avoided if there is any chance at all that the women may be pregnant, and none of them should be used once pregnancy is established until after at least the fifth month when risk of miscarriage is diminished.

Some women suffer from periods that are always abnormally heavy. For them, either Cypress, Geranium or Rose can have a regulating effect. Rose, indeed, can be beneficial for all kinds of menstrual problems, since it does not intrinsically reduce or increase the flow or frequency, but has a regulating effect on the cycle, and is a uterine tonic.

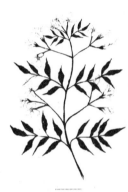

If the cycle is very erratic and unpredictable, an alternative would be to use oils with oestrogen-like properties in the first half of the cycle only. When the cycle is regular, the body produces more oestrogen in the first half of the cycle and more progesterone in the second half, and we need to work with this to re-establish a normal rhythm. The use of oestrogenic oils should be limited to 10 days (from day 4 to day 14) as longer use could shorten the cycle to as little as 20 days. There are no essential oils with progesterone-like properties, so in the second half of the cycle it's best to use tonic, cleansing oils combined with a herbal remedy that provides a progesterone equivalent.

A good regime would be to massage Clary Sage into the tummy each day from day 4 to day 14 of the cycle, and then switch to a blend of Juniper, Pine and Bergamot from day 15 to day 28. During the second two weeks a herb such as Agnus Castus should be taken in the form of tablets or tincture. This treatment would be very appropriate for women who have stopped taking the contraceptive Pill and are trying to conceive, and in fact any woman hoping to conceive as it makes it possible to predict the time of ovulation more accurately. The same treatment is equally helpful for painful and/or heavy periods.

If the cycle is extremely irregular or there are no periods at all (and it has been established that the client is not pregnant, and there is no serious disease of the ovaries, etc.) it is possible to time the treatment by counting the day of the New Moon as day 1 of the cycle and then continuing as above. If no bleeding takes place after day 28, wait 4 days and start again. If no improvement has been noted after three cycles of this treatment, it would be advisable to consult a gynaecologist.

In fact, any abnormality of the menstrual cycle which is prolonged or severe, such as extremely heavy or painful periods, absence of menstruation or bleeding between periods, must be checked by a gynaecologist to make quite sure that there is no serious medical condition that needs treatment. If such a condition is found, there is

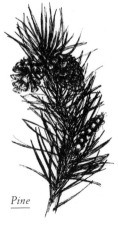

Pine

no need to discontinue aromatherapy treatment, which will almost always be a valuable adjunct to any treatment advised by the gynaecologist, but obviously this must be discussed with the doctor concerned.

see also **HORMONES, MENOPAUSE, OESTROGENS** *and* **PRE-MENSTRUAL TENSION.**

Mental Fatigue

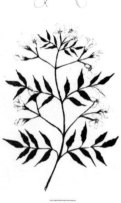

Any of the essential oils classified as stimulant or cephalic can help to reduce mental fatigue, though it would be very unwise to over-use any of them. You might sensibly use one of them to tide you over a crisis, or some short period of time when you really need to think clearly in spite of being tired, but in the long run, it is better to take adequate rest and breaks from mentally-demanding work.

Basil, Peppermint and Rosemary are the oils most often used for this purpose, and of these I have always found Rosemary the most helpful, though I know people who swear by Basil. A bath with 6 drops of Rosemary is wonderful if you have woken exhausted in the morning and know that you face another tough day. Peppermint is best used in the form of peppermint tea, which is far safer than using strong tea or coffee to help you through a long stint of work.

One of my favourite ways of keeping myself alert and clear-headed is to put 8 drops of Rosemary oil in an essential oil burner on my desk. In circumstances where this is not possible, such as when driving on a long journey, you could put a single drop of Rosemary on each wrist, so that as you move your hands the vapour will be released for you to inhale. I sometimes do this when writing.

see **STIMULANTS.**

Migraine

Aromatherapy is better used as a preventative measure than as an attempted treatment for migraine. Once a migraine attack has begun, many sufferers are unable to tolerate the smell of essential oils or anybody touching their heads.

If the person can bear to be touched, and is not troubled by smells, it is sometimes possible to avert a full-blown migraine by using the following measures at the first onset of an attack:

Cold compresses made with equal proportions of Lavender and Peppermint oils should be placed across the forehead and temples and changed frequently as soon as they begin to warm up. Extremely light massage of the temples with Lavender oil might be helpful if touching the head does not make the pain worse. Many migraines seem to be due to restricted blood supply to the brain, and hot or at least warm compresses with oil of Marjoram on the back of the neck will increase the flow of blood to the head. Marjoram is a vasodilator (it causes the blood vessels to expand slightly), and the warmth itself also helps.

As migraine is often associated with stress, regular massage with emphasis on any muscular tension in the shoulders and neck, is the best preventative measure. Self-massage, including light tapping on the scalp (obviously at times when there is no pain) is advisable.

Most people with migraine will have had any links with trigger-foods investigated, but if they have not, this should be an urgent priority. Cheese, chocolate and red wine are among the most common triggers but all sorts of foods may be involved. It is also worth looking at other, non-food factors which may trigger an attack, such as bad lighting, industrial and household chemicals etc.

Milk

Milk is a good medium in which to dilute essential oils before adding them to the bath, but it needs to be full-cream milk, as it is the fatty portion of the milk with which the essential oil can combine. Pour off the cream from the top of a bottle of milk and add 5 or 6 drops of your chosen oil to blend to this, stir and add to the bath just before getting into the water. This is a very suitable dilutant for people with sensitive skins and for young children.

You can also use the top of milk, or single cream, with a few drops of essential oil added, as a nourishing lotion for dry skin. To each tablespoon of milk-top or single cream, add between 8 and 10 drops of essential oil. Use at once or keep in the fridge for a day or two.

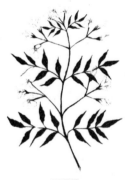

Mimosa
Acacia dealbata

203

I have to admit straight away to being in love with Mimosa! I cannot resist buying a bunch when it first appears in the florist's shop – usually late in winter. The fluffy yellow flowers bring a smile and remind me that spring is not far away. The oil has just the same effect, though it is extracted from a different variety of Mimosa, the Australian 'wattle', which now grows both wild and cultivated in southern Europe since being introduced here in the 19th century.

The 'oil' is, in fact, not an oil but an absolute, which is obtained from the flowers and flowering twigs by solvent extraction. It contains mainly palmic aldehyde, enanthic acid and anisic acid. It is a thick, dark yellow liquid, with a very sweet, floral scent with a woody undernote. It is a very complex aroma and smells more like a blend than a single oil, though it does, in fact, blend very well with a number of other oils.

Mimosa is used in top-class perfumery for its perfume and as a fixative. It is completely safe in use, being non-toxic and non-irritant. Its main physical properties are astringent and antiseptic, which makes it a possible choice for treating oily skin, and skin care in general. However, Mimosa is relatively expensive and there are plenty of other oils that will serve the same purposes.

I include Mimosa here because it is such a wonderful antidepressant and de-stressing oil (and because I like it so much!). It is deeply calming, excellent for helping with anxiety – you might like to use it sometimes blended with Neroli, or as an alternative where Neroli has not been as effective as you could wish.

Mimosa is perhaps best suited to very sensitive people. It is fascinating to note that one variety from S. America *(Mimosa humilis)* known as the 'sensitive plant', folds up its leaves at the lightest touch. Perhaps we can see something of the Mediaeval Doctrine of Signatures at work here?

The Mind

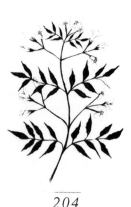

Have you ever wondered why smell is so strongly linked to memory? Why does a certain perfume always conjure up memories of a favourite aunt, or the smell of a particular flower transport you vividly back to the garden of your childhood home? Or, indeed, why and how essential oils can affect the mind and emotions?

This aspect of smell and our reaction to it is even less well understood than the physical process of olfaction, but the known facts are enough to make some sense of these phenomena.

Smell is registered in one of the oldest areas of the brain. That is to say, a part of the brain which was already developed in our very earliest ancestors. Before early humans had developed speech, or the making of tools, with the increase in brain size that went hand in hand with these steps forward, the Limbic Area of the brain was well developed. This part of our brain is concerned with many activities vital to survival: sleep, sexual response, hunger, thirst, memory and also smell. For, to the earliest humans, smell was essential for both individual survival and the survival of the clan, and the race. Scent led hunter/gatherers to their dinner, whether it was a wild animal or an edible plant. Smell gave the first warnings of predators, or rival clans, waiting to attack, and smell was involved in finding a mate. Although 'civilised' modern people depend far more on the areas of the brain which developed later, to co-ordinate speech, intellectual, creative and mechanical activities, the ancient knowledge is still there.

However, it seems that in modern humans, the association of ideas and memories with smells is partly associated with conscious learning. For example, although a reaction of disgust and even nausea to the smell of rotten food may be innate, and exists to protect us from harming ourselves from eating such food, the association of a perfume with a person or place is learnt, and to a certain extent is controlled by conscious processes. However, this is not entirely so, for the scent-memory, once learnt, is very hard to alter by conscious reasoning. For example, if you were afraid of a school teacher who wore a distinctive perfume, you will be likely to feel anxious whenever you encounter that smell, even though you are perfectly well aware that the present situation poses no threat to you. You may feel irrationally prejudiced towards any person who wears that perfume, however well you know intellectually that he or she is a good, likeable person. Conversely, smells associated with happy times of our life, or people we liked very much, make us feel relaxed and happy by association.

Rose

It is no accident that so many of the essential oils regarded as antidepressant are the product of summer flowers: Rose and Jasmine, Lavender and Geranium, for example. At a deep unconscious level they evoke warm sunny days, gardens, perhaps holidays, and for most people these are happy associations. One of the reasons why aromatherapists should always ascertain that the client likes the oil, or blend of oils, to be used in treatment is that the client will almost always select the oils that have the happiest associations, even if he or she has no idea that this is why he or she likes that smell best and this facilitates relaxation.

The association of aromas and situations can be put to good use in aromatherapy. Massage almost always brings about muscular relaxation, even without the use of essential oils. If a pleasing oil or a blend of oils is used for the massage, the smell will be associated with feelings of relaxation. Each time that oil is smelt in future, whether in the bath, in room perfumes or in another massage, it will invoke feelings of relaxation, and of course this is very helpful for people who are tense, stressed or anxious.

Experiments have been conducted quite recently by psychologists using synthesised 'sea'-smells which combined salt, seaweed and so forth. When volunteers were played recordings of seaside sounds, while the sea-smells compound was blown towards them by a fan, various physiological measurements showed how much they were relaxed. The more often each volunteer repeated the experiment, the faster and more deeply they relaxed. This isn't exactly aromatherapy, and elements other than smell are involved, but it does illustrate how pleasant associations induce relaxation, and how repetition strengthens that effect.

Another aspect of essential oils and their effect on the mind is the balance between the right and left hemispheres of the brain. We know that the right side of the brain is associated with intuitive thought and behaviour, while the left side of the brain relates more to logical and intellectual processes. When both hemispheres are in harmony with each other, we experience feelings of calm and wellbeing. Some experiments done with volunteers whose brain-activity was monitored with E.E.G. equipment, showed that when they inhaled essential oils, the activity of the two sides of the brain came into closer symmetry with each other. This effect appeared almost immediately after the volunteers had smelt the essential oils. The same group of tests also showed that such oils as Basil and Rosemary, which we associate with mental clarity, produced brain-rhythm patterns showing alertness, while the calming antidepressants, such as Jasmine, Rose and Neroli induced rhythms which showed the mind approaching a state of meditation.

A great deal of importance is attached in aromatherapy to the relationship of mind and body, particularly in psychosomatic or stress-related illness. How can the effect that essential oils undoubtedly have on the mind, help to heal the body? Again, we do not know all the answers but we do know that the hypothalamus is involved. The hypothalamus is a structure at the base of the brain which is often described as the place where mind and body meet. It regulates both the endocrine and nervous systems, and through them can influence every organ of the body and a very wide range of body processes. The hypothalamus is connected by nerve pathways to the various parts of the brain, and the connection between it and the Limbic Area of the brain is particularly strong. Once again, we can trace the importance of this link back to early humans: it would have been of little use for the nose to give warning of approaching danger if the rest of the body was not put on the alert and ready for action. A typical sequence of events might be: nose smells wolves; Limbic Area of

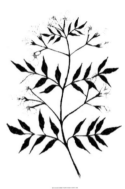

205

brain registers danger; impulses signalling danger pass to the hypothalamus; hypothalamus transmits these signals to the Pituitary Gland that governs the whole endocrine system; adrenal glands at once begin to pump out adrenalin; adrenalin enters the bloodstream; the adrenalin causes the heart to beat faster and harder, and the rate of breathing to increase so that extra blood and oxygen can be pumped to the muscles, making them better able to either fight or run away. At the same time, blood is diverted from the skin and digestive organs to the heart and muscles (digesting your last meal is less important than ensuring that you don't become the wolf's next one!). All this takes place in less time than it has taken you to read it.

The adrenalin-surge reaction takes place in all kinds of stressful situations, even though now physically running away, or fighting, is no longer the response that is needed to the threat. The source of anxiety may be somebody hundreds of miles away, but you will still feel your head pounding and the blood draining from your face as you take a crucial phone call. The body doesn't burn off the extra adrenalin with the kind of physical activity it is designed to fuel, so you may feel disturbed and even a bit ill for some hours. When this kind of situation is repeated often, the adrenal glands approach exhaustion, the body may start to display physical symptoms and we refer to such states as stress-related illness.

Sending pleasing, relaxing messages to the brain reverses this process. The hypothalamus receives impulses that signal safety, so it maintains body systems in a balanced state in which all organs and processes can function efficiently. The psychologists with their 'canned seaside' have demonstrated this in laboratory conditions. Aromatherapists, masseurs, meditators, yoga practitioners and many others have known it for thousands of years.

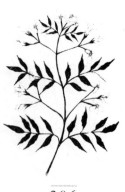

Monoterpenes

❧

Monoterpenes are the most commonly occurring of the organic molecules that make up essential oils, limonene and pinene being the most frequently occurring of all. They are antiseptic, analgesic and rubefacient (i.e. warming to the skin) but if used over a period of time they can cause skin and mucous membrane irritation. They are found in a very wide range of essential oils, for example: camphene, in Juniper, Petitgrain, Pine, etc.; dipentene, in Bergamot, Coriander, Fennel, Lemon, etc.; limonene, in Bergamot, Caraway, Carrot, Fennel, Lemon, Neroli, Orange, etc.; pinene, in Coriander, Cypress, Eucalyptus, Fennel, Pine, Rosemary, etc.: sylvestrene, in Cypress, Pine and many other tree oils.

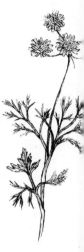

Coriander

Moods

❧

Essential oils can be used to affect mood, particularly those which are antidepressant and cheering such as Bergamot, Grapefruit, Orange and the other citrus oils; though calming, stimulating, balancing or other actions might be appropriate at various times.

Virtually any of the uses of essential oils, in massage, baths, perfumes and so forth will have this effect, but a very simple and effective way to influence the mood of anybody using a particular room is to choose one of the ways of diffusing essential oils into the air – an airspray, aerosol generator, burner or fragrancer.

see entries under the individual oils for their effects on mental *and* emotional states.

Mouth Ulcers

Mouth ulcers may result from a variety of causes varying from friction from a denture or rough tooth, poor circulation, bacterial or fungal infection (candida) or possibly an undetected food allergy. With the exception of those caused accidentally, for example through inadvertently biting the tongue or inside of the cheek, they almost always occur in people who are 'run down' physically, or under mental or emotional stress. Lack of sleep, poor diet, Vitamin C deficiency and antibiotics are some of the most common causative factors.

Several essential oils are useful in treating mouth ulcers, and ensuring the health of the mouth and gums generally. Myrrh has been used for thousands of years for its healing properties, especially where the skin is damp. It is also fungicidal, which makes it the only practicable aromatherapy treatment where the ulcers are due to candida. The most convenient form in which to use Myrrh is as a tincture, which you can buy from herbalists' shops. This can either be dabbed directly onto the ulcer with a cotton-bud or scrupulously clean fingertip, or made into a mouthwash by further diluting it in half a tumbler of warm water. Direct application will sting for a few moments, but is the most effective way to heal a mouth ulcer. A mouthwash is a good preventative measure. Fennel, Mandarin and Peppermint can also help, and you might mix a drop or two of any of these in brandy or vodka to dab on ulcers or dilute with water for a mouthwash.

High doses of Vitamin C (preferably in combination with bioflavonoids) will help to heal mouth ulcers. At least 3 grams a day should be taken until the ulcers are healed, and some people need and can tolerate as high as 9 grams. If the ulcers are a recurrent problem, it is important to ensure that the diet is rich in Vitamin C and B-complex. Occasionally a food allergy or intolerance may be responsible, so if ulcers persist in spite of all efforts to treat them with essential oils, vitamins and a good diet, it may be necessary to rotate the diet or have some food tests carried out to identify the guilty food or foods.

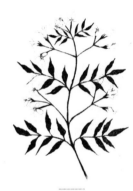

207

Mugwort
Artemisia vulgaris

The essential oil of Mugwort, sometimes sold under its French name of Armoise, contains a very high proportion of thujone, which makes is both toxic and abortifacient. It should not be used at all in aromatherapy.

Another variety of Artemisia, *A. arborescens* is sometimes described as Blue Camomile, and has many of the properties associated with Camomiles, due to the presence of azulene, but it is also an abortifacient and must be avoided in pregnancy.

Muscles

When we speak of muscles, we are usually referring to the Skeletal or Voluntary muscles, i.e., those near the surface of the body, identifiable beneath the skin, by means of which we move about. The less obvious but even more vital groups of Cardiac Muscle and Visceral, or Involuntary smooth muscle are concerned with the unceasing function of heart and internal organs.

Essential oils used in massage and baths have an almost immediate effect on the Voluntary muscles, which is heightened by the relaxing effects of the massage movements, and of hot water. Analgesic oils such as Camomile, Lavender, Marjoram and Rosemary will ease pain in muscles, especially where this is due to over exertion. Clary Sage and Jasmine have a relaxing effect on the muscles, while several oils, most notably Black Pepper, Juniper and Rosemary will increase muscle tone and help to prepare the muscles for action. These various actions can be used to good effect in increasing the muscular efficiency of athletes, dancers, etc., when used before and after training and performance.

These short lists of oils are by no means exhaustive and virtually any and every essential oil used in combination with massage will be beneficial to the Voluntary muscles.

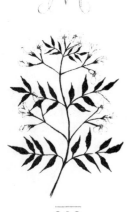

Quite a large number of essential oils, described as antispasmodic, have a relaxing effect on the smooth muscle of the internal organs and can be used to relieve such problems as indigestion, colic, diarrhoea, menstrual cramps, etc., which involve spasm of the smooth muscle. These oils include Bergamot, Black Pepper, Camomile, Clary Sage, Cypress, Fennel, Juniper, Lavender, Marjoram, Melissa, Neroli, Peppermint, Rosemary and Sandalwood. You will see that there is quite a lot of overlap between these and the oils which affect the Voluntary muscles. The best way to use these oils to relieve smooth muscle spasm is in a hot compress over the affected area.

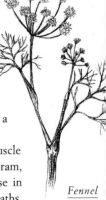

Fennel

A handful of oils are reputed to have a tonic effect on the muscle of the heart (Cardiac Muscle). These include Lavender, Marjoram, Neroli, Peppermint, Rose and Rosemary. It is best to use these in conjunction with massage whenever possible, or otherwise in baths. Here again you will see that there is some overlap, and that some oils benefit all three types of muscle.

Myrrh

Commiphora myrrha, C. molmol, etc.

Myrrh is a resin produced by a small, tough, spiny tree which grows in semi-desert in regions of Libya, Iran, along the Red Sea and various areas in Northeast Africa. Commiphora myrrha is the main source, though several other varieties of Commiphora are sometimes used. The trees belong to the same botanical genus as Frankincense: the Burseraceae, and it is perhaps no accident that these two are commonly spoken of in one breath. They do have a number of features in common, though Myrrh has certain properties not attributable to Frankincense, and vice versa. The name Myrrh comes from the Arabic 'murr', meaning 'bitter'.

The liquid resin is exuded from natural cracks or cuts in the trunk and sets into irregularly shaped brownish-red lumps. Legend has it that shepherds whose goats browsed and rubbed against the tree trunks, collected the resin that stuck to the goats' beards! Modern harvesting owes less to chance, and is carried out both by making systematic cuts in wild trees, and to a small extent from cultivated trees.

An essential oil is extracted from the resin by steam distillation, though most of the Myrrh available for aromatherapy is a resinoid, extracted from the raw resin with solvents. The essential oil ranges from pale to dark amber in colour and the active principles include limonene, dipentene, pinene, eugenol, cinnamaldehyde, cadinene, acetic acid, myrrholic acid and a number of resins. The resinoid is the same deep reddish-brown as the raw resin and is very thick and sticky and may need to be warmed before it is possible to pour it from the bottle. It is sometimes dissolved in alcohol to make this easier. Both the resinoid and the essential oil have a hot, smoky, bitter aromatic smell, reminiscent perhaps, of the climate in which the tough little tree survives.

In common with Frankincense, Myrrh was used in all the ancient civilisations as a perfume, incense and in medicine. It was highly valued as a healing ointment for wounds and it is said that no soldier of ancient Greece went into battle without a paste of Myrrh in his pouch. This use is well justified by what we know of Myrrh's properties: antiseptic, healing, and anti-inflammatory. It is specially valuable for wounds that are slow to heal, and for 'weepy' skin conditions, including weepy eczema and athlete's foot. For the latter, the fact that Myrrh is fungicidal is a double benefit. It heals cracked and chapped skin, and I often put just a little Myrrh in creams for deep cracks on the heels, and heavy-duty handcreams.

Because of the antifungal action of Myrrh, it can be used in a vaginal douche against thrush. It will eliminate the itch and discharge effectively, but thought should also be given to the underlying candida infection which leads to these symptoms, and Ti-tree oil, with perhaps a special dietary regime, used.

Myrrh is good for the gums, and quickly heals mouth ulcers and gum disorders. The most convenient form in which to use it in the mouth is as Tincture of Myrrh: it does sting momentarily and tastes extremely bitter, but the healing effect is so marked that it is worth suffering these inconveniences. It is used in many brands of toothpaste for its beneficial effects on the gums, with oil of Peppermint added to mask the bitterness.

The area in which Myrrh overlaps most with its 'cousin' Frankincense is in treating chest infections, catarrh, chronic bronchitis, colds and sore throats. It is a very good pulmonary antiseptic, expectorant and astringent (i.e. it has a drying action on excess mucus). It can be used as a massage oil or in inhalations. It is less useful as a bath oil, since it is very difficult indeed to dissolve, even in alcohol.

It is said to have tonic and stimulating actions on the stomach and the whole digestive tract, and is a remedy for diarrhoea. Gently massage the stomach and abdomen (always in a clockwise direction).

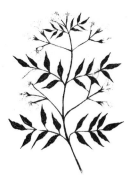

209

CAUTION
**Myrrh must not be
used during pregnancy.**

Myrtle

Myrtis communis

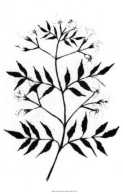

This large bush or small tree is a native of North Africa, but grows freely all around the Mediterranean and as a cultivated garden plant throughout most of Europe. In France it is sometimes called 'poivrier corse' (Corsican pepper).

It has been known for its antiseptic properties at least since the time of the ancient Greeks, and Dioscorides prescribed it for lung and bladder infections in the form of an extract made by macerating the leaves in wine.

The essential oil is distilled from the young leaves, and is pale yellow in colour. It has a pleasant, clear, fresh smell, resembling Eucalyptus (which belongs to the same plant genus, the Myrtaceae) but more delicate and less penetrating. The main constituent is cineol, with myrtenol, pinene, geraniol, linalol and camphene.

Its most important properties are antiseptic and bactericidal, particularly in pulmonary and urinary infections, as illustrated by Dioscorides. It is especially valuable in chronic conditions of the lungs, and where there is a lot of bronchial catarrh.

Because of its relative mildness, this is a very suitable oil to use for children's coughs and chest complaints. It is very well tolerated when used in normal 3% dilution as a chest rub, and because of the unobtrusive smell, children will accept it where they may dislike Eucalyptus. Used in small amounts, it is slightly sedative, unlike the stimulant Eucalyptus, so it is a good choice for use on the chest, in inhalations or burners at night.

I have also found it a good oil for elderly people both as a treatment and a preventative measure against chest infections.

Myrtle oil is astringent, and has been used to reduce haemorrhoids. Because of this astringent quality, the leaves and flowers used to be used in skincare, and were a major ingredient of 'Angel's Water', a popular 16th century skin lotion. With this in mind, we might consider adding Myrtle to the range of oils used to combat acne.

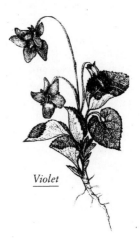

Violet

Nature-Identical Oils

The term 'nature-identical' has been coined to describe some of the more sophisticated synthetics which are made by taking organic molecules from cheap and plentiful essential oils and re-combining them in the proportions that approximate another oil. The result is never truly 'identical' to a naturally occurring oil. For example, there are over 300 known natural chemicals in Rose oil, some of them in only miniscule traces, and there are some parts of Rose oil that still remain to be identified, but even the tiniest of these components is vital to the fragrance and healing properties of Rose. Even if chemists were able to copy every single particle of a true oil, it would still lack the life force, or 'soul' of the Rose.

The same is true of any other 'nature-identical' oil and they have no place at all in aromatherapy. Avoid such oils like the plague!

Naturopathy

The underlying principle of naturopathy is that the body heals itself, given the right conditions. To help bring about the conditions for healing, the naturopath uses dietary means, especially fasting, hydrotherapy, relaxation techniques and sometimes manipulation. (A large number of naturopaths in Great Britain are also trained osteopaths.) Modern naturopathy has expanded to include the use of vitamin and mineral supplements.

This system ideally complements aromatherapy, especially when dealing with chronic illness. Massage, aromatic baths, etc., will help to stimulate the body's own healing processes, while aromatherapists may wish to refer clients to a naturopath for skilled dietary advice, etc.

The methods and principles of naturopathy have been embraced by many different complementary therapists, especially by those offering nutritional counselling.

see also **OSTEOPATHY** *and* **NUTRITION.**

Nausea

see **VOMITING.**

Nephritis

Nephritis, or inflammation of the kidneys, may be acute or chronic, but in every instance it is a very serious condition, and nobody should contemplate treating it by means of aromatherapy alone. A doctor, homoeopath or acupuncturist must be consulted, and essential oils used in conjunction with the treatment prescribed (remembering that with homoeopathy, essential oils might antidote the remedies, so the approval of the homoeopath must be sought before using them).

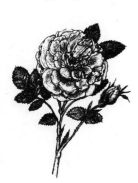

Oils which are generally tonic or cleansing for the kidneys may be helpful, with Camomile the most effective. Cedarwood and Juniper are both cleansing and detoxifying, but need to be used in very small amounts indeed, preferably simply as bath oils. Massage over the small of the back, where the kidneys are located, is recommended.

Herb teas which are beneficial to the kidneys, especially camomile and nettle, are a very good back up to any other treatment that is undertaken.

see also **KIDNEYS.**

Neroli

Citrus aurantium, var. *amara*

Oil of Neroli is obtained from the flowers of the Bitter Orange or Seville Orange, and it takes its name from that of an Italian princess who used it as her favourite perfume. The active principles of the oil include linalol, linalyl acetate, limonene, nerol, nerolidol, geraniol, indol, jasmone, and anthranilic, enzoic and phenylacetic esters.

The essential oil is usually produced by the enfleurage method, though sometimes steam distillation is used, and it is thick and deep brown in colour. The scent is of a bitter-sweet nature, as one might expect from its origins, and is not always liked in the concentrated form of the essential oil. However, once it has been suitably diluted as a massage oil, bath oil or in skin creams, etc., it is one of the most hauntingly beautiful of all those used in aromatherapy. It is widely used in commercial perfumery, and is another of the ingredients of true eau de cologne.

It is antidepressant, antiseptic, antispasmodic and aphrodisiac and a gentle sedative. It has one or two very important physical uses, though I find that by far the most important use of Neroli is in helping with problems of emotional origin. It is especially valuable for states of anxiety. On a fairly simplistic level, it can be used effectively to reduce anxiety before any stressful event, such as an interview, examination, driving test or public appearance, though obviously its greatest value lies in treating more serious and long-term anxiety states.

It is also valuable in the treatment of shock and – theoretically at least – hysteria, though I have to state that I have not had an opportunity of trying it for the latter. It is a very valuable oil for insomnia, particularly when the sleeplessness arises from anxiety. It is best used as a bath essence before bedtime.

Neroli is particularly valuable in skin care for it has the special property of stimulating the growth of healthy new cells, and has therefore certain rejuvenating effects. It can be used for all skin types, but is perhaps most useful for dry or sensitive skins. The delicate perfume makes it highly acceptable in all skin and toilet preparations, even for the most delicate skins.

It can safely be used during pregnancy, and I have often incorporated it with Mandarin in a cream to prevent stretch marks.

One of the physical actions of Neroli is to relieve spasms in the smooth muscle, especially that of the intestines. It is extremely helpful in chronic diarrhoea, especially where this arises from nervous tension.

Neroli blends well with almost any other floral oil, especially Rose, and for the ultimate in luxury you might try mixing it with both Rose and Jasmine.

The reputed aphrodisiac quality of Neroli stems not from a directly hormonal or stimulant effect, as with some oils, but rather from its ability to calm any nervous apprehension that may be felt before a sexual encounter; and as many sexual difficulties arise from a state of tension and anxiety, and in turn give rise to further anxiety and depression, Neroli can be one of the means of overcoming them. The traditional use of orange blossom in bridal wreaths arose from this property of the perfume, though this has long been forgotten now that the fresh flowers have been replaced, first by fabric and later by plastic imitations.

Recent studies suggest that Neroli can help P.M.T., probably because of its calming, anti-stress action and I have found it a particularly good oil for depression in older, menopausal and post-menopausal, women.

Neroli

Nerves

Oils which are helpful in conditions that are sometimes described as 'Nerves' are discussed under **ANXIETY**, **DEPRESSION** and **STRESS**.

The physical nervous system of the body and essential oils which relate to it are discussed under **NERVOUS SYSTEM**.

The Nervous System

It is helpful to consider the nervous system as a number of identifiable but inter-related parts: the Central Nervous System, consisting of the brain and spinal cord; the Peripheral Nervous System, which transmits sensations of heat, cold, pressure, pain, etc., from all over the body to the Central Nervous System (C.N.S.) and receives impulses from the C.N.S. to set the Voluntary muscles in motion; the Autonomic Nervous System which relays nerve impulses to and from the organs and also the specialised sensory nerves involved in sight, hearing, taste and smell.

The action of essential oils and of massage on the various activities of the nervous system form a major part of aromatherapy. For example, analgesic oils relieve pain because they damp down the activity of the pain-transmitting nerve endings, antispasmodic oils have a calming effect on the nerves which trigger muscle activity, sedative oils act partly by reducing over-activity in the nervous system. There is a great deal of overlap in these properties, and many analgesic oils are also sedative and/or antispasmodic. For example, Bergamot, Camomile, Lavender and Marjoram share all three of these properties, while Eucalyptus, Peppermint and Rosemary are both analgesic and antispasmodic though not sedative. Not surprisingly, these are among the most valuable and often-used oils in aromatherapy and we call on them repeatedly for all conditions where there is pain or spasm in the Voluntary muscles or internal organs.

Rosemary

Some other oils which combine sedative and antispasmodic effects are Clary Sage, Cypress, Juniper, Melissa, Neroli, Rose and Sandalwood. Of these, Neroli has a marked effect on the autonomic nerves governing the intestines and is very helpful for nervous diarrhoea and 'butterflies in the tummy'. Sandalwood is particularly active on the nerves of the bronchial passages and is one of the best oils to calm down a cough which is caused by nervous reflex action.

Nervine oils are those which have a beneficial tonic action on the nervous system as a whole and include Camomile, Clary Sage, Juniper, Lavender, Marjoram, Melissa and Rosemary. As you can see, all of these have already been mentioned for their other actions on the nervous system.

Nettlerash

෯

see entry *for* **URTICARIA.**

Neuralgia

෯

Neuralgia means a pain originating in a nerve. It can apply to any part of the Peripheral Nervous System (for example, sciatica, which is pain originating in the sciatic nerve, is a form of neuralgia) but the word is most commonly used to mean facial neuralgia.

The pain from this can be very intense, and orthodox medicine sometimes employs drastic measures, such as severing the affected nerve, to give relief.

Powerfully analgesic (i.e. pain-killing) essential oils offer a better alternative, and the most effective way of using them is in hot compresses over the affected part of the body. Camomile, Clary Sage, Lavender, Marjoram and Rosemary are the most effective, and can be alternated or blended with each other to give the maximum pain relief.

Niaouli
Melaleuca viridiflora

Niaouli is so very closely related to Cajeput *(Melaleuca leucodendron)* that the two are sometimes confused. However there are sufficient differences in the composition, odour and properties of the two oils to make such confusion inexcusable, and no good supplier will substitute one for the other. Both belong to the same family as Ti-tree and share some of its properties. You may occasionally find this oil sold under the name of Gomenol which originated from the fact that it used to be distilled near, and shipped from, the port of Gomen in the French East Indies, hence 'Gomen-oil'. Now most supplies come from Australia.

The oil is obtained from the leaves and young twigs, and varies from pale to dark yellow. It has a very strong, hot, camphorous odour and contains between 50% and 60% of cineol, eucalyptol, terpineol, pinene, limonene and various esters.

The reason why it is so important to distinguish clearly between this oil and its 'cousin' is that unlike Cajeput which is a skin irritant, Niaouli is well tolerated by the skin and mucous membranes when used in suitable dilutions. It can therefore be safely used for massage, as a gargle and even as a vaginal douche. It is good for cystitis and other urinary infections and has been used in hospitals in France as an antiseptic in obstetrics and gynaecology.

It is also suitable for cleaning minor wounds and burns. For cuts and grazes, especially if any dirt has got into them at the time of injury, mix 5 or 6 drops of Niaouli in 1/2 pint (250 mls) of boiled and cooled water and wash out repeatedly. For burns, the oil can be sprinkled neat on a sterile gauze and fastened over the burn. It is a powerful tissue-stimulant and will therefore help healing.

215

Because it is non-irritant and powerfully antiseptic, this is a good oil for the treatment of acne and similar skin conditions such as boils. This would not be my first choice of an oil for acne, but because treatment so often needs to be continued over a long period of time, it is important to have some alternatives and vary the oil used every few weeks.

Niaouli is good for all respiratory tract infections, whether they affect the nose, throat or chest, and is used in chest rubs as well as inhalations. It is quite a powerful stimulant, so it is better not to use it late in the evening, unless mixed with more sedative oils such as Lavender, or sleep may be disturbed.

A little-known but very valuable use of Niaouli is in conjunction with radiation therapy for cancer. A thin layer of Niaouli applied to the skin before each session of cobalt therapy gives some protection against burning of the skin and has been shown to reduce the severity of such burns. The tissue-stimulating properties probably help the burns to heal faster.

see also the entries for **TI-TREE** *and for* **CAJEPUT.**

Nose

Without this relatively small organ, there could be no aromatherapy, for the nose is involved in the two most important processes by which essential oils interact with the body and mind.

1. The nose forms the first part of the respiratory system, through which essential oils taken in with the breath reach the bloodstream.
2. In the upper part of the nose are the olfactory nerves, which transmit information about all smells to the brain.

Disorders affecting the nose are discussed in detail in the entries for CATARRH, COLDS, HAYFEVER, INFLUENZA and SINUSITIS.

see also entries for **RESPIRATORY SYSTEM** *and* **SENSE OF SMELL.**

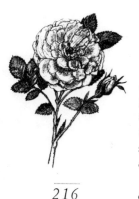

Nosebleeds

A nosebleed can be stopped simply and effectively by soaking a plug of gauze or cottonwool in cold water (iced if possible) with a drop or two of essential oil of Lemon, and inserting this as far up the nostril as possible. Oil of Lemon is haemostatic (i.e. it stops bleeding by speeding up the rate at which blood forms clots).

Get the victim to lie down in a quiet place, and put an icy-cold compress at the back of the neck – maybe with a few drops of oil of Lavender added. If the bleeding continues, get more qualified help, as the amount of blood lost can be serious.

Most nosebleeds result from minor injuries, but they may also be a symptom of high blood pressure or other serious disorders, so anybody who has nosebleeds frequently needs more than the first-aid help described here, and the cause of the bleeding must be sought and treated.

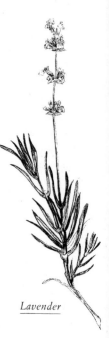

Lavender

Nutmeg
Myristica fragrans

Nutmeg is the kernel of the fruit of a tree native to India, Java and Sumatra, and which is also grown in the West Indies. The outer layer of the same fruit also yields a spice, mace, and you can sometimes buy nutmegs complete with the outer layer of mace surrounding them. The oil is extracted from the 'nut' by steam distillation, and its active principles include camphene, dipentene, sabinene, borneol, geraniol, linalol, eugenol, safrol and myristicin.

There is a great deal of overlap in the properties and uses of all the oils derived from warming spices, and in many respects Nutmeg duplicates the properties of Cinnamon. I use it less than Cinnamon, as caution is needed because Nutmeg in high doses, or over a long period of time, can cause mental or nervous disturbances. It is said that you can kill somebody with one whole nutmeg – but the intended victim would probably start vomiting long before the fatal dose was reached. I use Nutmeg mainly as an alternative to Cinnamon, when I wish to vary the oils being used.

Jean Valnet recommends Nutmeg combined with Clove and Rosemary for relieving rheumatic pain. This is certainly a powerful and effective blend, but it should be used with care, as it is very stimulating. Nutmeg is also a stimulant of the heart and circulation, another reason for caution.

Nutmeg makes an agreeable addition to winter blends of oils for warming and generally toning up the body, and strengthening its resistance to cold. In the bath 3 drops is enough, and more can give rise to skin problems.

This is another oil which I like to diffuse in the air by evaporating it in an essential oil burner or diffuser, especially during the winter. It makes a particularly enjoyable scent when used with oil of Orange, or Clove and Orange. The latter blend virtually reproduces the perfume of traditional pomanders, which have been used for centuries to perfume rooms and ward off infection.

Nutrition

The importance of a healthy diet in conjunction with aromatherapy treatments cannot be repeated too often. However potent the essential oils, and however skilled the therapist, healing will be slow in a body that is malnourished or overloaded with toxic wastes.

Many aromatherapists now combine nutritional advice with essential oil treatment, or refer clients to a nutritional therapist.

More than 2,000 years ago Hippocrates, the 'Father of Medicine' put forward the theory that bad diet causes disease and said, 'Let your medicine be your food and your food your medicine.' The foods available to most of us now are far less nutritious and more likely to be contaminated than those eaten in the predominantly agrarian society of Greece in the 5th century B.C.

Dietary needs vary enormously from one person to another, and there can be no hard and fast rules about a good diet, though there are certain useful guidelines. For example, while a simple vegetarian wholefood diet is usually regarded as the ideal, some people find they cannot keep really well without a little meat. Their bodies may be deficient in the enzymes needed to convert vegetable proteins into the forms in which the body can utilise them. Calorie requirements are just as hard to define because the efficiency with which we metabolise food varies so much from one individual to another. Daily needs of vitamins and minerals vary too, and the recommended daily intake of some vitamins calculated by government departments in several countries, are in many cases far below most people's real needs.

One point on which the same advice is valid for everybody is the need to avoid chemical additives. Chemicals are applied to foodstuffs at every stage from the seed to the finished product in the shop – fertilisers, pesticides and herbicides, colourings, flavourings and preservatives enter into almost all food that is marketed, and many of them are known or suspected carcinogens.

Others, which are officially considered harmless in small amounts, can build up in the body until they reach toxic levels, and still others, while not producing any detectable damage, add to the load of alien matter that the body has to process. During hundreds of thousands of years of evolution, our bodies have been 'programmed' to recognise certain organic substances, whether animal or vegetable, as foods. The few decades during which ever-increasing amounts of chemicals have been added to our food represent less than a blink in this massive time scale, and our bodies are not able to adapt to all the new substances they are expected to deal with. When the body rejects any substance as 'foreign', it mobilises various mechanisms to neutralise the substance. It may produce a quantity of histamine in response to the unfamiliar substance, triggering off symptoms of various allergies. It may make a massive effort to eliminate the foreign matter via the skin, giving rise to eczema or psoriasis, or it may try to inactivate it by literally wrapping it up to insulate it from the body tissues. In this case, large amounts of mucus are produced to surround the foreign material, and the lungs, nose, sinuses, and colon become very clogged. As a last resort, the body may simply store chemicals away in one of the organs, most often the liver, where they may do no harm for a while, but can lead to disease as they build up over a period of time.

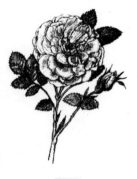

Hormones and antibiotics are fed in large amounts to animals reared for food, and these too have harmful effects on the body. Premature sexual maturity (menstruation beginning at 5 years of age, for example) and the growth of breasts on men have been produced by regular consumption of hormone-fed chicken, and small but repeated amounts of antibiotics may mean that if you really need an antibiotic in an emergency, it will be ineffective.

The simplest advice is to eat foods in as near their natural state as possible. Avoid foods that have been processed in any way – tinned, frozen, pre-cooked, packeted, etc. You may read that freezing foods conserves their vitamins far better than canning or other methods of preservation, but many frozen foods have colouring added.

Eat foods as near the beginning of the food chain as possible. Animals are reared on plants that have been grown in artificially fertilised soil and sprayed. The animals retain traces of chemicals from those plants and concentrate them within their bodies. If we then eat the animals, we take in a number of chemicals in concentrated form. This is true of eggs, milk and cheese, too, if they have been produced by commercially reared animals, so vegetarians need to be aware of these problems as well as meat eaters.

Grow as many of your own fruit and vegetables as you can, or try to find a source of supply of organically grown, unsprayed vegetables and fruit. If this is really impossible, thoroughly wash everything before you eat it. This will not remove all chemicals, but will reduce the total.

If you feel you need to eat meats, try to obtain them from farmers who rear their animals naturally, without hormones or antibiotics. Even if you can obtain naturally reared meat, red meats (pork and beef) are best avoided for they are high in fats and acids, with pork being the most toxic meat of all. Pork in particular, and beef to a lesser extent, produce an acid reaction in the body, which contributes to many diseases.

Eat as much of your food as possible raw. Cooking destroys or changes some of the most important nutritional elements. Eat 'living foods' – freshly sprouted grains, beans and pulses. It is very

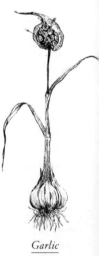

Garlic

easy to sprout beans, grains and other seeds on a kitchen shelf, and these foods are exceptionally nutritious. The growing seed really does represent the beginning of the food chain.

The bulk of our food intake should be complex carbohydrates, which provide warmth and energy and the fibre which is essential to healthy functioning of the digestive tract. Refined carbohydrates, such as white sugar, white flour and all foods made with them, clog up the body because the necessary fibre has been removed from them during processing. They provide fuel (calories) without bulk or nutritional value.

Refined sugars also increase the amount of sugar in the blood to dangerous levels, and the pancreas has to work overtime pumping out insulin to process this excess sugar. The insulin quite soon lowers the amount of sugar in circulation to a dangerously low level, where the person feels tired, irritable and possibly giddy or faint, and certainly hungry. Another snack of refined sugary food quickly relieves these symptoms, but sets up a see-saw process where the blood-sugar level is constantly swinging between too high and too low. It is *Thyme* far safer to eat unrefined carbohydrates, such as whole grains, unrefined sugar in small amounts, a little honey and dried fruits, to provide sugars and starches in a form that the body can cope with in a more efficient and balanced way. Whole grains and fruits and vegetables also provide the bulky fibre needed to ensure that food passes through the digestive tract at a reasonable speed. Food which is deficient in fibre tends to stay too long in the colon, setting up fermentation processes which can lead to various forms of disease, including diverticulitis and cancer of the colon.

Protein can be obtained from both animal and vegetable sources. The basic 'building bricks' of protein, which the human body needs for buildings and repairing its structure, are amino acids. These structures – bones, muscle, internal organs, hair and nails, for example, involve 20 amino acids, but not all of these can be manufactured in the body. There are 8 amino acids that we cannot make in our own bodies and need to obtain from food sources. Foods which contain all 8 are called prime or first-class proteins, and meat, eggs and soya come into this category. The main vegetable sources of protein need to be combined together in one meal to provide all 8 of the essential amino acids. Grains combined with pulses, grains with nuts, or pulses with nuts will give the equivalent of prime protein quite simply. Brazil nuts are an important ingredient in such combinations, as they provide an amino acid not found in many vegetable sources.

Most of us in the West eat too much protein, and this is potentially very damaging, especially if that protein is meat. Uric acid is one of the results of the breakdown of protein during digestion and is normally excreted without trouble. However, if there is too much of it, the body may not be able to cope, and the uric acid will be deposited in the joints, or maybe the kidneys, giving rise to gout, arthritis or kidney disease. Some people are deficient in the enzymes needed to dispose of uric acid. High blood pressure is another condition to which too high a protein intake contributes.

Animal proteins are often very high in fat, and this has been shown to contribute to high blood pressure and coronary heart disease. The body needs a certain amount of fats, but these are better obtained from vegetable sources. The brain and spinal cord, the heart, lungs, liver and other vital organs, as well as muscles, need certain fatty acids known as essential fatty acids (EFAs) and indeed these make up about 50% of the brain. Some of these, like the amino acids, can be made and combined within the body, but

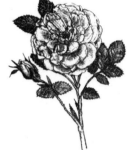

219

there are two – linoleic acid and linolenic acid which the body cannot manufacture, and which can only be obtained from plants. Evening Primrose oil is one of the most valuable sources.

Apart from the major constituents of foodstuffs, which we need to eat each day in reasonable amounts, there are the substances which we need in minute quantities, but which are vital to health: vitamins, minerals and trace elements.

Vitamins A, D, E and F are fat-soluble and can be stored in the liver for a time, but Vitamin C and the B group are water-soluble and are not stored in the body, so fresh supplies are needed each day. Ideally, all our requirements of vitamins and other trace nutrients should come from our food, but in a less-than-perfect world, relatively few people in developed countries get an adequate supply from their food. (And this is without considering the millions of people in the world who simply do not get enough to eat.)

In addition, individual requirements may vary widely. Government departments in many countries set out to recommend daily minimum requirements of various vitamins and minerals, but these are often so low that they are only just enough to prevent gross deficiency symptoms, such as scurvy. Individual needs for Vitamin C, for example, may be 400 times as much as the recommended intake, and in exceptional cases, as much as 1,000 times more. Illness, stress, food additives, environmental pollution, alcohol and smoking are all factors which increase the body's need for various nutrients and often, at the same time, decrease its ability to absorb them, making supplementation necessary, though maybe only for a short period.

Some aromatherapists advise avoiding meat on any day when you receive a treatment with essential oils, and in fact you may be given similar advice by acupuncturists and other natural therapists. They feel that the chemical reactions in the body when meat is being digested inhibit the subtler action of the essential oils. You may also be advised to drink copious amounts of water during the 24 hours following a treatment.

Certainly, meat eating alters the smell of essential oils (and perfumes) when they are applied to the body, and many aromatherapists can differentiate between the smell of meat eaters, and vegetarians. Many people have found that their own sensitivity to aromas has been heightened when they have stopped eating meat.

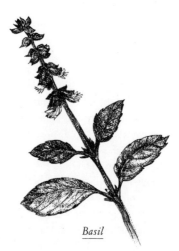

Basil

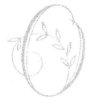

Obesity

❧

A small number of essential oils are sometimes described as being helpful in losing weight. The most notable of these is Fennel, which has had the reputation of suppressing hunger since at least the time of Julius Caesar. Roman soldiers on long marches carried Fennel seeds in their pouches to chew until they could make a meal at the next stopping place. Throughout the Middle Ages and well into the Tudor era, devout Christians used Fennel in the same way to help them through the various fast days of the church calendar. Fennel is also a mild diuretic which would help if fluid retention was involved, and a detoxifier, which could be valuable, if previous poor diet had created a build up of toxins in the body, but would not contribute directly to weight loss.

Fennel

Garlic and Onion are mentioned by some French authors, and both these oils have a strong stimulant action on the thyroid gland. If an underactive thyroid, leading to slow metabolism, is the cause, either of these could help, preferably in capsule form, or simply by including plenty of garlic and onion in meals.

Rosemary is a general stimulant and tonic which can help to get a sluggish metabolism on the move, and Geranium is a hormone balancer which could be taken into consideration if it seems likely that an imbalance is part of the problem.

However, the root causes of obesity are seldom simple physiological ones, and the most important role of the aromatherapist in helping overweight people is to look at the often complex emotional states underlying the gain of excess weight. As these may be immensely varied, so the choice of oils can be very wide, taking in all those which help in situations of stress, depression, anxiety, lack of confidence and so on. Here, I would like to mention Bergamot in particular because my experience of it is somewhat different from the generally accepted use. It is often used to stimulate appetite, but I have used it successfully to help compulsive eaters. This suggests that either it has a normalising effect, rather than a stimulating one, on the appetite centre in the brain, or that it is not working directly on the appetite at all, but rather on the mental or emotional state that has caused the appetite to go awry, and in view of everything else we know about Bergamot, I suspect the latter.

Many fat people intensely dislike their own bodies, so the mere fact of receiving a massage regularly can be a tremendous revelation. Treating the body with respect, nurturing and pampering it may be a completely new experience, and can help to build up a more positive self-image. Once this has been achieved, it becomes easier to tackle such questions as exercise and long-term changes in eating habits (I shun the emotive word 'diet' because for most fat people this suggests deprivation and failure).

Weight loss, especially if it has been fairly rapid, can leave the previously fat person looking and feeling rather 'saggy', so later massages might be geared to improving skin and muscle tone, which will once again give a boost to confidence as the appearance improves.

Counselling, mutual-support groups or even psychotherapy may help some people, but aromatherapy will certainly reinforce any other therapy or treatment.

Oedema

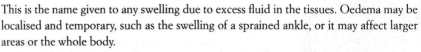

This is the name given to any swelling due to excess fluid in the tissues. Oedema may be localised and temporary, such as the swelling of a sprained ankle, or it may affect larger areas or the whole body.

Generalised oedema is often a symptom of serious illness, such as progressive heart failure or severe kidney malfunction, so no aromatherapist (unless he or she is also medically trained) should attempt to treat this except in collaboration with a doctor, acupuncturist or medically-trained homoeopath.

However, there are many other forms of oedema which can be effectively treated with essential oils, especially premenstrual fluid retention, which responds very well to massage in the week to ten days preceding each period. Appropriate oils include Geranium, Juniper and Rosemary.

Pine is effective in reducing the puffiness of legs and ankles that can occur after prolonged standing, and in the latter months of pregnancy. Massaging the legs with long strokes, always moving from the ankles upwards, will really reduce the swelling and although it is always more effective to have the massage carried out by a trained therapist, the legs are one of the areas of the body where self-massage is possible, and this can be carried out every day between visits to an aromatherapist. I like to make up the oils into a cream, rather than a massage oil for this use, as they are easier to handle in this form.

Some people also experience this kind of swelling on long flights for which Cypress, Geranium, Myrtle, or Pine are helpful. These oils have a stimulant action on the lymphatic system, which is responsible for draining excess fluid from the body tissues, and a specialised form of lymphatic massage is best in treating any form of oedema, though any kind of massage with appropriate oils will help.

Fluid accumulation is often associated with toxic wastes in the body, for example in cellulite: it is one of the body's ways of trying to render toxins less dangerous by diluting them. Detoxifying oils such as Fennel, Juniper and Lemon are very helpful in such cases.

Sometimes, fluid retention, either in the abdominal area or affecting the whole body, can be a sign of food allergy. Again, the body is trying to minimalise the harmful affects of the allergen by surrounding it with a lot of water. If aromatherapy treatment does not seem to help much, and the possibility of serious illness has been ruled out, it would be worth investigating this aspect. A nutritional counsellor or clinical ecologist will be able to advise.

see also **CELLULITIS, LYMPH** *and* **PREMENSTRUAL TENSION.**

Oestrogens

Oestrogens are the primary female sex hormones, mainly produced by the ovaries, though smaller amounts are made in the adrenal cortex. They are needed for various body processes apart from reproduction, and are found in both men and women, though in different proportions. Deficiencies are involved in various menstrual and reproductive problems, and the lowering of oestrogen levels after the menopause contributes to the ageing process, particularly to osteoporosis (thinning of the bones) which is becoming increasingly common among older people.

Some plants are known to contain plant oestrogens which are valuable in supplementing the body's own hormones. Anethol is a plant oestrogen found in Fennel, Ravensara, Tarragon and several other plants of the Umbelliferae family, etc. Sclareol is another, found in Clary Sage. The safest way to use these oils is to 'kick-start' the body's own processes rather than to rely on them long-term. There are also oestrogen-rich plants used in medical herbalism which don't yield essential oils, and these can be used alongside the oestrogenic oils. The most important are catkins, hops and liquorice.

Clary Sage

Fennel and liquorice can both be used to make pleasant herb teas which are helpful in premenstrual tension and menopausal disturbances, and I would strongly recommend older women to use one or other of these teas regularly to minimise loss of elasticity of the skin and other connective tissues, as well as the serious bone degeneration already mentioned.

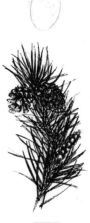

223

Oily Skin

Excessive oiliness of the skin is caused by too much sebum being produced in tiny glands just under the surface of the skin. Sebum is a natural lubricant which everybody needs for the health and good appearance of their skin, but too much produces a greasy appearance which is often associated with spots, blackheads and a tendency to acne. This is often most marked in adolescence because sebum production is linked to the activity of the whole endocrine system, which is in a state of flux following puberty. At this vulnerable stage in life, when appearances seem to be very important, it is small comfort to be told that a skin which is too oily in youth will age far more slowly than one which is relatively dry.

Essential oils can help these problems directly by reducing the amount of sebum produced, and indirectly by controlling the bacteria which thrive on the surface of an oily skin. Several oils combine both these actions, and are obviously the most effective. Cedarwood, Cypress, Geranium, Grapefruit and Sandalwood are the best examples, partly because of their real effectiveness, and partly because they have aromas which are acceptable to men and women alike and are often familiar because they are used in commercial toiletries.

My first choice of oils for an oily skin is Geranium and Lavender, blended in equal proportions. Geranium directly reduces sebum production and Lavender has a balancing effect: both are antiseptic and will control bacteria on the surface of the skin. As it is not good to use the same oil for more than a week or two, I vary this blend with Cedar, Grapefruit or Sandalwood in successive treatments. Any of these oils and various blends of them can be made up into cleansing and toning lotions for use at home. Most commercial toners sold for oily skins have a high alcohol content and remove all, or almost all, sebum from the skin. This improves the appearance temporarily, but has the effect of eventually increasing sebum output, since the glands respond to the absence of sebum on the surface by making more.

Some people are puzzled by the idea of using oils to treat an oily skin, but of course essential oils are non-greasy by nature, and all traces of carrier oil should be carefully removed after a treatment.

Geranium oil has a balancing effect on the endocrine system and on the sebaceous glands. It is another good alternative to the oils already mentioned, or can be blended with one or more of them (Geranium, Grapefruit and Lavender is a delightfully perfumed mixture as well as being very effective). Because of its balancing nature, this is also a good oil to use for 'combination' skins where most of the face is dry, but there are oily areas, usually around the nose and chin, where the sebaceous glands are more numerous.

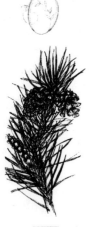

see also **ACNE, SKIN** *and* **SKINCARE.**

Ointments

❧

see entry for **CREAMS.**

Orange

Citrus aurantium, var. *amara, or* var. *bigaradia*
Citrus vulgaris, C. sinensis or *C. aurantium,* var. *dulcis*

Lavender

❧

The Orange tree was originally a native of the Far East, particularly China and India, and was not used medicinally in Europe until late in the 17th century, as it was considered both rare and expensive. It is probable that the legendary golden 'apples' in the Garden of the Hesperides were, in fact, oranges. The orange adapted well to the climate of the Mediterranean, where, of course, it grows abundantly, as well as in California, Israel and South America.

Essential oils are extracted by simple pressure from the outer, coloured part of the peel, from both the Bitter Orange *(Citrus aurantium,* var *amara* or *bigaradia)* and the Sweet Orange *(Citrus aurantium,* var *dulcis).* The Bitter, or Seville Orange, is also sometimes called *Citrus vulgaris* or *Citrus bigaradia.* The oil is a deep golden yellow with the characteristic orange peel aroma. The active constituents are mainly limonene with smaller amounts of bergaptene, citral, citronellal, myrcene, etc.: the composition and proportions varying somewhat between the sweet and bitter varieties. The Bitter Orange gives an oil with a slightly more delicate aroma than the Sweet Orange.

The properties of Orange overlap to a large extent with those of the closely-related oil of Neroli (obtained from the orange blossoms), being antidepressant, antispasmodic, stomachic and mildly sedative, and it is recommended for several purposes for which Neroli may often be used. Orange appears to have a normalising effect on the peristaltic action of the intestines, for it is recommended for the treatment of constipation by Paul Duraffourd in 'En Forme Tous Les Jours', while Dominique Sibe in '70 Huiles Essentielles' mentions the value of oil of Orange in helping chronic diarrhoea.

Despite its obvious overlapping with Neroli, Orange has quite a definite character of its own, reflecting the difference you might expect between the flower oil and that from the fruit, for the oil of Orange is warmer and more rounded in aroma, with a feeling of jollity about it. It seems to carry with it some of the sunshine needed for its ripening, and for this reason is a wonderful oil to use in the winter. It is very cheering as a winter bath oil – with the important proviso that more than 4 drops in an average bath can cause skin irritation. It blends well with almost any of the spice oils: Cinnamon, Nutmeg or Clove especially, and also, surprisingly, with Lavender and Frankincense.

Orange is a good oil to combat insomnia, and can be alternated with Lavender or Neroli or blended with either of them if there is a need for long-term treatment, since it is always wise to vary the oils used over a period of time.

The association of Orange with Cloves and Cinnamon is also found in such traditional drinks as mulled wines, and these (in moderation!) can be a good and enjoyable antidote to winters chills.

The same combination of aromas is found in the pomander – originally an orange stuck with cloves and dried in a mixture which includes powdered cinnamon – and the oils can be used to revive a pomander that has lost some of its aroma with age. I often use Orange in burners during the winter, usually with one or more of the spices.

Mixed in equal amounts with oil of Lemon, and diluted, Orange is a useful mouthwash, used as a gum tonic and a treatment for mouth ulcers.

see also **MANDARIN, NEROLI** *and* **PETITGRAIN.**

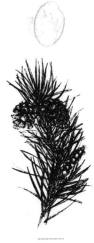

225

Orange Blossom, Orange-Flower or Orange-Flower Absolute

see the entry for **NEROLI.**

Orange-Flower Water

❧

Orange-flower water bears the same relationship to oil of Neroli that rosewater does to oil of Rose, being obtained by distillation from the orange blossom petals that also yield Neroli oil.

The major use of orange-flower water in aromatherapy is in skincare, as a tonic or aromatic wash, particularly if used in conjunction with creams or massage oils containing Neroli.

Orange-flower water is slightly more astringent than rosewater, so whereas the latter is used primarily for dry or sensitive skins, orange-flower is the better choice for oily skins. I often use it as a base for making a treatment lotion for young people with acne. Its delicate odour is so far removed from the over-harsh, medicinal-smelling preparations obtainable from chemists that it positively encourages regular use.

It is sometimes used in cooking, particularly around the Mediterranean, to give a delicate savour to cakes and biscuits, and you may find a good quality orange-flower water in Greek or other Mediterranean grocers' shops but it is too often a reconstituted version, so read labels carefully.

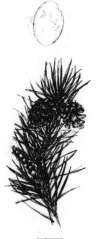

Oregano
Origanum vulgare

❧

Oregano is also known as 'Wild Marjoram' and is in fact very closely related botanically to Marjoram *(Origanum majorana)*. The plant is a native of the Mediterranean, and gives a characteristic flavour to local cookery.

The essential oil has a variety of therapeutic properties, but too many hazards are attached to it to make this a good oil for general use in aromatherapy. It is a powerful emmenagogue, which must be scrupulously avoided during pregnancy, and it is a fairly severe skin irritant and a very severe mucous membrane irritant. As this virtually rules out use in massage and baths, and as this is not an oil which is particularly useful in burners, vaporisations or inhalation, it is better to use Marjoram for most applications where Origanum may be described in texts.

Osteopathy

❧

Oregano

Of all other systems of healing, Osteopathy is perhaps the one with which an aromatherapist will most often have dealings. A significant proportion of people consulting an aromatherapist for the first time do so because of back pain and although essential oil massage is wonderfully effective in relieving muscular pain, the cause of the pain is often displacement of a joint, and referral to an osteopath is the only responsible course of action.

Osteopathy is based on the principle that the structure and function of the body are interdependent. If the structure becomes abnormal or is altered in any way – such as by a fall or accident – then the function will be impaired. When the structure (and the bony structure in particular) is in correct alignment, the various systems of the body are free to work normally. The osteopath therefore works to correct faults in the structure, whether these have arisen as the result of an accident, poor posture, abnormal muscular tension or other causes. He or she does so by manipulating displaced joints through their full range of movements to enable them to return to their correct position. This is done by using both the patient's body and that of the therapist to apply various kinds of leverage.

Where a joint is incorrectly placed, the surrounding muscles may often be in spasm and if the problem is of long standing, many nodules of fibrous tissue will often have built up in the muscles. Massage carried out before the manipulation helps to soften, warm and loosen the muscles so that the manipulation can be done more easily and effectively. Depending on their background and training osteopaths may give preliminary massage, or employ a masseur/masseuse in their practice to do so. In a few practices, the masseuse uses essential oils, and these certainly enhance the massage and prepare the muscles more effectively for the manipulation to follow, particularly those oils known as 'rubefacient', i.e. those which have a locally warming effect. Marjoram is probably the most effective oil here, and small amounts of Black Pepper in a blend with Lavender or Rosemary are a good alternative. Clary Sage is a good muscle relaxant, but not to be used if the patient is going to be driving after the treatment.

Where facilities for receiving massage at the osteopath's own premises are not available, a wise patient might make his or her own arrangements to have a massage before visiting the osteopath. Many of my own clients have done this with excellent results, which have been confirmed by their osteopaths.

An osteopath may sometimes have to exert quite a strong pull on the muscles to get a joint back into its correct position, and this can give rise to some superficial soreness for a day or two after treatment. Here again, massage can help. It should be fairly gentle, and essential oils can be chosen from Camomile, Lavender, Marjoram, Clary Sage or any other analgesic oil. Aromatic baths with any of these oils are comforting, but osteopaths advise that these should be neither too hot, nor prolonged for two or three days after manipulative treatment. Long hot baths may relax the muscles too much, and after treatment it is necessary for the muscles to regain their normal tone as quickly as possible to provide proper support for the joints.

In the case of long-standing problems, a series of aromatherapy massages alternating with manipulation can be far more effective than either massage or manipulation alone.

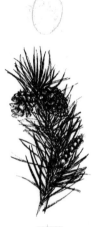

227

Otitis

This is the medical term used to describe ear infections of various kinds, and is subdivided according to the part of the ear involved – otitis externa affecting the outer ear, otitis media (by far the most common cause of earache) the middle ear, and otitis interna the inner ear. Infection spreads very easily from one part of the ear to another, and also from the nose to the ear via the Eustachian tubes, and from the inner ear into the skull cavity.

Because of this, and the potentially dangerous nature of the possible complications, no earache should ever be neglected. Essential oils can be used at the first sign of pain, to help relieve this and to combat the infection, but if there is no improvement within 24 hours, or if the pain is acute, or there is fever with it, or if pus is seen coming from the ear, a doctor should be consulted at once. This really is one of the situations in which antibiotics should not be despised, though it is possible and advisable to continue with aromatherapy treatments at the same time. Neglect of an apparently simple earache can lead to permanent deafness.

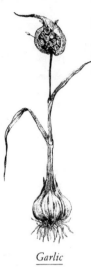

Garlic

Most earaches are secondary infections originating with a cold, sinusitis or other nasal problems, so the original nose infection should be treated as well.

Hot compresses of Camomile and/or Lavender will soothe pain, and reduce the risk of middle ear infections spreading to the inner ear through the action of heat in 'drawing' infection and pus to the surface. You can also try gentle massage all around the ear with the same oils. Camomile is the classic earache remedy, but I find it more effective combined with Lavender than either of them alone. I have sometimes used Birch oil, a more powerful analgesic, but if the pain is that bad, you should consult a doctor. To counteract infection you can put 3 drops of either Lavender or Ti-tree into a teaspoon of almond or olive oil warmed to blood heat, and trickle a little of this into the ear cavity. Gently insert a small plug of cottonwool to help keep the oil in the ear. However this should ONLY be done after medical examination has shown that the ear-drum is not perforated.

Frequently recurring earache indicates a congested and infected state in the ear and nasal passages, and, especially if there is a lot of catarrh present, such infections can be very slow to clear up. Garlic capsules, steam inhalations and a diet that is rich in raw fruits and vegetables, and low in dairy products and refined starches, will usually reduce the amount of mucus and enable the infection to be eradicated, so that the earache will no longer be a problem.

see also, **CATARRH**, **COLDS** *and* **SINUSITIS.**

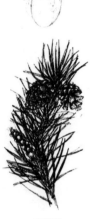

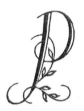

Palmarosa
Cympobogon martinii, var. *Motia*

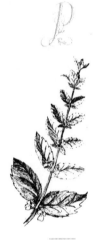

Palmarosa is a scented grass of the same family as Lemongrass (*Cymbopogon citratus*) and Citronella (*Cymbopogon nardus*). It is native to the Indian sub-continent, although now cultivated in Africa, South America and elsewhere. The whole family might well be regarded as nature's copycats, for they all contain a number of elements which are found in rarer and more costly plants and give them their characteristic odour. Their oils are often used commercially to adulterate more expensive ones. Where the last two mimic the scent of lemon, Palmarosa contains a high proportion of geraniol and has a gentle perfume somewhere between those of Geranium and Rose. It is found as an adulterant in Rose oil although nobody with a sensitive nose would confuse the two.

The oil is obtained by steam distillation and is usually pale yellow, sometimes with a greenish tint. Its active constituents are mainly geraniol (between 75% and 95%) with traces of citronellol, farnesol, geranyl acetate, etc.

In traditional Indian medicine, Palmarosa oil has a long history of use against fevers and infectious diseases. It is a very powerful, wide-spectrum bactericide but particularly active against various bacteria responsible for intestinal infections, such as gastro-enteritis: for example it will kill *Escherichia coli* bacteria in 5 minutes. Another traditional use is as a digestive stimulant, excellent for loss of appetite and sluggish digestion.

Palmarosa is probably best known as a valuable skincare oil, hydrating and stimulating and helping to balance sebum production. Like Lavender and Neroli, Palmarosa stimulates cellular regeneration. Its use in skin treatments is enhanced by its antiseptic properties which make it useful for acne and many minor skin infections, also some forms of dermatitis. Used regularly, it may even help to smooth out wrinkles, and tones up crepey skin on the neck. It is used in hand creams, moisturisers and all types of skin care preparations, as much for its delightful fragrance as for its active properties.

It blends well with a very wide range of other oils: floral, woody, citrus, etc., though its fragrance is sufficiently complex to stand alone without blending. This makes it a lovely massage or bath oil, and it is valuable for stress and stress-related conditions.

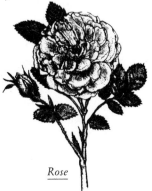

Rose

Palpitations

A strictly medical definition of palpitations is an awareness of the heartbeat, either because the person concerned is paying greater attention to it, or because the heart is actually beating more forcibly than usual. This may be experienced when the person is frightened, shocked or anxious, and essential oils such as Neroli, which have a profoundly calming effect, are the most effective. As an emergency measure, simply give some of the oil to smell straight from the bottle or on a tissue or handkerchief. A person who is subject to palpitations would benefit from regular massage with any one of a wide range of essential oils with calming properties, including Camomile, Lavender, Neroli, Rose and Ylang-Ylang.

The term palpitations is very often used (incorrectly) to describe the over-rapid heartbeat often experienced in similar circumstances. This should more correctly be called tachycardia, but this is really an academic distinction, since the same essential oils and methods of use will be helpful,with Ylang-Ylang being the oil most often found helpful for slowing the excessively rapid beating.

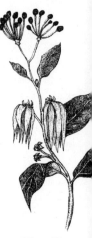

Ylang-Ylang

Parsley

Petroselinum sativum

Although the pretty, curly green Parsley will grow anywhere with a temperate climate, it is a native of Greece, and the Greeks very early on recognised it as a medicinal herb. The inclusion of the word 'sativum' in its botanical name tells us that it has been a culinary herb for a very long time, too. They considered that the best Parsley was that grown in Macedonia. Nowadays it is widely cultivated in Europe, Asia and the U.S.A.

An essential oil is obtained from the leaves and, occasionally, the roots, but mainly from the seeds, which are far richer in oil than any other part of the plant. The principal constituent of Parsley Leaf oil is apiol, (sometimes called Parsley Camphor) with apiolic aldehyde and pinene, while that from the seeds has much less apiol: myristicin is the largest component with small amounts of phellandrene, myrcene, pinene, etc. The Parsley Seed is the most useful in aromatherapy. The oil varies from yellow to deep amber, and has a nutty, spicy aroma.

Greek and Roman physicians, including Dioscorides and Pliny recommended Parsley seed for kidney and bladder disorders, including bladder and kidney stones and retention of urine, also as an emmenagogue and to treat sterility. The essential oil has been known and used since the beginning of the 16th century for the same purposes, as well as a mild stimulant, a digestive aid, to reduce fevers and as a tonic for the circulatory system.

The principal uses of Parsley Seed oil at the present day are still those for which it has always been known.

One of its main uses is as a diuretic, and in the treatment of urinary tract problems. (You may recognise here an affinity between many oils from the Umbelliferae family.)

Hot compresses over the bladder are comforting and helpful in cystitis and can be used for kidney problems, providing it is well understood that medical help should be sought as well. The diuretic action makes Parsley helpful in all situations where there is fluid retention: P.M.T., oedema due to standing for long periods (but NOT in pregnancy), and cellulite.

Parsley has a tonic effect on the smooth muscles, particularly those of the reproductive system. As a uterine tonic it is sometimes used as an aid to labour, but should not be used earlier in pregnancy as it is a potent emmenagogue. This, of course, makes it useful for missing, scanty or irregular periods, and this may be why it was considered a cure for sterility in antiquity: if menstruation is absent or erratic, conception becomes problematical. Among Frenchmen it has the reputation of increasing their sexual prowess – perhaps that is the other half of the story.

It is also tonic in its effect on the blood vessels and is sometimes used externally in the treatment of piles (haemorrhoids). Applied to bruises it helps to shrink the broken blood-vessels immediately below the skin, and so reduce the amount of blood seeping into the surrounding tissues. This same action of shrinking small blood-vessels can be used to help thread-veins in the face, if it is used consistently over a period of several months.

Parsley Seed is a digestive aid, and a good tonic where the digestion is sluggish. When I lived in France, we used to chew a few Parsley seeds after a meal to help it digest and to freshen the breath (useful, as the meals were so often rich in Garlic!). Massage over the stomach would be a good treatment for anybody with impaired digestion.

Patchouli

Pogostemon patchouli or *P. cablin*

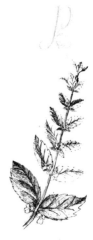

231

Patchouli is a native of Malaysia, now cultivated in a number of S.E. Asian countries, the West Indies and Paraguay. It is a bushy plant, growing to as much as a metre in height, with large, soft, furry leaves. Although it is a member of the same plant family as many of the Mediterranean herbs (Basil, Hyssop, Lavender, Marjoram, Melissa, Peppermint, Rosemary, Thyme, etc.) it is unlike most of them in its appearance, habitat and medicinal properties.

The essential oil is thick and dark brown, often with a green tinge. The odour is not easy to describe: hot, musty and pungent, strong, penetrating and so persistent that I have known it to linger on clothes for as much as two weeks, even after laundering. This is perhaps unfortunate, given the fact that quite a lot of people find the smell unpleasant. In many places in this book I have stressed that the client's choice should guide your selection of oils, and this is particularly important when dealing with Patchouli. It has perhaps a more animal than plant quality to it. Even so, it is widely used in the perfumery trade as a fixative due to its long-lasting character, and in fact very small proportions in a blend can give a mysterious, oriental characteristic. I have used as little as 0.5% in blends with very pleasing results.

The active principles are mainly patchoulene, patchoulol, and norpatchoulol with traces of eugenol, cadinene, carvone, caryophyllene, etc. Of these, it is interesting to note that patchoulene is very similar in structure to azulene (found in Camomile) and has the same anti-inflammatory properties.

The plant, which is known as Pucha-pot in its native habitats, has a long history of use in the traditional medicine of China, Japan and Malaysia as a stimulant, tonic, antiseptic and febrifuge, as well as in treating snake-bites and the stings of poisonous insects, and it has always been used as a perfume, insecticide and antiseptic in the countries of origin.

In aromatherapy, Patchouli has some valuable uses in skincare and the treatment of skin disorders. As mentioned already, it is anti-inflammatory and antiseptic in effect. It is also fungicidal and is a cell-regenerator in much the same way as Lavender and Neroli and this combination of properties makes it useful in treating acne, cracked skin, certain types of eczema, fungal infections such as athlete's foot, some skin allergies and dandruff.

It has been used in treatments for obesity, possibly because of (unsubstantiated) reports that it induces loss of appetite and possibly because it reduces fluid retention. However, it is an antidepressant and I think it is more likely that Patchouli may help with weight loss because it helps the underlying anxiety and depression from which so many fat people suffer. In fact, it is helpful for all forms of depression, anxiety and stress-related conditions.

Some writers consider Patchouli an aphrodisiac, but this would certainly depend a great deal on whether both partners found the perfume pleasing.

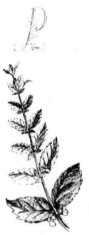

Pepper, Black
Piper nigrum

Pepper is a woody climbing plant, native to East Asia. In its natural state it can climb as high as 20 feet, but when grown commercially it is usually pruned to a maximum of 12 feet for convenience. It has been known as both a medicinal and a culinary spice in the Far East for over 4,000 years, and in Europe from at least the 5th century. Like many spices, it was highly prized, and Attila the Hun is reputed to have demanded 3,000 lbs of pepper as part of the ransom for the city of Rome.

The essential oil may vary from almost colourless to pale green, yellowing with age. Its principal constituent is piperine, and the odour is pleasantly warm, resembling fresh peppercorns, with a characteristic 'kick' in the after-taste.

It is, as you would expect, a very warming oil and a fairly strong rubefacient, though strangely it can be used to bring down high temperatures, when used in very small amounts.

It is particularly valuable in treating disorders of the digestive tract, for it is an antispasmodic, carminative, tonic and stimulant. This means, for example, that it can be used to help a sluggish digestive system, without causing griping pains, as the antispasmodic action will soothe the smooth muscle of the gut.

It also stimulates the kidneys, and is sometimes used as a diuretic, but this is a very questionable practice as the distinction between stimulating and irritating is a very fine one, and over-use of this oil could damage the kidneys. It is also described as an aphrodisiac, but I would be inclined to advise against such use, since the amount needed to have a stimulant effect could produce kidney damage.

Oil of Black Pepper can be valuable in anaemia, as it is a stimulant of the spleen, which is involved in the production of new blood cells. This action is also of great use following heavy bleeding or severe bruising.

The main use to which I put Black Pepper is in massage blends for muscular pain, stiffness and fatigue, but it is important to keep the proportion of Black Pepper in a blend very low, as it is possible to produce local irritation by overdoing it. Because of its stimulant and tonic properties, I often include this oil in massage oils to be used by dancers and athletes. Used before training or performance, it seems to prevent pain and stiffness and possibly improves performance. Combined with Rosemary for use before running, it has been used by marathon runners, who report improved times and far less muscular fatigue and pain. Their training schedule also included massage as soon as possible after running, with a variety of blends based mainly on Lavender and Marjoram. Black Pepper can also be used with discretion in massage to help rheumatic and arthritic pain.

From the purely aesthetic point of view, in blending oils, a little Black Pepper can give an intriguing 'lift' to many blends. There is also a Green Pepper oil, with a subtler, more elusive aroma, which has the same properties and is even more interesting in blends.

Peppermint
Mentha piperata

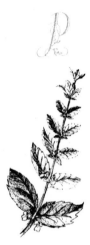

Peppermint is another plant native to Europe (although the U.S.A. now produces more essential oil than any other country) and has been widely used for thousands of years. It was used for its digestive properties by the Romans, and probably by the Egyptians before them.

The active principles of Peppermint oil include menthol – the most important element – mentone, limonene, menthene and phellandrene. English plants are said to produce the best quality oil because of our moderate climate. Although menthol is extracted and extensively used in pharmaceutical products, it is more effective when used in its 'whole' state, i.e., as an integral part of the essential oil. Commercially the oil is used in flavouring toothpaste, various medicines and, of course, in confectionery.

Peppermint is best known as a remedy for digestive upsets and has a beneficial action on the stomach, liver and intestines. It is valuable in colic, diarrhoea, indigestion, vomiting and stomach pain because of its antispasmodic action which will relieve the smooth muscles of the stomach and gut. Use it, well diluted, to massage the stomach and abdomen in a clockwise direction. Drinking Peppermint tea augments the effects of massage.

Peppermint helps colds and 'flu, particularly used in conjunction with Lavender, Marjoram and some of the other oils that are used in these conditions. Its warming and stimulating properties are particularly valuable at the onset of a cold, to combat the chilly and depressed feelings that often precede the sneezing, runny nose and feverishness. In a bath, do not use more than 3 drops, as more than this will produce a curious tingling which is more pronounced on people with sensitive skins.

Peppermint can also be used for its cooling effect in feverish conditions. This is not as paradoxical as it may seem, for the 'warming' effect is, in fact, due to the body's vigorous reaction to the cooling action of Peppermint. Peppermint also induces sweating, which reduces a fever in a natural way. It can also be used in steam inhalations to clear the nasal passages and sinuses. I like to use it combined with Lavender as each of these oils enhances the action of the other.

Steaming can also be used to cleanse and decongest the skin, especially in acne. Peppermint has a mildly antiseptic effect which helps to control the bacteria on the surface of the skin.

Cold compresses of Peppermint, or Peppermint and Lavender, applied to the forehead and temples will relieve headache, and sometimes migraine, though not all migraine sufferers can tolerate the smell once an attack has begun. The compresses are most effective if they can be applied at the first sign of pain. Both these oils are effective painkillers, but while Peppermint is stimulant, Lavender is sedative. The combination of stimulant and sedative is found in many commercial pain-killing preparations (aspirin, phenatacin and caffeine, for example), but with the important difference that essential oils do not merely suppress the pain, but work on its causes, such as blocked sinuses, a congested liver, or mental fatigue.

Peppermint is one of the oils described as 'cephalic', that is, it stimulates the brain and aids clear thinking. (Rosemary and Basil are others.) Any of these oils will physically clear the head, leaving the user feeling fresh and bright and ready for mental effort.

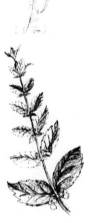

Peppermint is sometimes used as an emergency treatment for shock, because of its stimulant properties. Just put a few drops on a tissue, or inhale directly from the bottle. This can also help to relieve nausea.

Vermin, both six-legged and four-legged, dislike the strong odour of Peppermint, so it is a useful deterrent. Peppermint sprinkled on the runs of mice, rats, ants or cockroaches will offend them, and they will usually go away. You could combine the Peppermint with another strong-smelling oil, Eucalyptus for example. If you wish to get rid of pests, but do not want to take another creature's life, this offers a pleasing alternative to poisons, as well as presenting no risk to domestic animals or young children.

234

Finally, two warnings:

Peppermint should not be used if any homoeopathic remedies are being taken, and must be stored far away from such remedies, as it can antidote them.

Do not use Peppermint in the evening, as it can cause wakefulness. It is unwise to use it over long periods, as the stimulant effect is cumulative and it may cause considerable disturbance of the normal sleep pattern.

Percolation

Percolation is a relatively recently invented method of extracting essential oil from plants. It can be described as resembling distillation, with the difference that the steam is produced in a steam generator above the plant material, and percolates downwards through this. The steam and vapours are collected into a pipe which passes through a series of cooling tanks, each one of which is progressively colder than the one before. The distillate is collected and drawn off at the end of the process in a similar manner to that used in distilling.

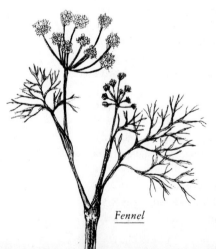

Fennel

This method is not as yet widely used, but is valuable for extracting essential oils from woody and tough material, such as the seeds from plants of the Umbelliferae family (Aniseed, Dill, Fennel, etc.). Using normal distillation methods, these take up to 12 hours to extract, but can be obtained in 4 hours using percolation. The shorter time involved also means that the plant materials are in contact with the steam for shorter periods, and this produces a better quality oil.

see also **DISTILLATION.**

Perfume

Essential oils, and other plant substances, are the oldest form of perfume known. Shakespeare's 'perfumes of Arabia' were essential oils, principally Rose, Jasmine and other flowers, which had been distilled in the Arab countries since the 10th century. Earlier cultures, without the knowledge of distillation, made infused oils from flowers and other sweet-scented plant material or pounded the plant matter with animal fats to make a perfumed pomade.

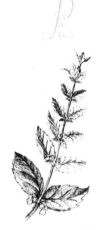

The manufacture of perfume as we know it today, using refined alcohols to dissolve the aromatic oils, has been widespread since the 17th century, with Germany and France being the most important influences. By the 19th century the commercial manufacture of perfumes was centred around the town of Grasse, which lies in the middle of a region that produces huge amounts of flowers and other aromatic plants. Because of this, Grasse has also become a centre of trade for essential oils, both for perfumery and aromatherapy, and those which are not produced in France are often imported and exported via Grasse.

235

Some of the greatest, world class classic perfumes still use essential oils as their principal perfuming
Jasmine
ingredients, especially those which were formulated in the last part of the 19th century and the early years of the 20th. More recently created perfumes are likely to be largely or wholly perfumed with synthetic substances. The synthesising of aromatic molecules has become extremely sophisticated and can match, or at least approximate, thousands of naturally occurring odours, sometimes by extracting certain constituents from several essential oils and putting them together in a different combination. We can be glad, at least, that synthetics have almost totally replaced the extracts of animal origin, such as musk and civet, which were previously used as fixatives in a great number of perfumes.

Certain aromas, of which Jasmine is one, have never been successfully synthesised, and commercial manufacturers will use a little true Jasmine absolute along with the synthetic Jasmine to give it a more authentic odour.

Although the creation of synthetic aromatic particles may be satisfactory from the perfumery point of view, they have no therapeutic application, even when these copies are made from parts of various essential oils pieced together.

Some manufacturers, usually on a relatively small scale, make a point of only using natural plant oils in their perfumes, and these are to be welcomed, as if we wish to buy commercial perfumes, we can at least feel that they are compatible with the materials of aromatherapy.

Many aromatherapists enjoy blending oils to create a perfume and such blends can be carefully made for their therapeutic value, as well as for pleasure. Virtually the whole gamut of therapeutically valuable oils are pleasing to smell, and even some of those which are not generally liked in their neat state, can contribute to a blend when used in very tiny proportions.

It is not possible to buy the kind of alcohol used in perfumery without a customs and excise licence, so a home made perfume will usually be an undiluted blend of pure essential oils. This has some advantages over an alcohol-based perfume in terms of lasting power, since the pure oils will last far longer on the skin. Only apply such perfumes to very small areas of the skin. Some of the exquisite flower absolutes make wonderful perfumes when used unblended.

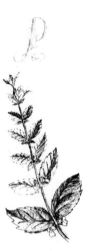

In commercial perfumery, the end product is classified according to how much aromatic material (essential oil or other) it includes in relation to the alcohol content. A perfume contains 15% to 20%, an 'eau de parfum' about 10%, eau de toilette between 4% and 6% and eau de cologne from 2% to 3%.

Theories on blending abound, including one devised by the 19th century French perfumier, Piesse, in which odours are arranged in a scale corresponding to notes on the musical stave. From this arose the very widely used notion of Top, Middle and Base notes in perfuming. The top note is what you are first aware of when you smell an essential oil, a blend, or a perfume. The middle note, or notes, give the oil, blend or perfume its main characteristics, while the base note is the longest-lasting element. There are a few essential oils which can easily be recognised as base notes, such as Patchouli, Myrrh, Jasmine and Sandalwood, but neither aromatherapists nor perfumiers are always in agreement as to which essential oils can be described as top and middle notes. Seasonal variations in the oils are partly responsible for this: for example, oil extracted from the very same plant may be described as a top note after a very sunny, dry growing season, and as a middle note when the summer has been overcast. However, these definitions are to a large degree subjective.

The best guide to blending essential oils is your own nose. Develop its sensitivity by working with very good quality oils, and excluding synthetic perfumes from your home and working environment. This is not always as easily done as might be wished, for synthetic perfumes are used in virtually all domestic products, from shampoos and washing up liquids, to floor polishes, detergents, air 'fresheners' (who needs them when we have nature's beautiful oils at our disposal?) and every imaginable kind of cosmetic.

However, alternatives do exist for all of these things, either unperfumed, or perfumed with natural plant extracts only, and it is well worth seeking them out and paying the little extra that they may cost. Your health will benefit as well as your ability to perceive perfumes and essential oils with greater subtlety.

Petitgrain

Citrus aurantium bigaradia, and other Citrus varieties.

Petitgrain oil is obtained from the bitter orange tree which also gives us Neroli, and in fact there is a 'family' resemblance between the two oils. Petitgrain is distilled from leaves and sometimes the tips of young twigs but in earlier centuries it was extracted from unripe oranges, picked when they were still green and no bigger than a cherry, hence the name 'Petit Grains', meaning little grains. This was uneconomic, as to produce enough oil to warrant the effort reduced the crop of mature oranges drastically, and the old name was gradually transferred to the oil from the leaves. Different varieties of Petitgrain are made from the Sweet Orange *(Citrus aurantium,* var. *dulce),* Lemon *(Citrus limonum),* Bergamot *(Citrus bergamia)* and Mandarin *(Citrus reticulata)* etc., and it is useful sometimes to have alternatives to the Bitter Orange variety. The best Petitgrain comes from the Mediterranean region and a cheaper grade is imported from Paraguay.

Good Petitgrain oil has a fresh, flowery, light perfume, resembling that of Neroli although less bitter. It has been compared to a good Eau de Cologne, and in fact Petitgrain enters into the formulae of some colognes. Chemically, it shares many of the constituents of Neroli, though with a higher proportion of linalol and linalyl acetate with some variation between the different types.

Most people like the aroma very much and it blends well with a wide range of other oils. I once smelt a delicious blend of Neroli, Orange and Petitgrain oils, which the therapist explained she had made because she liked the idea of bringing together the fruit, flowers and leaves of the orange.

Therapeutically, Petitgrain also resembles Neroli, though it is slightly less sedative. Even so, Petitgrain is valuable for insomnia, more so if the sleeplessness is linked to loneliness and unhappiness, rather than anxiety or an over-active mind. There is, though, one less common variety of Petitgrain – that from the Combava tree *(Citrus hystrix)* – which is very sedative and seems to help all sleeplessness, whatever the cause.

Petitgrain is decidedly antidepressant and it is good to have this alternative to Bergamot and the other antidepressant citrus oils where help is needed over a long period. (It is also worth remembering that Petitgrain is not a photosensitiser, so you can consider using it when Bergamot would be a problem.) Also, of course, tastes and needs vary and Petitgrain may be more appropriate or more acceptable to some people than some other antidepressants. I have found it particularly helpful for lonely people, those who perhaps feel a little 'down' a lot of the time, also for 'winter blues' (Seasonal Affective Disorder).

It is perhaps misleading, though, to think of Petitgrain only as an alternative to Neroli or other oils, for it is a useful aromatherapy oil in its own right. It has several applications in skin care as it helps to reduce over-production of sebum and is a gentle but effective antiseptic. This makes is a good oil for acne, also for oily dandruff: put a few drops in the final rinse after shampooing greasy hair. It is a wonderfully refreshing bath oil, with deodorant properties. It blends well with Lavender for evening baths, but I like it even more mixed with Rosemary for a 'wake up' bath in the morning.

It is a comforting oil in convalescence, and can help anybody who is run down, especially – as I have suggested above – when this is accompanied by mild but long-term depression.

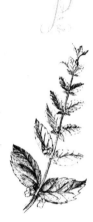

237

see also entry for **NEROLI.**

Phenols

Phenols are a class of aromatic molecules which are highly antibacterial and antiviral, also immunostimulant and tonic, but they are severely irritant to the skin and mucous membranes. If used in large amounts, or over a period of time they can damage the liver, so caution must be used with any oils containing them. Never use such oils undiluted. They include Carvacrol (the most toxic) found in Oregano, Thyme, etc.; Eugenol in Clove, Cinnamon Leaf, Black Pepper, Nutmeg, etc. and Thymol, in Thyme (large amounts) and some other oils.

Phenyl Methyl Ethers

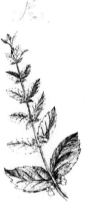

Phenyl Methyl Ethers are found occasionally in essential oils, often in traces so small they are not listed. They have similar properties to Esters but are more powerful in their action. They are usually very sedative, antispasmodic and antidepressant. They include anethol, in Fennel, Star Anise, etc.; chavicol methyl ether, in Basil, Fennel, Tarragon, etc., and eugenol methyl ether in Clove.

Photosensitisation

A small number of essential oils increase the skin's sensitivity to ultra-violet light (i.e. strong sunlight, sunbeds and other tanning devices). The combination of oil-plus-exposure can cause severe burns which are very slow to heal – taking several weeks in some cases. In a very few individuals there may be an allergic reaction.

The best-known example is oil of Bergamot, and several other oils from the Citrus group, including Lemon, Lime and Bitter Orange. Other citrus oils, such as Grapefruit, Sweet Orange and Tangerine have not been shown conclusively to be photosensitisers, but should perhaps be treated with caution. Verbena, is another oil known to have this effect, as are Rue, Angelica Root, Cumin and Opoponax. These last four are not commonly used oils while Bergamot and most of the other citrus oils have many valuable applications.

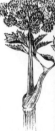

Care should be taken not to use any of these oils before exposure to strong sunshine, or using sunbeds or other sources of ultra violet light. Cases that I have seen personally indicate that the photosensitising effect lasts much longer than previously thought so do not use any of these oils on skin that is likely to be exposed to the sun or UV light within the next day or two.

Angelica

Bergamot oil has in the past been used in commercial suntanning preparations but its use was discontinued because of some evidence that it might be a cause of skin cancer. Any sunburn increases the risk of skin cancer, though it can take twenty or thirty years to develop. Damage to the ozone layer is increasing the risk of skin cancer even in temperate climates.

The photosensitising effect does not appear to operate when these oils are diluted to less than 2% so if there is a real therapeutic need for any of these oils, they could be considered provided that they are diluted to that degree.

Phytohormone

A word derived from the Greek, meaning plant hormone. Plants, like human beings, produce hormones, which can be described as 'chemical messengers'. These substances travel in the plant's sap, just as human hormones travel in the blood stream, and influence functions in another part of the organism. They are involved in growth, reproduction and many other functions.

Some plant hormones are similar to human hormones in structure and function, and plants containing them can be used to help the hormone function in our own bodies. Notable among these are fennel, hops, liquorice and willow-catkins, which all contain forms of the female hormone, oestrogen, and sarsaparilla which contains the male hormone, testosterone.

Some of the essential oils which have an aphrodisiac effect may contain plant hormones too, but there is still a great deal to be learnt about these substances and their uses. When we know more about them, the actions of certain essential oils will probably be better understood. It could well be that the oils which balance the menstrual cycle, increase the flow of breast milk, or strengthen contractions during childbirth, do so because of the presence of plant hormones.

Many of the oils which influence the female reproductive system are known to contain compounds which closely resemble oestrogen. There are no essential oils with progesterone-like compounds, but these can be found in a number of medicinal herbs, most notably Agnus Castus. Ginseng and other plants contain equivalents of the male hormone, testosterone.

see also the section on **OESTROGENS.**

Phytols

see under **INFUSED OILS.**

Phytotherapy

This term is a compound of two Greek words meaning 'plant' and 'healing' and is used to describe all forms of treatments using plants. In France, this term is used to describe what we would call Medical Herbalism, but aromatherapy is often included under the same heading. Few aromatherapists in France practise with essential oils alone, but more often combine this with the use of other herbal or plant treatments.

Pimento
Pimenta dioica (syn. P. officinalis)

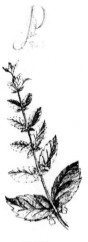

The Pimento tree is native to the West Indies and South America where its berries are widely used as a culinary spice. It is sometimes called Allspice, because the flavour is reminiscent of several other spices combined. In local folk medicine it is used for digestive problems and rheumatism. The essential oil is distilled from the leaves or berries and smells somewhat like Clove oil. Eugenol is the main constituent – up to 80% in Pimento Berry oil and as much as 96% in the oil from the leaves – with some cineol, phellandrene and caryophyllene. (Caryophyllene is also found in Clove oil, and accounts for the resemblance in smell.) The oil from the berries is preferable in aromatherapy, as it is less irritant than that from the leaves.

Pimento is not an oil I use often, but when I do the effect can be almost magic. I think of it as a 'crisis' oil, to be used in tiny amounts (often just a single drop) when dramatic help is needed very quickly. For example, one drop, well diluted and massaged clockwise over the abdomen will rapidly relieve vomiting and intestinal spasm, especially when this is associated with an emotional crisis or acute anxiety.

The effect is deeply warming, but not as 'fiery' as with some of the other spice oils. Rather, in suitably low concentrations, it produces a comforting sensation of warmth gradually penetrating the body. I never use more than 1% in a massage blend, as it is a potential skin irritant. Sometimes I add a single drop to a blend that I have already prepared if, during the course of a massage, I come across an area of the body that is cold to the touch, or which seems to be the seat of great tension or stored emotion. The rapid heating can help to disperse the cold and tightness in quite a dramatic way, though this is no substitute for paying attention to the cause of such tensions.

The same warming effect is very comforting in arthritis and rheumatism and for tired, aching muscles. In muscle spasm, Pimento will help to restore mobility quickly and I have used it to massage dancers and athletes. Massaging the chest with Pimento can calm an exhausting cough.

Not surprisingly, this is a tonic and stimulant oil, and would be helpful for extreme fatigue as long as its role as a 'crisis' oil is respected and it is not used over too long a period.

Some people have noticed an aphrodisiac effect with Pimento, not uncommon with the spice oils, but here again it should not be used to excess. The tonic/stimulant aphrodisiacs can have unwanted side effects if used repeatedly. Be that as it may, a single drop of Pimento added to Jasmine in a carrier oil is enough to make Don Juan stir in his grave!

CAUTION
Pimento is a mucous membrane irritant and must be kept well away from the mouth, nose and genitals.

Pine

Pinus sylvestris, Pinus pinaster (maritima), Abies siberica

❧

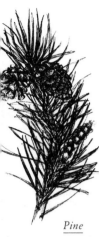

Pine

Essential oil of Pine is obtained from several species of Pine and it is very important to know the source of the oil, with its botanical name, as there are other species and varieties of Pine with very different properties and uses, and at least one, Dwarf Pine *(Pinus pumilio* or *P. mugo)* is classed as a hazardous oil. The best quality is considered to be that from trees grown as far north as possible. The oil is produced by dry distillation of the needles and sometimes the young twigs and cones. An inferior oil can be made from the wood but should not be used in aromatherapy.

The essential oil is very pale yellow with a strong, fresh, resinous aroma. The main constituent of all varieties is pinene, with carvene, sylvestrene, borneol, camphene, dipentene, phellandrene and other elements. The exact composition depends on the variety used, and to some extent the region of origin.

The chief uses of Pine are in the treatment of respiratory and urinary tract infections and muscular pain. Avicenna regarded it as a specific for pneumonia and other lung infections (though pneumonia must always be treated by a doctor). It is expectorant and a very powerful pulmonary antiseptic, helpful for bronchitis and all coughs. Use it several times a day, preferably in steam inhalations.

Inhalations of Pine are good for colds, catarrh, sinusitis and sore throats and it can either be used alone, or mixed with Eucalyptus or Ti-tree. Many people find the smell of Pine preferable to some of the other oils, so it will be welcome as an alternative.

In the bath it needs to be used with care, as some skin irritation might be experienced if the neat oil is added to the water. Pine is, of course, an ingredient of countless commercial bath preparations, but remember that in these it is presented in some form of carrier. As almost everyone will be aware from these commercial uses, Pine is refreshing, deodorant, stimulating and relieves muscular pain.

Pine has a stimulating effect on the circulation, and is sometimes used to relieve the pain of rheumatism and arthritis, as well as muscular aches from over-exertion. If you want to use it as a massage oil, blend it and use in small proportions and well diluted as higher concentrations could cause skin irritation in some people.

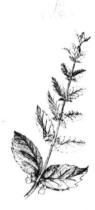

Plague

❧

The great epidemics that swept across Europe at intervals from the Black Death in the 14th century, to the Great Plague in the 17th, may not all have been of the same disease, but the major outbreaks can be identified by eye-witness accounts of the symptoms, particularly those written by contemporary physicians. The successive waves of pneumonic and bubonic plague were caused by the bacteria *Pasteurella pestis,* carried by rat-fleas. The severe fever is a disease of rodents, but it can be transmitted to humans whenever they live in close proximity to rats. As an epidemic strikes a colony of rats and the rats die, the fleas leave them to seek new host-bodies, and carry the plague with them.

The expression 'Black Death' arose from the slate-blue colour of the face which occurs in the pneumonic form of the plague, where the lungs are affected by the bacteria, and also from the dark patches caused by blood seeping underneath the skin in the bubonic form of the fever.

Stories abound of individuals or groups of people who escaped the plague due to the action of aromatic plants. Labourers who worked in the lavender fields escaped infection, and so did tanners, who used essential oils in the preparation of perfumed leathers. Gardeners working with herbs in 'Physick Gardens' were also protected from the infection, and in Toulouse a band of thieves is alleged to have stripped and robbed the bodies of plague victims without coming to harm themselves, thanks to an aromatic compound of vinegar, cloves, sage, marjoram, rosemary, juniper and camphor – all known and used in aromatherapy for their antibacterial properties – with wormwood, meadowsweet, horehound and angelica.

The cloves used in the 'Four Thieves Vinegar' are one of the most powerful antiseptics used in aromatherapy, and in the 16th and 17th centuries, an orange stuck with cloves was often used as a protection from infection. The practices of strewing floors with aromatic herbs, which gave off their volatile oils when crushed underfoot, and of carrying aromatic posies in the evil-smelling streets, were also sensible precautions, for the herbs that composed them are among some of the best bactericides known.

This information is far from being merely of historical interest, for although there has been no great outbreak of the plague since the 17th century, it is not unknown in tropical areas – there was an outbreak in India in 1994 – and a major epidemic is always a possibility if sanitation breaks down in a time of war, or after such disasters as floods or earthquakes.

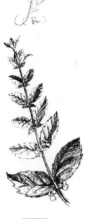

Pneumonia

Many authorities list essential oils which can be used in the treatment of pneumonia, but it would be grossly irresponsible to do so without a doctor being consulted. I know of at least one death attributable to self-treatment with essential oils for pneumonia. An acute infection of this kind is one of the situations in which the use of antibiotics can be fully justified and has dramatically reduced the death-toll from pneumonia among the young and middle-aged. Many elderly people still die from pneumonia, but this is frequently a secondary infection following other illnesses, operations or fractures, when the elderly person's powers of resistance are lowered.

Pneumonia can be a response to both bacterial and viral infection, and may follow a milder respiratory infection, such as a common cold, or may appear with no prior infection. The alveoli (see entry for LUNGS) fill with fluid, which makes breathing very difficult and reduces the efficiency of the process by which oxygen passes into the bloodstream. Indeed, from this fluid the infection can spread outside the lungs.

While medical treatment is absolutely necessary, this can be reinforced with careful use of essential oils. Eucalyptus, Lavender, Pine and Ti-tree are among those which have been used effectively, also Cajeput and Niaouli (both closely related to Ti-tree). If the patient can sit up and take steam inhalations, this would be the most effective form of treatment. Any of these oils, or a blend of two or three of them, should be gently rubbed onto the chest and back at frequent intervals – as often as half-hourly if possible. Massage should not be attempted while there is any fever present. If the patient feels well enough, a bath with one or more of these oils is a good alternative. Once all trace of fever has disappeared, vigorous massage, with tapottage, especially on the sides of the torso, can help to loosen and expel fluid from the lungs.

Pomade

see under **ENFLEURAGE.**

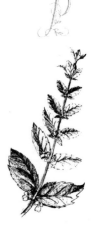

Pregnancy

When considering the use of aromatherapy during pregnancy, we should first put aside a small group of essential oils which should never be used in the first few months of pregnancy, either because they are toxic, and could possibly harm the mother and foetus, or because they involve some risk of miscarriage. Provided these oils are carefully avoided, aromatherapy techniques can be used very safely and beneficially to maintain the general health of the expectant mother, and to help minimise the various discomforts of pregnancy, such as nausea, backache, swollen legs and ankles. ,

The oils which must be avoided during the first three or four months of pregnancy include those which are described as 'emmenagogue', i.e., they induce menstrual flow, those which are recommended for use during labour to strengthen contractions, and a few rather toxic oils which could harm both the mother and the foetus. (There is some degree of overlap between these three categories.)

The oils which should NOT be used at this time are: Aniseed, Armoise (Mugwort), Arnica, Basil, Birch, Camphor, Cedarwood, Clary Sage, Cypress, Fennel, Hyssop, Jasmine, Juniper, Marjoram, Myrrh, Origanum, Pennyroyal, Peppermint, Rose, Rosemary, Sage, Savoury, Thyme and Wintergreen plus any other oil described as toxic.

Camomile and Lavender are also described as emmenagogue, but can be used with care in small amounts and well diluted (1% to 1.5%) except where the mother has reason to fear a possible miscarriage, e.g. if she has miscarried previously, there is a history of miscarriages in her family, if she has had any abnormal bleeding or other symptoms, or has been told by her doctor that there is some risk. Later in pregnancy, from about the sixth month, I have often used Lavender as it is so good at relieving backache, and Rose diluted to 1% or 1.5% as it corresponds so much to the emotional needs of many pregnant women.

A great many women experience some low back pain as their pregnancy advances, due not only to the increased weight of the baby, but to the changing shape of her own body, and the way this increases the lumbar curve of the spine. Gentle exercise, such as yoga and specific ante-natal exercises, are important, and it is also a great help to rest for at least 20 minutes each day lying flat on the back with the legs bent at the knees and supported on a chair. The thighs should be at right angles to the body, and the calves at right angles to the thighs. This position straightens out the lumbar curve and deeply relaxes the overworked muscles of the lower back. However, massage with essential oils will give a tremendous amount of relief from pain, and help to tone the muscles which are carrying the increased load. Obviously, as the baby grows, it will not be possible to lie the mother on her tummy to be massaged. It is possible to give back massage with the woman lying on her side, but I have found it more comfortable for the mother and more efficient for the masseuse if the woman sits on a stool alongside the massage couch, rests her folded forearms against the couch and leans her forehead against her arms. The masseuse then kneels on the floor behind her and can apply an effective amount of pressure to the back muscles, which is quite difficult with the mother lying on one side. The lower (lumbar) area of the back should only be massaged lightly during the first four months, but at this stage, backache is seldom a problem. By the time it is becoming a real discomfort (say, from the sixth month onwards) it is perfectly safe to massage well in this area.

The same comments apply to massage of the abdomen – work very lightly in this area – or not at all if the expectant mother has any hesitations about it – for the first four months, but after this massage is not only beneficial but very enjoyable. Very often, the developing child responds to the massage given to its mother. A lively baby which may be causing its mother some discomfort through the amount it kicks and moves around, will calm down and be still for quite a while when its mother has been massaged with a soothing, calming oil and babies whose mothers have received regular massage throughout their pregnancy are generally very peaceful when they are born.

As well as massage from a therapist or friend, the expectant mother should massage oil into her own tummy and hips each day from about the fifth month, to prevent stretch marks. Even massage with unperfumed oil, such as almond, will be helpful, but it will be both more effective and more enjoyable if 1% to 2% of essential oil is added. See the separate entry for **STRETCHMARKS** for a special formula.

For the nausea which often accompanies the first few months, ginger tea is a safe and effective remedy. Peppermint tea is better avoided, as is Peppermint oil.

Oedema (swelling) of the ankles or legs is often a problem in the latter months of pregnancy. If this is severe and persistent, a doctor or other qualified practitioner must be consulted, in case there is a serious underlying problem, but mild oedema, or puffiness of the ankles after standing or at the end of the day, can be effectively relieved by massage of the legs with oil of Geranium. This should preferably be carried out regularly by an aromatherapist, but it is also possible for the mother to apply the oils to her own legs in smooth, firm strokes, moving always from the ankles towards the thighs. Resting with the feet higher than the head is a classic remedy that should not be overlooked, and this can be carried out in the position described above, so helping backache at the same time. Avoidance of salt, coffee and strong tea will also help to reduce swelling, and it is also advisable to drink plenty of plain water (bottled or filtered).

Sometimes, the bulk and weight of the growing baby cause pressure on the veins and arteries of the lower abdomen, and give rise to circulatory problems, such as varicose veins, haemorrhoids, and (very rarely) vulvar varicosity. Resting with the legs raised, as described above, is very important, and so is the avoidance of constipation, but aromatherapy treatment is somewhat complicated by the fact that many of the oils usually used in the treatment of circulatory problems are among those to be avoided in pregnancy. However, oil of Lemon diluted to 2% can be used in gentle massage, and plenty of fresh garlic or garlic perles should be included in the diet.

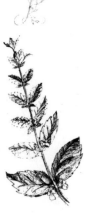

Other health problems which may arise during pregnancy, such as high blood pressure, cystitis, fainting, are dealt with under the individual entries for these subjects, and can be treated as described there, provided that the list of hazardous oils is borne in mind.

Aromatic baths can be enjoyed right throughout pregnancy, and can in fact be one of the expectant mother's greatest luxuries and forms of relaxation – once again, avoid the risky oils and also avoid over-hot water.

see also entries for **CHILDBIRTH, BABIES, BREASTFEEDING,** *etc.*

Pre-Menstrual Tension

The expression pre-menstrual tension, or pre-menstrual syndrome, is applied to a variety of disturbances experienced by many women in the week to ten days before a period is due. In extreme cases this may extend for two weeks – or half the entire menstrual cycle, beginning at mid-cycle when ovulation takes place and continuing until the start of the next period.

Physical symptoms can include mild to severe fluid retention, tenderness of the breasts, swollen abdomen, headaches and nausea, while on the emotional level many women experience depression or weepiness, irritability, food cravings, loss of concentration, while a few become violent, exhibiting dramatic personality changes.

Various essential oils and aromatherapy techniques have been very successful in reducing the severity of the problem and sometimes overcoming it altogether, though for maximum benefit it is best to combine these with a nutritional approach.

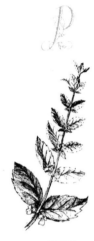

245

Lymphatic drainage massage, preferably with oils of Geranium and Rosemary, can minimise or completely prevent fluid retention. It is most effective if this type of massage is carried out twice a week for two or three weeks initially, and once a month thereafter. The timing of the monthly massage should be a day or two before the time when fluid retention is usually experienced. Women with very severe fluid retention may need two lymphatic massages a month, but this technique has been extremely successful in a large proportion of cases. Quite often, eradication of the fluid retention will make other physical symptoms disappear too, and many women have found that depression or irritability will also be less after such treatment, even though it is designed purely to treat a physical aspect of the syndrome.

Bergamot, Camomile, Petitgrain and Rose oils are very effective in reducing depression and irritability. As with so many other situations that can be helped by aromatherapy, massage is the best form of treatment, but baths are a valuable addition.

Supplementation with Evening Primrose oil and with Vitamin B6 and B complex have been very successful, but a much wider nutritional approach has been developed in the past few years with excellent results. This consists of removing all refined starches, processed foods and additives, reducing sugar, tea, coffee and alcohol intake drastically and aiming at a balanced wholefood diet, with the emphasis on fresh fruit and vegetables.

Camomile

Reducing or preferably stopping smoking also helps enormously. Ironically, the very items that need to be removed or cut down are the very ones a woman is most likely to turn to for comfort when feeling tense or low, but if she can manage without the tea, coffee, sugar, cigarette or drink she longs for, the severity of her pre-menstrual tension can be greatly reduced.

Gentle exercise, such as dancing, swimming, yoga or just going for a walk when depression or irrational anger threaten, can also be a big help.

The regime using oestrogenic oils and progesterone-like herbal remedies, which is described in the section on menstruation, has been effective for some women with pre-menstrual problems.

Pruritis

This simply means itching, but is almost always used to describe itching of the mucous membrane, especially in the genital area. Soothing and anti-inflammatory oils will ease itching in any part of the body, but it is very important indeed to remember how concentrated and potent the oils are, and that they need to be considerably diluted before being applied to such delicate tissues.

Using about 6 drops of Camomile or Lavender in the bath is the safest and most effective treatment though they can also be used as a local wash for use at intervals throughout the day if needed. The safest and most effective method is to dilute the oil in vodka, and then add a teaspoon of this mixture to one pint of boiled and cooled water.

If the itching is possibly due to thrush (candida albicans) oil of Myrrh is one of the most effective used on its own or mixed with Lavender or Ti-tree, as these are all anti-fungal oils. (Of course, it is important to treat the thrush, as well as the symptoms.) Avoid synthetic underwear or trousers as these do not allow circulation of air and will aggravate any tendency to itch.

Psoriasis

This disfiguring and distressing skin disorder is, unfortunately, one of the most intractable. Neither orthodox nor complementary medicine has had much success in doing more than alleviating symptoms temporarily and cases treated by aromatherapists have seldom shown more than slight improvement.

However, there have been some successful outcomes, so it is worth discussing what can be done to help.

The outer layer of the skin is made up of dead cells, and as these are shed in the normal wear and tear of daily living, they are replaced by cells from the layer beneath. These in turn are replaced by new cells growing in the third layer. In people with psoriasis, the new cells grow faster than the dead cells can be sloughed off, the skin appears red and thickened with a scaly appearance. The affected areas may be large or small: in the people worst affected the scaly skin may cover almost the whole body. It is not usually itchy or painful, and the distress caused to the sufferer is due to a feeling of being unclean, different or unattractive.

Psoriasis does not seem to be connected with allergies, and is not contagious. There is a hereditary factor predisposing certain people to this disorder. Stress certainly plays a very important part in the onset of psoriasis, and symptoms may come and go as the individual is more or less relaxed. For example, people who experience a great deal of stress connected with their work will improve noticeably on holiday. Sunlight has a beneficial effect on psoriasis but improvement on holiday is not connected only to this fact, as improvement has been noted after holidays in rainy or cloudy weather.

Aromatherapy is a very valuable de-stressing technique, so in this area at least can be a great help. All the sedative and antidepressant oils are suitable, though Bergamot has been reported by several therapists as being most beneficial.

Emollient creams help to reduce scaliness and improve the appearance of the skin, and rubbing the skin with a gentle exfoliant such as fine oatmeal, slightly moistened, increases the shedding of dead cells from the surface.

Naturopathic techniques for cleansing the whole body of toxins have been successful combined with aromatherapy, usually beginning with a fast on fruit juices and water and following this with a period of eating nothing but fresh, raw fruits and vegetables. Lightly cooked vegetables are introduced later and eventually a simple, wholefood eating pattern. The exclusion of alcohol, coffee, red meat and all food additives has produced very real improvement in psoriasis sufferers who have tried this. A good level of vitamin and mineral intake, with emphasis on Vitamins C, B complex and E, together with Zinc is also important, and another valuable supplement is Evening Primrose Oil (or any equivalent source of gamma linoleic acid). This can be taken in capsules or as the pure oil, also applied to the skin in the form of a cream or lotion.

The Bach Flower Remedy Crab Apple is strongly indicated, and other flower remedies can be chosen according to individual needs.

247

Psychosomatic Illness

The term psychosomatic is taken from two Greek words, 'psyche' meaning mind, and 'soma', meaning body, and is used to describe physical symptoms which are a direct result of a person's mental or emotional state.

Psychosomatic illness is not imaginary illness or 'all in the mind'. The physical illness is very real, and may manifest in such diverse forms as back pain, loss of voice, migraine, nausea, colitis, stomach ulcers and even temporary paralysis. Asthma, eczema and other allergic responses often come into this category as well, for although there may be an external trigger which provokes an asthma attack or a flare-up of eczema, it often happens that a person will have allergic reactions when under stress, but can be exposed to the same allergens without reacting when unstressed.

Anxiety about a physical symptom – particularly if a doctor has said that there is no apparent reason for it – often adds to the original stress and a vicious circle is created.

Aromatherapy is ideally suited to the treatment of psychosomatic illness, because the essential oils work on many levels, some of them very subtle. It is possible for the aromatherapist to choose oils which give some immediate relief from the physical symptoms, while acting in a more subtle way on the emotional or mental factors that have given rise to these symptoms in the first place. As virtually all forms of aromatherapy treatment are profoundly relaxing, it is possible to create a situation which is the opposite of a vicious circle. The treatment alleviates the physical discomfort and this in itself is enough to reduce the level of anxiety being experienced: the reduction of anxiety will in turn help to lessen the symptoms in the long-term.

The caring relationship between the giver and receiver of massage makes massage with essential oils the best form of treatment. Great sensitivity is needed in choosing the most suitable oils to help with the underlying stresses, but all the relaxing, anti-depressant oils offer themselves as possibilities. The physical symptoms may be a guide to the choice of oil or oils for many of them have specific actions that will be helpful on the physical plane while acting on an emotional level at the same time.

To give a few examples, Neroli has been found to help with nausea and diarrhoea where these are associated with stress, Camomile and Melissa are the two oils most commonly used to help skin allergies and both of them are deeply soothing and antidepressant too. Rose has profound effects on the emotions, and at the same time is one of the finest oils for treatment of menstrual, menopausal and other reproductive problems. Asthma attacks often respond well to oils that have subtle emotional and even spiritual connotations. Frankincense, for instance, has the physical effect of deepening and slowing the breathing – exactly what is needed physically at the moment of an asthma attack, but Frankincense is also a meditational aid and is thought to help break links with the past, particularly with painful events, and past trauma is often the root cause of asthma. Many other such parallels exist, and often less obvious ones, which the sensitive therapist will discover for him or herself in the course of working with each individual.

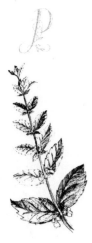

Pyelitis

❧

Pyelitis is an inflammation of the kidney, in the area where the urine drains into the ureter (the tube that carries it to the bladder). The bacteria which cause it most frequently travel up this tube as a complication of bladder infections, which is one reason why the latter must never be neglected. Like all kidney diseases, pyelitis should be treated by a doctor or other suitably qualified person, but aromatherapy treatments can be a valuable back-up. Camomile, Cedarwood, Juniper or Thyme oils should be massaged gently into the small of the back over the area where the kidneys are situated, and used in hot compresses and as bath oils. Pyelitis can often occur as a complication of cystitis, and early treatment of cystitis with essential oils is a valuable preventative measure.

Pyorrhoea

❧

An infection of the gums with discharge of pus. See the entry under **GINGIVITIS** for suitable treatment.

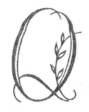

Quality

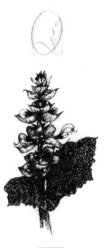

The quality of essential oils which are to be used therapeutically is of prime importance. If they are to be used for perfumery the following criteria are less important, but it remains true that to make fine perfumes, you also need fine essential oils. Unfortunately, it is not difficult to adulterate essential oils, to reproduce them synthetically, or to make 'reconstituted' oils from elements extracted from a variety of plant sources. These oils may be satisfactory for some perfuming requirements but the therapist, and anybody who wishes to use essential oils to promote their own health, must be sure that the materials they use have not been tampered with in any way.

The best way to be certain of this is to buy from suppliers who know the sources of the oils they sell, either by importing directly or by dealing through a very reputable importer who can give them the necessary guarantees. Alternatively, a supplier or importer may have samples of each batch tested in a laboratory by means of gas chromo-spectography, which identifies any 'foreign' element in the sample.

An essential oil which has not been altered in any way since distillation, may also carry traces of chemical contaminants if the plants from which it was extracted were grown with artificial pesticides, herbicides or fertilisers. The best safeguard against this is to buy only oils which have been extracted from wild or organically grown plants. Fortunately, an increasing number of growers, importers and suppliers are aware of these factors, and can provide essential oils of guaranteed origin.

Another problem is that confusion may arise over the botanical species from which the oil has been obtained. Closely related plants, those with similar names, and the use of local names in different countries contribute to this. It is, obviously, very important to be sure that the oil you are using is indeed obtained from the plant whose therapeutic properties you had in mind when choosing that oil, and the only way to be certain of this is to use the Latin botanical names for the plants. By doing so, you will avoid such pitfalls as Spanish Marjoram, which is a variety of Thyme; Moroccan Camomile (*Camomile Maroc*) which is not a camomile at all, although it has similar properties; and the use of 'Marigold' to describe both the common marigold of English gardens (*Calendula officinalis*) which has valuable skin-healing virtues, and the French and African marigolds (several varieties of Tagetes) whose properties and smell are entirely different. Even more serious is the fact that some producers and exporters of essential oils resort to various mixtures and adulterations of oils for economic reasons.

It is also important to know from which part of the plant the oil has been extracted, since the active constituents, or the proportions in which they are present, may vary from one part of the plant to another, with consequent variations in the usefulness or safety of the oil. Juniper oil, for example, must be extracted from the berries though a lower-grade oil can be obtained from the twigs.

Even an oil which is quite truthfully described as pure may be of poor quality, and therefore of less value therapeutically. If an essential oil costs much less than you would normally expect to pay for it, the oil may well be a third or fourth distillate from a batch of plant material which has already yielded the greater part of its properties to the first or second distillation. Some of the more volatile elements in an oil will all be extracted in the first distillation, meaning that the chemical composition of a second or subsequent extraction will be different.

The best safeguard is to buy from suppliers who can unequivocally tell you:

The country or region of origin.

The botanical name of the plant.

The part of the plant used, where relevant.

The method of extraction.

Whether the plant is wild or organically grown.

The supplier should know the 'chain' of supply, i.e. through whose hands each batch of oil has passed between the plant and the bottle to ensure that no skullduggery has taken place en route. Some suppliers will be able to give you specific guarantees on these points. They may use laboratory testing (gas chromo-spectography) to be certain of the composition and purity of the oils, or they may buy only from exporters who test in this way, or direct from organic growers. They should also understand the proper conditions for storing and handling essential oils, and not keep them in stock for excessively long periods, so that the oils reach you in optimum condition.

As a rough-and-ready guide, especially if you are buying retail and cannot question the supplier, look for simple but informative labelling (botanical name, part of plant, country of origin, organic or wild grown). Compare price-lists of a number of suppliers so that you have a good idea of the normal price for any particular oil, and do not buy anything that is very much cheaper.

The best quality oils will, not surprisingly, cost more than those without the safeguards outlined above, but when we bear in mind the very small amounts used in each treatment, and the great responsibility we have towards the people we treat, the difference falls into perspective. As therapists, we must have oils we can use with a clear conscience and complete confidence.

A list of reliable suppliers is given in **APPENDIX D**.

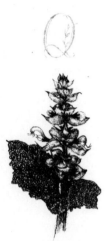

Quantities

The quantity of essential oil used in any form of treatment is very small, and modern practice tends towards the use of even less than was common even a decade ago. Dr. Jean Valnet has said that 'While not speaking here of homeopathy, I have found that the smaller amount of essential oils used, the more potent are its effects.'

For massage, it is most usual to use a dilution of 3% essential oil in a vegetable carrier oil, i.e. 3 drops of essential oil to every 100 drops of carrier, so it is very easy to remember 3 drops to each teaspoon (but be sure it is a full 5 ml measuring teaspoon, as domestic spoons may hold much less). 5 mls of carrier oil will be quite enough to do a face massage and 20 to 25 mls will suffice for a full body massage.

In the bath, great care needs to be taken over the quantities used, since the oil is NOT DILUTED IN THE WATER but floats on top in an ultra-thin film. Too much can irritate the skin. How much is too much, will of course vary according to the oil, and because some people have more sensitive skins, but a safe maximum is 6 drops of most oils. Citrus oils, and those which have a 'lemon' scent, even though not from the citrus family, such as Lemongrass, Lemon Verbena and Melissa, need to be restricted to 2 or 3 drops only; and oils from spice plants, such as Cinnamon, Clove, Nutmeg, etc. avoided altogether in the bath. 10 drops is often given as a maximum, and this may be safe for oils which are non-irritant and non-sensitising. Photo-sensitising oils should always be diluted before adding to bath water. If preparing a bath for a baby or young child, it is very important to DILUTE THE OIL BEFORE ADDING IT TO THE BATH, and to use not more than 2 or 3 drops in total.

For other applications to the skin, such as in creams and lotions, the dilution is usually similar to that used in massage.

In steam inhalations, a single drop to a bowl of hot water may be enough, and 3 or 4 drops is the maximum. Try one drop only the first time you prepare an inhalation, and if this is well tolerated, you can try increasing the amount to 2 or 3 drops if you feel a stronger inhalation would be more helpful. If using an electric steamer, a single drop of oil is plenty.

Ginger

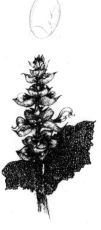

see also *under the* INDIVIDUAL FORMS OF TREATMENT *mentioned.*

Quinsy

An old name for an abscess surrounding the tonsil, although in some old books this is confused with diphtheria.

Such abscesses are rare now, as tonsillitis and other throat infections are usually treated promptly before such complications arise.

Inhalations and frequent gargles, especially with oils of Thyme, Lemon or Ginger, are an effective treatment for all kinds of sore and infected throats. Thyme is perhaps the most important because it is not only a very powerful antiseptic, but is also a mild local anaesthetic, which will ease the pain in the throat at the same time.

High doses of Vitamin C for a few days are usually very effective in clearing up throat infections quickly.

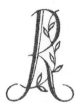

Radiation

❧

We are all subject to various forms of radiation all the time, from the sun, radioactive minerals in the earth's crust, and other natural sources. This has always been so, long before radiation or the nature of radioactive substances was understood. This 'background' radiation is probably not enough to be harmful, but human inventions, from nuclear weapons and power plants to microwaves and T.V. screens are adding to it all the time, and I am sure that nobody reading this book needs to be told the frightening implications of this.

The following formula is not, in fact, aromatherapy, but incorporates Bach Flower Remedies, and I feel it is well worth including in this book as it can be used to counteract side-effects by cancer patients who have received radiation therapy.

DR. WESTLAKE'S FORMULA
Mix 3.5 gms of sea salt with 100 mls of distilled water. Put into a 10 ml dropper bottle 2 drops of each of the following Bach Flower Remedies: Cherry Plum, Gentian, Rock Rose, Star of Bethlehem, Vine, Walnut and Wild Oat, and top up the bottle with the sea salt solution.

Take 2 drops, 3 or 4 times a day, or add 10 to 15 drops to a bath.

People who have been exposed to a radiation source, such as X-rays, cobalt therapy or other medical radiation therapies, or have been contaminated in an escape from a nuclear power station or processing plant, should follow this treatment for two weeks. Those who regularly use office or domestic equipment that gives out low-level radiation, such as colour television sets, microwaves, and visual display units, would do well to use this formula in a bath once or twice a week.

see also the entries for **CANCER** *and* **X-RAYS**.

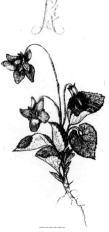

Ravensara
Ravensara aromatica

❧

Ravensara is a tall forest tree native to Madagascar, also found in cultivation on the island of Reunion and in Mauritius. Its name is compounded from two Malagassy words: 'ravina' meaning leaf, and 'tsara' meaning good. All parts of the tree are strongly aromatic and the local people have used the bark, leaves and fruit as flavourings and medicines since time immemorial. The French scientist, Baumé, distilled an oil from the bark as long ago as the 18th century, but Ravensara has only really come into use in aromatherapy since the 1980s.

The oil is extracted from the leaves by a very long, slow steam distillation and it contains principally cineol (between 60% and 75%), with some pinene, terpineol, linalol and eugenol. The oil is almost colourless with an aroma that I can best describe as a more delicate version of Rosemary.

Ravensara is a multi-action oil, to the extent that it could be compared with Lavender and, like Lavender, it is often more effective in blends than when used alone. It is a completely safe oil and can be used for anybody, including children.

It is, above all, antiviral and immunostimulant. It is particularly effective against 'flu and 'flu-like virus infections, especially if used at the first sign of shivering, etc. A few drops in the bath immediately before going to bed will often avert an attack of 'flu and if that is not possible, Ravensara used intensively (in massage, baths and inhalations) can often stop 'flu in one day. It is used by medically-trained aromatherapists (mainly in France) to treat viral hepatitis and viral enteritis. This is not something the non-medical aromatherapist should attempt to do: I mention it here to demonstrate the high antiviral activity of Ravensara. It is active against some bacteria, but the action is not as consistently successful as it is against viruses. I have used Ravensara in my vaporiser during a particularly virulent 'flu epidemic and remained well throughout. It has a much pleasanter smell than some of the antiviral oils.

It is good for all respiratory tract infections, such as sinusitis and catarrh (also earache when it has originated with nasal catarrh), and where the infection affects the chest, as in bronchitis, whooping cough, etc., the fact that Ravensara is a good expectorant is useful. It is even more so if used in blends with other suitable oils such as Myrtle, Pine, Thyme, etc.

The strong antiviral action and the fact that Ravensara is safe on the skin, make it a good oil for cold sores, shingles and genital herpes. For genital herpes it is best in a blend with Helichrysum in a base of St. John's Wort oil and for shingles in a blend with Lavender and Camomile to help the pain.

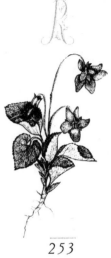

253

It is a muscle relaxant and analgesic, good for joint pains and muscular tension, especially when this is linked to anxiety. It is both mentally and physically stimulating, and could be a good oil to help people who are overtired, or depressed and lethargic.

Reflexology

Many aromatherapists use reflexology in conjunction with essential oil treatments, and the two therapies are certainly very compatible.

Reflexology is based on the principle that various reflex points or zones on the feet affect, and are affected by, different parts and organs of the body. A knowledge of these zones allows the therapist to use them both to identify and to treat areas of weakness. The theory and method were first codified by an American therapist, Eunice Ingham earlier this century, drawing on traditions going back to ancient Egypt.

Firm but gentle pressure with a thumb or finger is applied systematically over the whole surface of each foot in turn. Where a problem or weakness exists in any organ or area of the body a trained reflexologist can feel tiny granules or crystals in the corresponding reflex zone. Continuing to apply pressure until any initial discomfort has dispersed has a beneficial effect on the organ.

No essential oil or carrier oil is used in a reflexology treatment, so it cannot be considered as an integral part of aromatherapy treatment, though some therapists use modified reflexology movements during an oil massage. Many use reflexology either to diagnose areas of possible weakness to guide them in their choice of oils and treatment, or to reinforce the effect of the general treatment with essential oils.

It is also possible to apply essential oils to specific reflex points in order to treat the areas connected with these points, although this is not strictly speaking reflexology. This can be a very useful form of self-treatment, as it allows treatment of areas that would be difficult to reach for self-massage, such as the neck and back.

Rejuvenation

The idea of restoring lost youth has appealed to mankind since the earliest times, and many attempts have been made to find an elixir which will either prolong life, or make the old become young.

There is no evidence that aromatherapy can prolong the expectation of life, but if we accept that 'Death is certain: the time of death uncertain' we can, with essential oils, maintain health, appearance and activity, both mental and physical, well beyond the point at which slow decline is usually regarded as inevitable.

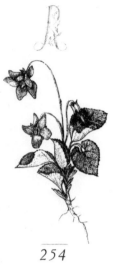

It may be more accurate to speak of delaying the ageing process than of rejuvenation, and certainly the best time to tackle the question of ageing is while still relatively young and vigorous. However, both Dr. Jean Valnet and Marguerite Maury relate impressive case histories in which senility – both mental and physical – has been reversed, and their patients continued in an active and enjoyable life to an advanced age. Maury also refers to young people – even children – who are 'old' in terms of physical debility, and applies the term rejuvenation to their treatment.

All essential oils are, to a certain extent, cytophylactic, i.e. they promote the growth of healthy new cells, and it is at the cellular level that degeneration, which we tend to think of as inevitable with age, begins. Individual cells of the body may live for a few days, or for several months, depending on the type of cell and the work it does, and continuing health and vitality depend on these cells being replaced all the time. Infection, poor nutrition, environmental and other factors, as well as increasing age, all lead to a slowing down of cell reproduction. Worse, new cells may be formed in a damaged or distorted form, and the organs and systems of the body function less efficiently. This diminishing efficiency of the body is often thought of as unavoidable, but in fact much can be done to prevent it.

The most powerfully cytophylactic oils are Lavender and Neroli, and regular use of such oils, particularly in baths and massage, can help to maintain cellular reproduction at the levels which occur naturally in youth, and in this way vigour and healthy functioning follow.

The daily use of essential oils in the home, in baths, diffusers, burners or other means, is an excellent way of keeping infection at bay, and increasing resistance to infection, and this alone can be an important contribution to maintaining a healthy, and therefore 'youthful' body.

Essential oils can also be used to treat many of the degenerative diseases associated with age – arthritis and rheumatism, sciatica and chronic bronchitis to name but a few.

Other oils balance hormone levels, and can be very helpful for women at and after the menopause. Yet others can calm or stimulate the central nervous system, or individual organs – heart, stomach, lungs, liver, etc., or have a toning and stimulating effect on the mind, helping to prevent such problems as loss of memory or concentration.

The outward signs of ageing, in particular wrinkles and sagging skin, can be reduced, and to a certain degree even reversed, by skin treatments with oils such as Frankincense, Sandalwood, Jasmine and Rose, as well as Lavender and Neroli which have already been mentioned.

We should not overlook the importance of really good nutrition. The cells cannot function and reproduce efficiently without a wide range of nutrients, including proteins and the amino acids found in them, and the whole range of vitamins, minerals and trace elements. A well trained aromatherapist will either be able to suggest an anti-ageing eating plan, or refer clients to a qualified nutritionist. Nobody knows for certain how much chemical additives and pollutants in our food, water and air contribute to premature ageing, but there is growing evidence that they do, and it makes good sense to avoid them as far as possible. This can be done by eating, as far as possible, foods which have been grown organically, are as fresh as possible, and have had nothing added to them or taken away from them. Cooking destroys many nutrients, and distorts others, so try to eat at least half of your food raw. A basic vegetarian diet, with a little white meat and fish added if you wish, is best. I would add a word of caution, though, about methods of meat production. Most animals reared for slaughter have been fed on chemically-sprayed plants and have had antibiotics routinely added to their foods: they may also have had growth or sex hormones injected or implanted, even though this is illegal in many countries. So, in eating their meat, you may be taking in a large load of unseen chemicals. If you do not object morally to meat eating, it is possible to find organically reared meat from a number of sources.

Exercise is essential, not only to maintain firm muscles but to ensure a good supply of oxygen to every cell in the body. Without oxygen we die. With a reduced oxygen supply cells function less efficiently. Exercise does more than anything else to ensure that we take in plenty of oxygen and that our heart pumps it effectively round the body, carried in our blood-stream.

Adequate rest and proper relaxation are important, too. Stress and tension reduce the body's efficiency faster than anything else. And here we come back to aromatherapy, for massage and essential oil baths are among some of the best de-stressing techniques available.

But, perhaps the most important thing of all is a young mind.

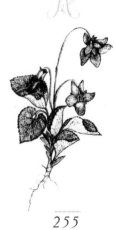

Lavender

255

Relaxation

A very high proportion of the people who turn to aromatherapy for help are suffering symptoms caused by stress. Massage is a wonderful way to help release stress, and bring the receiver into a state of deep relaxation, but unless the individual learns some method of controlling stress and letting go of tensions, the problems will be recurrent and massage will act only as a palliative.

Many aromatherapists now include some instruction in simple relaxation techniques as a regular part of treatment, while others may suggest a local teacher or centre where such techniques can be learned. Yoga, Autogenics and 'Relaxation for Living' are among the most effective methods, and all are easily available in most parts of the country.

Specially recorded tapes which take the listener through a relaxation sequence can also be a good back-up to aromatherapy massage, though I don't think they can be compared to working with a live teacher. They are helpful if a method has already been learned from a teacher, to help practice it at home.

Repetitive Strain Injury (R.S.I.)

Repetitive strain injury is a painful and disabling condition which is unfortunately becoming more and more prevalent. As the name implies, it it due to performing the same movement repeatedly. The joints most often affected are the wrists, or wrists and elbows. The people most at risk are typists and computer operators, though the worst case I have treated affected a young woman who spent hours each day pulling a lever on a machine that cut out soles for shoes. Any repetitive movement, though, can give rise to the condition. Little was heard of R.S.I. before computers and electronic typewriters became standard equipment in offices – and many homes. This is because many more strokes per minute can be made on these machines than on old-style manual typewriters.

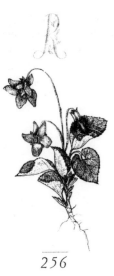

R.S.I. is sometimes confused with tenosynovitis (q.v.) but the two are not quite the same thing. Tenosynovitis (inflammation of the tendons and their surrounding sheath), most often affecting the wrist, is the major part of the problem, but in cases of R.S.I. that I have treated there has always been strain or damage to muscles as well. However, the treatment for tenosynovitis is the same as for R.S.I.

All anti-inflammatory oils can help, particularly German Camomile and Birch. Of the two, I have found Birch the most helpful. The fact that it is such a powerful analgesic makes it very welcome, but it is very important that it is not used to override pain and continue working. Rest is an essential part of any treatment, and the worst possible thing anybody with R.S.I. can do is to continue carrying out the same repetitive movements that caused it in the first place. To continue using the arm makes the inflammation worse, and can cause it to spread up the tendons until the upper arm is affected as well. The severity of many reported cases – often amounting to permanent disablement – is sadly due to the fact that many people affected by R.S.I. are afraid of losing their jobs, and try to carry on working, perhaps with the aid of elastic supports and painkillers.

Cold compresses of German Camomile should be used to reduce the inflammation as soon as possible after the first signs of trouble. The more often these are applied in the initial stages the better – not less than three or four times a day. Gentle massage with an analgesic oil, preferably Birch, will ease the pain. Later, many sufferers find hot compresses more comforting, and you might try alternate hot and cold compressing to stimulate healing. Deep massage, following the line of the tendon, is temporarily painful, but reduces pain and helps healing in the long run. I use Birch for this, too, as it makes the massage more bearable while its anti-inflammatory action works on the root cause.

Recovery is never quick, and treatment may need to be kept up for many months, so varying the oils will always be necessary. However, I would suggest returning to German Camomile and Birch as often as possible, since they seem to give far more relief than any other oils.

Aromatherapy alone may not be enough to bring about healing in every case and I would strongly recommend acupuncture as well. I have seen good recovery from R.S.I.

when these two systems were used in conjunction. Homoeopathic Arnica and Rhus Tox, taken internally and used in creams have been very effective for some people, though obviously a bit of juggling needs to be done if you want to use homeopathy and aromatherapy. One possible approach might be to use the homoeopathic creams for a week or so while taking a break from the oils. Arnica or Rhus Tox tablets can be taken concurrently with using essential oils provided they are not used within a hour or so of each other. Some people find one more effective than the other, and the only recommendation I can make is to try each in turn and observe the results.

Each person with a repetitive strain injury needs to be seen as an individual, in the context of their lifestyle and – especially – their work, and individual solutions found that work for them.

Respiratory System

This refers to the various organs and tubes through which air is taken in, processed and breathed out again. It comprises the nose, throat (divided into pharynx, larynx and trachea), the bronchial passages and lungs. In the lungs, the inhaled air gives up most of its oxygen to the blood, together with some other substances that are inhaled in the air. Carbon dioxide and other waste is extracted from the blood, also in the lungs, and exhaled.

This process, and its importance in understanding the effects of essential oils, is discussed in the entries for **LUNGS** and **NOSE**.

Disorders of the Respiratory System are discussed in the entries for **ASTHMA**, **BRONCHITIS**, **CATARRH**, **COLDS**, **COUGHS**, **INFLUENZA**, **LARYNGITIS**, **PNEUMONIA** and **SINUSITIS**.

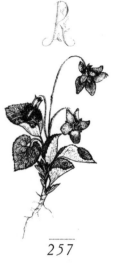

257

Rheumatism

The term rheumatism is used medically to include a whole group of disorders that involve pain in the muscles or joints, including rheumatism, the various forms of arthritis, gout and fibrositis. General use, however, distinguishes between those that involve joint pain (arthritis and gout) and those in which the pain is experienced mainly in the muscles (rheumatism and fibrositis) which are discussed here.

Anti-rheumatic essential oils include those which give local relief from pain and those which help to eliminate some of the toxins which are involved in rheumatic conditions as causes of pain. Any of the analgesic oils can be helpful locally, but those which have been found most effective are Camomile, Lavender, Marjoram and Rosemary. Hot compresses give considerable relief, but should not be relied on as the only, or main, form of treatment, as the repeated application of heat may lead to congestion in the area which will eventually make the condition worse. Massage should be given as often as possible, to stimulate local circulation and thus remove toxins more effectively. Baths are always a good back-up treatment, and this is perhaps the best way of using those oils which aid elimination of toxins. Juniper is the most important of these, but Cypress,

Marjoram

Lavender and Rosemary are almost as valuable.

If the sufferer can bear it, the application of alternate hot and cold compresses is very beneficial.

Dietary adjustment, such as described for arthritis, is important.

see also entry for **ARTHRITIS.**

Ringworm

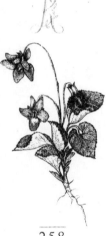

Ringworm is caused by a fungal infection, similar to athlete's foot. A number of different fungus organisms may be responsible. It can occur on any part of the body, but is particularly distressing when it affects the scalp, causing temporary patches of baldness.

An anti-fungal oil, such as Myrrh or Lavender should be prepared in a cream and applied to the infected area of skin four times a day. Some of the organisms respond better to Myrrh and others to Lavender, so you may wish to combine the two rather than wait to see which is the most effective. A fairly high proportion of the oils in a cream is needed: about 5% is usually effective.

Both these oils also have a healing action on the skin, so they will help to restore the dry flaky rings that persist after the fungus has been eradicated. If the ringworm has affected the scalp, you may need to replace the cream with a preparation including oil of Rosemary once there is no more sign of infection, to encourage new hair to grow. You could use small amounts of Rosemary oil neat rubbed into a small area, rosemary water as a friction for the whole scalp, or make up a mixture of Rosemary oil in alcohol and use this as a friction. Ti-tree can be used instead of Lavender and Myrrh, or alternated with them.

Rose
Rosa centifolia and Rosa damascena, var. Kazanlik

The rose was probably the first flower from which an essential oil was ever distilled, in 10th century Persia. The great Arab physician, Avicenna, is credited with having distilled the first Rose oil, possibly by chance during the course of alchemical experiments. The rose has considerable significance in the theoretical and metaphysical aspects of alchemy, with red and white roses each being thought appropriate to different stages of the alchemist's work, and for this reason they were placed in retorts and heated with a variety of different materials in the attempt to transmute base metals into gold, producing rosewater and essential oil almost accidentally in the process. Whether or not Avicenna himself did make this discovery (and he was an alchemist, as well as a physician, poet, astronomer and mathematician) rosewater and oil were known in Arab speaking countries by the end of that century.

At the present day, the major production of essential oil of Rose is not by distillation (which yields only very small amounts of essential oil as a secondary product during the extraction of rosewater) but by the enfleurage method or solvent extraction. The very high price of Rose oil is due to the huge quantity of rose petals needed to extract a tiny amount of oil, and the very high labour costs involved in this method of extraction. However the 'attar' or 'otto of roses' extracted in this way is so highly concentrated that only a very small amount is needed for each treatment. The attar is solid in the bottle at average room temperatures, only turning into a thick oil when the bottle is warmed in the hands. It is a deep reddish-brown, and needs to be used sparingly, for its perfuming power is very great indeed.

Two varieties of rose are used commercially for the production of oil of Rose: *Rosa centifolia* and *Rosa damascena,* and slight variations of aroma and colour will be found in the oils made from the different varieties, from a greenish-orange to a deep browny-red. *Rosa damascena*, var. *Kazanlik* is grown in huge quantities in Bulgaria for oil production while *Rosa centifolia* is grown in the area around Grasse, the heart of the French perfume industry, and in North Africa, the product from which is known as Rose Maroc.

Rose oil has an extraordinarily complex chemistry, with over 300 known constituents, which make up about 86% of the whole. The remaining 14% comprises a large number of different compounds, each in miniscule amounts, but they are vital to the whole oil, both from the point of view of its perfume and its therapeutic properties. There is a marked difference in the chemistry of the two types: *Rosa damascena,* (Bulgarian type) has between 35% and 55% of citronellol, 30% to 40% is made up of geraniol and nerol, 16% to 22% stearopten, 1.5% to 2.0% phenyl ethanol, 0.2% to 2% farnesol, plus traces of a very large number of other compounds. *Rosa centifolia* (French or Moroccan type) has up to 63% phenyl ethanol, 18% to 22% citronellol, 10% to 15% geraniol and nerol, 8% stearopten, up to 2% farnesol and, again, large numbers of traces. While the properties of the two types do overlap to a large extent, the differing chemistry accounts for some variations. The French type is more aphrodisiac, more sedative and more bactericidal than the Bulgarian.

The rose has traditionally been called the 'Queen of Flowers' and in aromatherapy, Rose oil is often thought of as the queen among essential oils. Nicholas Culpeper described the rose as being governed by Venus, and the area in which Rose oil is used in aromatherapy, in preference to all other oils, is in treating disorders of the female reproductive system. Many essential oils have a therapeutic affinity with a particular organ of the body, and it is not surprising that Rose, with its 'feminine' qualities, has a powerful effect on the uterus. It is cleansing, purifying, regulating and tonic, and is valuable where there is loss of uterine muscle tone; for example, in slight prolapse (combined with suitable exercises such as some of the inverted postures of yoga), or for women who have a tendency to miscarry.

However, women with serious gynaecological problems are less likely to seek help from an aromatherapist than those who have irregularities of the menstrual cycle, or who are tense, depressed or sad, and these are areas where oil of Rose is supremely valuable.

It can be used to regulate the menstrual cycle where this is irregular, and to reduce excessive loss. Rose is thought to aid conception, and it is certainly helpful where it is difficult to predict ovulation dates because of an irregular cycle. Rose also, perhaps surprisingly, appears to increase the production of semen.

However, the physical effects of Rose oil are perhaps less important than its effects on the mental/emotional level. It is a

Rose

259

gentle but potent antidepressant, and as you might expect from the preceding paragraphs, and from its generally 'feminine' qualities, it is especially helpful where an emotional disturbance is linked to female sexuality or the reproductive cycle. It is one of the oils which is valuable in helping women suffering from post-natal depression, or depression following the break-down of a relationship, particularly if the woman needing help is experiencing grief rather than anger at the situation.

From my own observation, this is a very valuable oil for any woman who is not secure in her own sexuality, whether her insecurity is expressed as a lack of confidence in her own desirability, reluctance to acknowledge herself as a sexually mature person (for example, in cases of anorexia) or difficulties within an established relationship.

Kazanlik Rose

Rose has long been renowned as an aphrodisiac, and the Romans used to scatter rose-petals on the bridal bed, a custom that has degenerated into throwing paper rose-petals at weddings. Given this, and the other properties discussed already, it is not surprising that oil of Rose is used to help women suffering from frigidity and to help with male impotence. Marguerite Maury distinguished between French and Bulgarian Rose in this respect, describing the French as a more powerful aphrodisiac, and in fact the differing chemistry of the two types confirms this.

Rose has a powerful tonic effect on the nervous system, and on the stomach, liver and spleen, but is generally less used for these purposes, as there are other essential oils which are equally effective and far less expensive. In the sphere of reproduction and sexuality, Rose is unique in its action and will always be the first choice of oil for treatment, in spite of its price.

It is also a very good oil for use in skincare. It can be used for all skin types, but it is especially valuable for dry, sensitive or ageing skins. It has a tonic and astringent effect on the capillaries and in fact on the circulation generally which makes it useful for diminishing the redness caused by enlarged capillaries (often known as 'thread-veins') in the cheeks, though treatment needs to be kept up every day for many weeks, or even months, before a real improvement can be expected.

Rosewater is soothing, antiseptic and tonic to the skin, a pleasing light perfume, and is also an effective antiseptic for eye infections.

The delicious perfume of Rose makes it popular in skin preparations, too, but unfortunately leads some commercial manufacturers to use synthetic rose perfumes in many bath and skincare products. When you are buying creams, lotions, perfumes, bath essences, etc., either for yourself or to use in treatments, it is unfortunately true that if the product is cheap, the perfume is almost certainly synthetic and totally lacking in any of the therapeutic properties of Rose. The perfume industry uses each year more than the world's annual production of Rose oil… so where does the rest come from? It is, unfortunately, quite difficult to detect adulterated Rose oil, even with gas chromo-spectography. Your nose is probably the best guide.

It is not difficult to make your own creams, etc., and perfume them with just a drop or two of the concentrated attar. Although it may be expensive to buy initially, very little needs to be used to produce both the perfuming and the healing effects, so your oil will last a very long time.

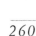

One final word of warning: most Rose absolute is now produced by solvent extraction and is likely to contain traces of chemical solvents that are potentially toxic. If you possibly can, try to find distilled Rose oil, or an absolute that has been extracted by the carbon dioxide method.

Rosehip

Rosa rubiginosa

The cold-pressed oil from Rosehip seeds contains between 30% and 40% gamma linoleic acid (G.L.A.), which has valuable uses in treating skin problems such as eczema and psoriasis, and is needed by the body to manufacture oestrogen. G.L.A. supplements are widely used to help menstrual and menopausal problems. Rosehip seed oil can be used as a carrier oil with very small amounts of essential oil added, as a massage oil in its own right, or added to other vegetable oils or infused oils in blends.

Rosemary

Rosmarinus officinalis and *R. pyramidalis*

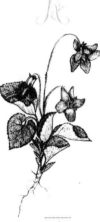

After Lavender, Rosemary is probably the most important plant of the Labiatae family used in aromatherapy. The bush, with its silver-green needle shaped leaves and pale blue flowers, grows freely all over Europe, but is most at home near the sea. This is reflected in its name, which is taken from two Latin words (ros + marinus) meaning 'dew of the sea', for the plant was originally a native of the Mediterranean coast. Legend says that the flowers were once white, but that they turned blue after the Virgin Mary hung her cloak on a rosemary bush when the Holy Family stopped to rest on the flight into Egypt.

Rosemary was one of the earliest plants to have been used in medicine, and this undoubtedly overlapped with its use in cooking and in religious rites. The country people in ancient Greece, who did not have access to prepared incense, burnt sprigs of Rosemary on their shrines, and it was often called the 'incense bush'. The Romans, too, revered it as a sacred plant, and traces have been found in Egyptian tombs. The perfume of Rosemary does bear some resemblance to that of Frankincense. Both are very penetrating. It was used throughout the Middle Ages to smoke out devils during exorcisms, and continued to be burnt in sickrooms as a fumigant for many centuries. The practice of burning Rosemary in hospital wards in France, persisted into the present century, ironically being abandoned at about the same time that modern research proved its antiseptic properties. Because of its strong antiseptic action, Rosemary can delay or prevent putrefaction in meat, but we shall never know whether it was first used in cooking for the flavour or to preserve meat in distant times, when there was no refrigeration or other means of keeping cooked meat fresh in a hot climate.

Rosemary

Rosemary oil may be distilled from the flowering tips or the leaves, though an inferior oil is sometimes extracted from the whole plant. Like Thyme, this is a plant with quite variable chemistry but a typical example would include camphor,

261

borneol, pinene and cineol though not necessarily in that order. Some samples of wild Rosemary have mostly cineol and pinene, and there is a chemotype with mainly verbenone. *R. pyramidalis* also has cineol and pinene as its main constituents. The essential oil is pale straw coloured, with a strong and piercing aroma. It is a stimulating oil, both warm and penetrating in its odour and its actions. Poor quality samples may be adulterated with Eucalyptus oil.

The stimulant effect of Rosemary on the central nervous system is very marked, and for this reason Rosemary is used where there is loss or reduction of functions, such as loss of smell; where the sensory nerves have been affected; for some kinds of speech impairment; and for temporary paralysis, where the motor nerves are affected. Of course, if the nerve cells are permanently damaged, as in injuries to the spinal cord, paralysis is irreversible. Rosemary is also an excellent brain stimulant (the brain being, of course, the most vital part of the central nervous system). Ophelia in 'Hamlet' says 'There's rosemary, that's for remembrance' and Rosemary has long had the reputation of improving memory. Inhaling a few drops of this oil certainly produces a feeling of great mental clarity, which undoubtedly aids all thought processes. Nicholas Culpeper wrote in his Herbal: 'The oil drawn from the leaves and flowers is a sovereign help . . . to touch the temples and nostrils with two or three drops for all the diseases of the brain spoken of before; as also to take one drop, two, or three as the case requires, for the inward disease; yet it must be done with discretion, for it is very quick and piercing, and therefore but little must be taken at a time.'

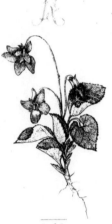

The piercing quality of Rosemary makes it valuable for respiratory problems, ranging from the common cold, catarrh and sinusitis, through to asthma. For these it is best used as a steam inhalation – its ability to 'clear the head' works on the physical as well as the mental plane.

The Rosemary Verbenone chemotype is even more effective at clearing catarrh than standard Rosemary. It is less stimulant generally, and especially less of a mental stimulant, so it can be used in the evening. It is, though, more likely to be skin irritant, so it would be wise to dilute it before adding to baths.

Culpeper also says that Rosemary is good for 'wasting' diseases, and this, combined with its known effects on the central nervous system, suggests that it might be of some help in degenerative conditions such as multiple sclerosis, though I have to emphasise that this is pure speculation. I have certainly seen some relief of pain resulting from aromatherapy treatment with this oil, but far more work would need to be done before anything more than that could be suggested.

Caution must be used with Rosemary, as it can cause epileptic-type fits, or even poisoning, though in very small amounts it is used to treat epilepsy. (Please refer to the entry for EPILEPSY for more detail.) We can see here something akin to homoeopathy; a substance which, in large amounts, would provoke a symptom, can be used in tiny amounts to treat it.

Rosemary is an excellent tonic for the heart, liver and gallbladder, and helps to lower cholesterol levels in the blood. It could be described as the middle-aged executive's best friend, though Rosemary alone would do little good unless diet and lifestyle were taken into account as well.

It is a good analgesic, without having the sedative effects of many of the other painkilling oils, and I often use it in massage, baths and compresses to relieve pain in rheumatism and arthritis. It is also a very good oil to use for tired, stiff and overworked muscles. I have used it very successfully in treating dancers and athletes, particularly long-distance runners, using Rosemary in combination with other oils before training or competitive events, and Lavender, usually combined with Marjoram, for massage after training or competing.

Rosemary has traditionally been used in skin and hair care for many hundreds of years. It is an ingredient of true eau de cologne, and a major ingredient of Hungary Water (or the Queen of Hungary's Water) which is reputed to have almost miraculous rejuvenating effects. It is used in rinsing water for dark hair, and as a scalp friction, which is valuable for excessive hair loss or poor condition, especially when these follow a period of illness or convalescence. It is reputed to restore colour to grey hair and even to cure baldness, but I am afraid that these actions are more or less mythical.

see also entries for **EAU DE COLOGNE, EPILEPSY** *and* **HUNGARY WATER.**

Rosewater

Rosewater is a useful adjunct to the use of essential oils, particularly in skin treatments and in the care of the eyes. It is obtained from rose petals by distillation. Steam is passed through the mass of rose petals, and collected in a tube which then passes through a cooling tank. The liquid which is obtained when the steam is cooled is rosewater.

Rosewater has soothing, cooling and anti-inflammatory properties. It is a gentle antiseptic, and mild astringent, all of which makes it useful in skincare. It is often incorporated with natural oils to make creams, both commercially and for home preparation, and can be used alone as a gentle skin toner, or mixed with alcohol and essential oils to make a somewhat more powerful preparation. Rosewater can be safely used on the most sensitive skins, and is the only toner recommended for dry skins. Oily skins are better treated with orange-flower water (q.v.).

In treating the eyes, it is important to remember that essential oils should never be used near them, and where Rose is mentioned in many books and herbals, rosewater should be chosen rather than oil of Rose. Pure rosewater on pads of cottonwool can be placed over the eyes to rest and refresh them, and rosewater is a very good treatment for conjunctivitis.

Many people love the aroma of roses, and rosewater can be used as a perfume, taking the place of the expensive essential oil.

see also **HYDROLATS.**

Rosewood
Aniba rosaeodora

The Rosewood tree is a native of the Amazon basin and many aromatherapists are, quite rightly, concerned that in using the oil they are contributing to the destruction of the rainforest. This is certainly true of any oil obtained from wild trees, but fortunately there are cultivated plantations where logging is well controlled. Some of these have existed since the 1930s and were established for purely commercial

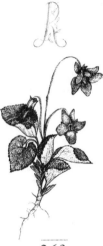

reasons: because of the cost of transporting wood from the interior to the ports, and because timber from the wild trees could only be collected between April and July – the flood season – this being the only time the heavy logs could be floated down to the main river. By making sure that any Rosewood oil you buy does come from such plantations, you can use it with a clear conscience.

The essential oil is extracted by steam distillation from wood chippings and contains between 80% and 97% of linalol, with small amounts of terpineol, nerol, geraniol and traces of various other substances. It is colourless or very pale yellow, with a rich and subtle odour that is both floral and woody, with slightly spicy tones. It is a complex fragrance which stands well on its own with no need of blending, though it does blend well with a wide range of other oils.

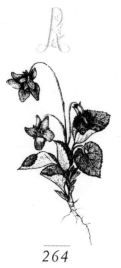

Rosewood is a very safe oil, being non-toxic, non-irritant and non-sensitizing in all its actions. It has a tonic effect on the body without being stimulant. At the same time, though, it is an immune system stimulant, so it would be a good oil for anybody with lowered immunity. I have not personally used Rosewood for anybody who was H.I.V. positive, but I have heard from aromatherapists working with people with A.I.D.S. that this oil is much preferred to the more 'medical' immunostimulants like Ti-tree. I have used Rosewood for chronic fatigue, and it suggests itself as a possible choice for people with M.E., glandular fever, etc.

It is mildly analgesic, and effective in clearing headaches, especially if these are allied to slight nausea. The effect on headaches is allied to a cephalic property, for Rosewood certainly clears the head. At the same time, it has a steadying effect on the nerves, and this combination is useful during exams, or when driving long distances. The same calming and steadying effect has been observed during crises, when its uplifting effect on the emotions is also valuable.

Many people find Rosewood aphrodisiac more, I think, through its actions on the mind and emotions than any physical/hormonal effect.

Rosewood has a range of useful properties in the area of skin care: being antiseptic and bactericidal makes it useful in treating acne, and its gentle, non-irritant nature means that it can be used on even the most sensitive skins. It is a cellular regenerator, which makes it valuable for older skin and it may even help to diminish wrinkles. I have sometimes included it in anti-stretch-mark creams. It is a good deodorant and is widely employed in the manufacture of commercial bath and skincare products. Its delightful fragrance makes it particularly well-suited to such uses.

However, there are plenty of other oils that fill all these needs and I think of Rosewood as a very precious oil and try to keep it for situations where something a little special is called for. I use it far more for its antidepressant and uplifting property than for any physical application. It is a wonderful oil for people who are stressed, depressed, dragged down by life. It has always seemed to me to be a very spiritual oil: in common with many other oils it can lift the mind and emotions, unlike some others Rosewood lifts the soul.

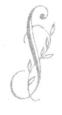

Sage

Salvia officinalis

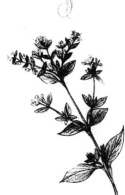

Common Sage originated in the Mediterranean basin, like most of our culinary herbs, but is hardy enough to grow almost all over the world, both wild and as a garden plant. It has been valued for its medicinal properties since ancient times, and indeed its Latin name derives from the same root as 'salvation', since Sage was considered able to save people from illness and death. It was also called 'herba sacra' – sacred herb – by the Romans.

Apart from its widespread use in cooking, flavouring cheeses, and, in the past, in brewing ales, it has been used in the folk medicine of many countries in the form of infusions (teas), gargles, vinegars and poultices, particularly for mouth and throat infections, to heal wounds, and clear headaches. It is often described in old herbals as a mental stimulant. For example, John Gerard says, 'Sage is singularly good for the head and brain, it quickeneth the senses and memory.' Sage has a powerful action on the female reproductive system, and was among the simples used by village 'wise-women' (so many of whom were burnt during witch-hunts from the Middle Ages to the 17th century) to help women in childbirth, to induce menstruation when it was late or scanty, or to normalise it during the menopause. Many of the folk uses of Sage are thoroughly vindicated by experience and by scientific testing, but others belong to the area where folk-medicine and folklore overlap. It may well be an antidote to snake-bites, but other claims such as that where Sage grows abundantly in the garden, the wife rules the roost, or that if your garden Sage collapses and dies your business will also collapse, can be regarded less seriously.

However, in spite of the undoubted value of Sage in the form of the fresh or dried plant, when we come to consider the essential oil, a great deal of caution is needed. The oil contains a high proportion of thujone which can provoke epileptic fits or convulsions, and, in larger amounts, is toxic to the central nervous system and capable of inducing paralysis.

I have collated first-hand experience of poisoning with essential oil of Sage from a number of women who attempted self-treatment based on information in books. The symptoms and severity of their experiences ranged from feeling slightly faint and shaking, through to such violent abdominal pain that the victim was admitted to hospital for three days. The most common experience, though, was moderate to severe uterine contractions and menstrual bleeding so excessive as to verge on haemorrhage. In every

Sage

CAUTION

Sage should be used
only with great caution
at all times, and not at
all during pregnancy,
for young children, or
anybody suffering
from epilepsy.

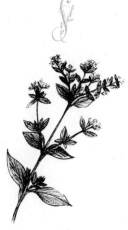

266

case except that of the girl who needed hospitalisation, the Sage oil was used externally only, either in a massage oil or in baths, and in amounts varying from 2 or 3 drops to about 10.

For these reasons, aromatherapists use the oil of Clary Sage (*Salvia sclarea*) in preference to the common Sage, as it shares many of the therapeutic properties of Sage oil, but contains only a very small proportion of thujone. The character and properties of CLARY SAGE can be found under the entry for that oil.

The few uses to which essential oil of Sage can be safely put, are in gargles and mouthwashes, for which it is diluted in alcohol and water to a very low concentration, and just occasionally in a massage blend for men with a very developed musculature. Sage oil is very warming and has a softening effect on muscles which have been perhaps over-developed by weight-training, or other sports involving short bursts of intensive effort, and when working with male athletes we can ignore the effect of Sage on the female reproductive system. Even here, though, there are other choices, such as Lavender, Marjoram or Rosemary, which are generally preferable to Sage.

Sandalwood
Santalum album

Sandalwood is a small, evergreen, parasitic tree, which obtains its nourishment by attaching suckers to the roots of other trees. It grows in India and various islands of the Indian Ocean, with the best quality being found in the province of Mysore. Despite rumours to the contrary, the Sandalwood trees in Mysore are in no danger of extinction and are protected by the State government. The trees are very slow-growing, and only very mature trees, which are nearing the end of their life, are cut. The trunks are left to lie in the forests until the outer wood has been eaten away by ants, and only the heartwood, which the insects will not attack, is then used for building, furniture making, incense and the extraction of essential oil by steam distillation.

The oil contains santalol (up to 90%), pinene, santalic acid, terasantalic acid and santalone, etc., and varies from yellowish to a deep brown. It is extremely thick and viscous, and the odour, although not initially strong, develops when applied to the skin, and is amazingly persistent. When buying Sandalwood oil, make sure that it is not Australian or West Indian. Australian Sandalwood is a related species (*Eucarya spicata*) from which an inferior oil is obtained while West Indian 'Sandalwood' is a totally unrelated species without therapeutic value. Vietnam and New Caledonia have well-controlled plantations of genuine Sandalwood.

Sandalwood has been used in India for many centuries as a perfume and incense and in traditional Ayurvedic medicine, its most important medicinal use being as a very powerful urinary antiseptic. It has been used for at least two and a half thousand years for the treatment of various infections of the urinary tract, such as cystitis, also for gonorrhoea, but it would be irresponsible and illegal for an aromatherapist without a medical training to use it in this context, unless medical advice and treatment was also sought and the doctor agreed to the use of aromatherapy.

It is also a very good pulmonary antiseptic, and I have found it good particularly for dry, persistent and irritating coughs, for it is also very sedative. It is one of the best essential oils to use in the treatment of chronic bronchitis, and can also be used for soothing sore throats. The best methods of use are inhalations and external application to the chest and throat. The taste is bitter in the extreme, which makes it very unpalatable for use as a gargle.

It is probably best known as a perfume, since it has been used in perfumes, toiletries and cosmetics, both in the East and in Europe, for longer than anybody has recorded.

As a cosmetic ingredient, Sandalwood is far more than a perfume, for it is beneficial to many different skin types and problems. It can be used for dry and dehydrated skins, especially in the form of warm compresses, but at the opposite end of the scale it is helpful for oily skins and acne, as it is slightly astringent and a powerful antiseptic. It is one of the perfumes that seems to be as popular for use by men as it is with women, and this can be a useful way of ensuring that a man, or perhaps more often a teenage boy, will regularly use any skin preparation you may prescribe, as he will feel assured that he will not smell 'funny', but more as if he had been using an expensive soap or aftershave. I have often used Sandalwood in aftershaves for young men with barber's rash, for it is extremely soothing, and relieves the itch as well as inhibiting the bacteria which cause the rash.

The widespread popularity of Sandalwood as a perfume may be due to its long-held reputation as an aphrodisiac, and unlike some of the essential oils and other substances believed to have such an effect, Sandalwood really does seem to live up to such expectations.

Scabies

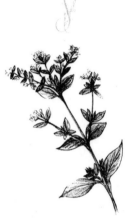

Scabies is a distressing condition, with intense itching, caused by a minute insect (*sarcoptes scabei*) which burrows just below the surface of the skin and lays its eggs. As these hatch out the movement of the mites beneath the skin causes itching and irritation. Infection of scratches can be a secondary problem. Scabies is very contagious, and is becoming more widespread. It is endemic in sheep farming areas, as the mite lives in the sheep's fleece and is easily transmitted to farm workers, and from them to other human contacts, but I have come across a number of cases of infection picked up in the changing rooms of dance and exercise centres, where the warmth encourages the mite.

Creams prescribed by doctors to kill the mites can be very damaging to the skin, especially if used repeatedly, as may often be needed.

Aromatherapy treatment usually combines external treatment with creams and garlic capsules to be taken several times a day until all the mites have gone. A combination of Lavender and Peppermint oils is one very effective treatment, alternatives being Cinnamon, Clove, Lemon and Rosemary. Jean Valnet quotes a formula (Helmerich's ointment) which combines Cinnamon, Clove, Lavender, Lemon and Peppermint in a cream, but I prefer to alternate two or three of these oils in successive jars of cream. They need to be added to the cream or ointment in a fairly high concentration: say a total of 5% by weight, but Cinnamon and Clove should form only a small proportion of the blend, to avoid further irritating the skin.

The cream should be applied to itching areas at least twice a day, preferably after bathing, and treatment will be more effective if essential oils are also added to the bath.

Lavender and Rosemary are the best oils for this, and Camomile can be added for its soothing properties. Do not use Cinnamon or Clove in the bath and use Lemon or Peppermint in very small amounts (up to 3 drops) only.

Once the scabies has been cleared, the skin is often dry and flaky in areas that were infected. This is a worse problem where orthodox medical prescriptions have been used before trying essential oils. Benzoin, Lavender, Myrrh and Neroli, in a carrier oil or cream with some wheatgerm oil added, will help to repair the damage and promote growth of healthy skin.

During treatment, scrupulous attention to hygiene is vital. The mites live in clothes and bedding, especially wool, so every single item of clothing and linen which the sufferer has used must be treated to remove the mites. Anything that can be washed at a high temperature is best treated that way, and a solution of Camphor and Lavender oils in alcohol (5% of each oil) should be used to clean mattresses, pillows and anything else that cannot be washed. In very bad infestations it has sometimes been necessary to burn clothing and other items as constant re-infection occurred.

Scalds

ॐ

see under **BURNS.**

Scarlet Fever

ॐ

Unlike most of the infectious illnesses of childhood, scarlet fever (scarlatina) is not a viral infection but due to a bacterium, Streptococcus pyogenes. It takes the form of a severe sore throat with a fever and the scarlet rash which gives the illness its name.

During the past fifty years, scarlet fever has changed from being a killer disease to being regarded as fairly innocuous (mainly due to the discovery of modern sulphonamide drugs and antibiotics), but in recent years it does seem that a more virulent strain has appeared. I have come across cases of children being very ill indeed. Never attempt to treat scarlet fever with aromatherapy alone, but be sure to call a doctor in every case.

The natural way to reduce the severity of an attack is basically the same as for measles and rather than describe it again in detail I would refer you to that entry, with the comment that in scarlet fever German Camomile seems to be the most effective oil in reducing the rash, fever and general discomfort.

Any child who has had scarlet fever needs to be carefully monitored for some months afterwards. The illness is very debilitating and rheumatic fever can sometimes occur as after-effects of streptococcal infections, also acute nephritis. I have known one child to develop haemolytic anaemia after a particularly severe attack of scarlet fever. Clearly, medical care should be urgently sought.

Sciatica

The term sciatica is often used incorrectly to mean pain very low in the back, but correctly used it indicates pain at any point along the sciatic nerve caused by pressure on, or irritation of, that nerve.

The sciatic nerve originates in the pelvis and travels below the sacroiliac joint to the buttocks, behind the hip joint, down the thigh, dividing at the knee into two branches, which continue down the calf to the foot. Pain may arise from pressure caused by an intervertebral disc, from badly designed chairs or from poor sitting posture. Even an overstuffed wallet kept in a back trouser pocket can be the origin of the pain (no, that is not a joke – such cases have actually been reported!). Some illnesses which give rise to irritation of the nerves, diabetes for example, can give rise to a form of sciatica, and so can alcoholism.

The pain of sciatica is a symptom, and treating the pain alone is no treatment. The cause must be found and treated, too. This will often involve examination and treatment from an osteopath where pressure is involved, and obviously chairs and posture need to be looked at. While the pain is bad, massage is not advisable, but cold compresses over the painful area with Camomile or Lavender will reduce the irritation and lessen the pain. Gentle massage with either of these oils at times when there is less or no pain can be very beneficial, and baths can help too – they should not be too hot.

Seasonal Affective Disorder (S.A.D.)

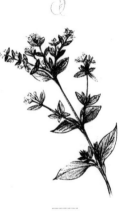

Seasonal Affective Disorder afflicts many thousands of people in northerly latitudes. Most people tend to feel a bit low in winter more often than in summer, but for S.A.D. sufferers, winter brings real depression, in some cases very severe. This is often linked to fatigue, lethargy, food cravings and weight increase, and other emotional and physical problems. It is usually easy to distinguish between S.A.D. and other forms of depression because of its very seasonal nature.

S.A.D. is directly linked to the reduction in sunlight when days get shorter and the weather is frequently overcast. The pineal gland, at the base of the brain, controls the balance of several brain chemicals, especially those that influence our patterns of sleeping and waking (and, in some other animals, hibernation). The pineal gland is strongly influenced by the amount of daylight available and as the days shorten it increases production of melatonin, which suppresses some of the hormones involved in activity, metabolism and reproduction. This may have been a useful function in our distant past, when food was short in winter, the tribe withdrew to a cave or winter encampment and the general level of activity declined, but it creates problems in the context of 20th century life.

An effective treatment has been developed using full-spectrum lights, which are a close approximation of natural daylight, but aromatherapy can certainly help as part of an overall treatment. We can use oils such as Basil, Black Pepper, Rosemary, Thyme, etc., to counteract fatigue and lethargy, the whole range of antidepressants and any other oils which meet the client's needs at the time.

The oils which I have found most effective tend to be those with a 'sunny' nature, particularly the Citrus family, and of these, the most helpful seem to be Grapefruit, Orange and Petitgrain. Of these, Grapefruit is often welcomed because it facilitates mental activity, and many S.A.D. sufferers feel as if their brain is half-asleep much of the time. Vaporising Grapefruit in the home or office seems to stimulate the mind as well as lifting the spirits. The fact that the smell is fresh and familiar makes it easy to use in the workplace without attracting adverse comment from colleagues. A blend of Petitgrain and Rosemary or Grapefruit and Rosemary in a morning bath has helped several people through the darkest weeks of the year, when getting up is really difficult. Occasionally, I have used Myrrh for its hot, dry, getting-things-moving character.

Good nutrition seems to reduce S.A.D. symptoms, including plenty of complex carbohydrates, as little as possible of sugary foods (which, unfortunately, are what sufferers crave) and a good vitamin and mineral supplement with plenty of Vitamin C, and the 'sunshine' vitamins A and D. Red and orange foods, such as dried apricots, red peppers, beetroot and red kidney beans all seem to help – and this is not just a fanciful association with sunny colours: they each contain nutrients that combat depression and are classed as Yang foods in terms of energy.

Finally, some S.A.D. sufferers have found acupuncture a great help in keeping their spirits and energy levels up during the winter. A point on the ear, called Shen Men, 'The Gate of Heaven', stimulates the release of endorphins, which are the brain's 'happy' chemicals. Shen Men is also used to help people with addictions, so it may reduce the food cravings.

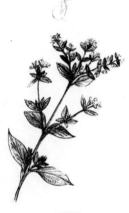

Sebum

Sebum is a wax-like oily substance produced in glands just below the surface of the skin. These are called sebaceous glands, and open into the hair follicle (the opening through which the hair grows). Sebum in normal amounts is a valuable secretion, which helps to lubricate the skin and keep it supple, and also gives some protection from the outer environment.

Sebum only becomes a problem when there is too little or too much of it, giving rise to dry or oily skin conditions. When the skin is excessively oily the hair follicles may become blocked by excess sebum combined with dirt and particles of dead skin cells flaking away at the surface. Bacteria feed on the plug of sebum and debris, and the hair follicle becomes inflamed and infected and a 'spot' is produced. When an area of skin is affected by a number of spots (more correctly called pustules) and this condition persists, it is known as acne.

Over production of sebum is common in adolescents, when the whole hormonal system is going through a stage of upheaval, though people whose skins are oily in youth will often retain a normal and attractive skin texture far longer than those whose skin was dry in youth, since sebum production declines with age.

Two or three oils, most notably Geranium and Lavender, have the property of balancing both over- and under-production of sebum, and so can be used to help both excessively dry and very greasy skins. Among the oils which are useful for correcting very oily skins, the most effective is Bergamot, followed by Cedarwood, Grapefruit and Juniper. To help with over-dry skins, lacking in natural lubrication, Camomile, Jasmine,

Neroli and Rose oils are all good choices, but the best of all is probably Sandalwood.

Any of these oils can be used, preferably as a facial massage oil, but also in creams and lotions for use between massage treatments. For dry skins a very emollient carrier oil, such as oil of avocado or peach kernel oil, is very helpful.

see also **SKIN.**

Sedative Oils

A good number of essential oils are sedative in effect – that is, they have a calming effect, particularly on the central nervous system.

Among the most effective sedative oils are Camomile, Lavender, Bergamot and Neroli. Others are Rose, Benzoin, Clary Sage, Jasmine, Marjoram, Melissa and Sandalwood, and there are still others, though these are less used. The most effective means of using these oils is in massage and in baths, most particularly before sleeping, when they will help to prevent insomnia.

The choice of a particular oil will depend very much on the individual for whom it is to be used: on that person's preferences for a particular aroma, and on their situation at the time. Every one of the oils mentioned has many other properties, in addition to being sedative, and one or more of these may determine the final choice from among the wide range of oils available.

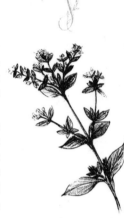

Jasmine

271

Sensitive Skin

Sensitive skin is often very youthful in appearance, and may be compared to the skin of babies and young children. It is often fair, delicate and almost translucent with scarcely visible pores and can be dry and fragile. It reacts strongly to both heat and cold, becoming dry and taut to such a degree that it is painful, with redness, blotches and itching. Cosmetics, soaps and other substances often produce irritation and the skin may burn very easily in the sun. Rubbing by shoulder straps, elastic and garment seams can cause redness, and in extreme examples even the normal amount of pressure exerted in massage will have this effect, so the therapist needs to use only the lightest of strokes.

Great care must be taken in selecting essential oils and testing them first on a very small area of skin. Use only the gentlest oils, such as Camomile, Neroli and Rose. Even Lavender has been known to cause irritation, redness and flaking on some sensitive skins. It is advisable to dilute the essential oils to much less than the usual 3% for massage: perhaps 2% for body massage and 1% for use on the face. Oils used in the bath should always be diluted in a carrier oil before being added to the water. In fact, the precautions to be taken are very similar to those observed when using essential oils for babies.

Lotions and very light creams are best for such skins, in preference to heavier and richer ones and light carrier oils such as sesame and grapeseed are best for massage. Soap should be avoided completely and all cosmetics and skincare products need to be carefully chosen to exclude all possible irritants. Toners should be alcohol-free (you will find a suitable formula in Appendix C). Pure natural cosmetics of exclusively vegetable origin are the safest. Honey mixed with ground almonds or fine oatmeal makes a good, non-irritant facepack.

Sesquiterpenes

Sesquiterpenes are a class of aromatic molecules which are predominantly soothing, calming and anti-inflammatory. The most strongly anti-inflammatory is azulene, found in Camomiles and some of the Artemisia family. Caryophyllene is the most common of the sesquiterpenes, found in Lavender, Marjoram, Clary Sage and most oils from the Labiatae family and others; cadinene occurs in Frankincense, Lemon, Patchouli, etc., and cedrene, in Cedar and Juniper.

Shiatsu

Shiatsu is a traditional Japanese system of massage based on similar principles to acupuncture. The word means 'finger pressure' and the practitioner uses pressure of the finger or thumb on specific points where an acupuncturist would use a needle to obtain a similar effect. However, this does not fully describe shiatsu, which also makes use of the whole hand, elbows, and even feet to relax or stimulate, so balancing the flow of Yin and Yang energies in the body's meridians. (See entry for ACUPUNCTURE for a fuller account of the theory of Yin and Yang and chi energy.)

Classic shiatsu is applied through the clothing, and so does not lend itself to use by an aromatherapist, but the system can be adapted for massage with oils and incorporated into an aromatherapy treatment with a great deal of benefit. By working along specific meridians during a massage with essential oils, and applying pressure to appropriate points on the meridians, the aromatherapist can help to balance the body energies, and heighten the effect of the essential oils.

see also entries for YIN/YANG and ACUPUNCTURE.

Shingles

see ZONA.

Shock

There are several essential oils which are useful in cases of shock. Inhaling Peppermint or Neroli directly from the bottle, or on a handkerchief or tissue can be a valuable first aid.

The best treatment for shock, in my experience, is Dr. Bach's Rescue Remedy, and four drops on the tongue should be given as quickly as possible, and can safely be repeated a little later if necessary. You can give essential oils to smell at the same time. Rescue Remedy is a compound of five of the Bach Flower Remedies: Rock Rose, Clematis, Impatiens, Cherry Plum and Star of Bethlehem. It can be given before any stressful event, as well as after any trauma, from the hearing of tragic news, to a road accident, a bad fall or an operation.

Arnica is used homoeopathically for shock, and can be used in the same way as Rescue Remedy, but in this case it is important not to use essential oils at the same time, as the very oil which is most useful for shock – Peppermint – is a powerful antidote to homoeopathic remedies.

Sinusitis

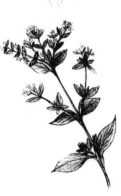

The sinuses are bony cavities behind, above and at each side of the nose and opening into the nasal cavity. They act as a sound-box to give resonance to the voice – this can perhaps be best understood by considering how flat the voice sounds when the nose and its associated cavities are blocked.

The sinuses are lined with mucous membrane similar to that lining the nose, and infection from the nose can easily spread into them. Because the openings from the nose into the sinuses are very narrow, they quickly become blocked when the mucous membrane of the nose becomes swollen during a cold, hayfever or catarrh, and then the infection is trapped inside the sinus.

Acute attacks of sinusitis may follow a cold, etc., or be brought on by cold, damp air. Acute attacks can be extremely painful, with headaches so severe that it is impossible to move the head without pain. The sufferer may feel quite ill, and possibly have a raised temperature. Acute sinusitis needs prompt treatment, as there is a risk, although admittedly very small, of the infection spreading inwards to cause meningitis.

Chronic (i.e. long-term) sinusitis gives rise to dull pain, in the forehead and/or the area between eyes and cheekbone, with a continually stuffy feeling in the nose. This, too, should be treated very thoroughly, to be sure of eradicating all traces of infection.

Frequent (up to 5 or 6 times a day) steam inhalations are the best treatment. Eucalyptus, Lavender, Peppermint, Pine, Thyme and Ti-tree oils are all effective, and I would recommend alternating several of these. Lavender and Thyme are the most effective when there is much pain; Eucalyptus, Peppermint and Pine are very good at relieving the blockage and stuffiness, while Ti-tree is the most powerful antiseptic of these – very important in eradicating the infection.

Lavender

273

Garlic decongests, detoxifies and disinfects, so include plenty of fresh garlic in the diet of anybody prone to sinusitis, and during an acute attack give garlic in the more concentrated form of tablets or capsules.

Certain foods, especially dairy produce and wheat, seem to pre-dispose people towards sinusitis, because they provoke excessive formation of mucus. During an acute attack of sinusitis all dairy and wheat-based foods must be excluded for several days, and people who have chronic or repeated attacks are advised to exclude these foods completely for several months, and then reintroduce them in very small amounts, if at all. Goat and sheep's milk products are sometimes better tolerated than cow's milk.

Special techniques of facial massage can be used to encourage drainage of mucus from the nose and sinuses, but during a severe attack these may be too uncomfortable for the patient. They can be introduced after a day or two, or whenever steam inhalations have reduced the congestion enough for massage to be tolerable. Very light drumming (tapottement) over the area of the affected sinuses is used, together with pressure on appropriate acupuncture points and sweeping circles round the eyebrow ridge and the cheekbones.

Acupuncture is a very effective therapy for sinusitis and can be used alongside aromatherapy.

---

see also the entry for **CATARRH.**

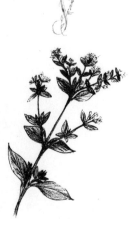

Skin

The skin is very much more than an outer covering wrapping up the 'parcel' that is your body. It is the body's largest organ. It is also vitally important in aromatherapy, because it is one of the two routes by which essential oils can get into the bloodstream and thus travel around the body (the other being via the lungs).

The skin is a giant organ of elimination, getting rid of the waste-products of many bodily processes carried in sweat through the pores. If the other organs of elimination (the kidneys and colon) are not working as efficiently as they should, a variety of skin diseases, ranging from eczema to acne and boils, may occur because the body is trying to push out through the skin more toxins than the skin can effectively cope with.

If the skin allows certain substances to pass out of the body, while safely containing others, it is equally true that it can absorb some substances into the body while excluding many that could harm the muscles and organs beneath it. Because of this, the skin is described as 'semi-permeable'. The factor which determines whether any particular substances will be able to pass through the skin or not, is the size of the molecules from which it is made up.

Essential oils have a molecular structure which is relatively small and simple, and they pass through the skin easily. This has been clearly demonstrated in an experiment in which oil of Garlic was rubbed into the skin of a volunteer's foot: ten minutes later the Garlic was measurable on his exhaled breath. This means that in ten minutes, the Garlic oil had passed through the skin, been absorbed into the bloodstream, and already reached the deoxygenated blood returning to the lungs.

Not all essential oils pass through the skin quite so quickly. It may take from 20 minutes to several hours for the oils used in a bath or massage to be completely

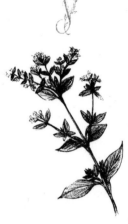

Garlic

absorbed into the body, but part of the oil will usually reach the bloodstream quite soon after first being applied to the skin.

A second factor which enables essential oils to be absorbed by the skin is the fact that they dissolve easily in fatty substances. The skin produces its own protective layer of an oily wax, called sebum, and essential oils can dissolve in this, making their absorption by the skin even easier.

Immediately below the skin, the particles of essential oil pass into the fluid that bathes every cell of the body, and from here they can pass through the ultra-thin walls of the lymph ducts and tiny blood-vessels (capillaries). In this way, the aromatic particles pass into the general circulation, and travel around the body.

This gives us a very effective, and very safe, method of getting essential oils into the body when needed. As you will read elsewhere in this book, I am one of the large number of therapists who oppose the practice of taking essential oils by mouth, and application to the skin allows us to by-pass the digestive system completely. In a crisis, such as an infectious illness, more essential oil can be absorbed into the body by massaging the back at half-hour intervals, than could be given by mouth in the same period of time without irritating the stomach lining.

A few sensible precautions are needed, such as diluting essential oils in a carrier, usually a 3% dilution, before massage, avoiding oils known to be irritant to the skin, and in the case of people with very sensitive skins, checking their reaction by trying an oil on a very small area first.

Essential oils can contribute enormously to the health and appearance of the skin itself, and this is discussed in the entries for **SKINCARE, DRY SKIN, OILY SKIN, DEHYDRATED SKIN, AGEING SKIN, WRINKLES,** etc.

Aromatherapy is also used very widely in the treatment of skin problems, and here again, you will find entries for **ACNE, ECZEMA, DERMATITIS** etc.

Skincare

Skincare is a very large and important branch of aromatherapy. (Indeed, some people are under the impression that it is the whole of aromatherapy!) Using essential oils, flower waters, fresh fruits, almonds, honey and other fresh natural substances, it is possible to provide a very wide range of treatments for every type of skin, and for a variety of skin disorders, such as acne, eczema and psoriasis.

A typical aromatherapy facial treatment (assuming that your skin is generally healthy and you are not suffering from a specific skin disease) will usually consist of a thorough cleansing of the face with a gentle plant-based cream or milk, followed by a careful and specialised massage of the face, neck and shoulders and often the scalp, too. This is, of course, the most important part of the treatment, for it is during the massage that the appropriate essential oil or oils for your particular skin, at that time (since our skins vary from day to day), will have the opportunity of penetrating the dead, outer layer of the skin and working on the living layers beneath. Part of the therapist's training will have been directed at equipping her to make the best possible choice of oils for each person's skin at any given time from among the considerable number of oils available.

Following the massage, she may cover your face with a warm compress to aid the absorption of the oils, or she may make you a face-pack from one or more of a wide range of natural plant substances, ranging from fresh strawberries or other fruits that are in season, to avocado pulp. Some therapists, especially those working in salons largely devoted to beauty treatments, may use commercially made preparations for the face-pack, but I consider this neither necessary nor desirable. Apart from the fact that such preparations increase the cost of a treatment, I feel that the maximum benefit can be derived from fruits and other plant products in their fresh state – the nearer to the plant, the more beneficial. After the pack has been on your face for about ten minutes, the therapist will clean it off, and gently wipe your face and neck with rosewater or orange-flower water. She may then apply a very light film of oil or appropriate cream to protect your skin against the environment before you leave, and she might also give you creams or other preparations made with essential oils to use at home.

Most treatments will follow approximately this outline, though of course there will be variations depending on the therapist's individual approach and your particular skin condition. For example, if you have a very oily skin or acne, the session might include a facial steam, with a few drops of essential oil added to the water.

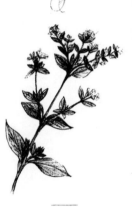

It is also relatively easy to make simple creams, lotions and aromatic waters for the skin at home, using essential oils, beeswax, cocoa butter and flower waters, and the methods and ingredients are described in full in other sections of this book. The ways of making such creams, and the products that go into them, have been in use for literally thousands of years and are known and proved by long experience to be safe and beneficial for the skin. Many of the formulae are very similar to those used by our great-great grandmothers, and also by commercial firms until fairly recent times, although commercial cosmetic preparations have often included some mineral and animal substances, too. Not all the minerals are completely harmless, and many of us prefer not to use animal derivatives for ethical reasons, so the possibility of making our own skincare preparations from essential oils and other plant products is very welcome. They also have the advantage of being very cheap when compared to the commercial equivalent, and you know, to the last drop, what ingredients have gone into each jar.

Of course, skincare is not confined to the facial skin, although more attention is lavished on that part of our skin than any other, partly because the face is constantly exposed to the weather, environmental pollution, central heating and other harmful elements, and partly because of the importance most of us attach to our facial appearance. Aromatherapy treatments, in the form of massage, creams, lotions and aromatic baths, can be applied with much benefit to the skin of the entire body. Next to the skin of the face, the hands are probably the area to which we give the most care, and it is very easy to produce good and effective handcreams.

Some aromatherapists are trained, or choose to specialise, in skincare only, rather than the wider clinical field and I think it is important that we should acknowledge the value of their work. The whole process of being looked after, massaged, pampered and made to feel good is wonderfully relaxing, and from that point of view can be seen as valuable therapy in its own right, quite apart from the direct physical benefit to the skin.

The essential oils which can be used in skin treatment are so many and varied, that for ease of reference they are described under the entries for various skin types, and different skin problems. You will find entries for DRY SKIN, OILY SKIN, DEHYDRATED SKIN, SENSITIVE SKIN, WRINKLES, THREAD VEINS, and also ACNE, ECZEMA and PSORIASIS as well as an entry under SKIN which gives a fuller account of the functions of the skin and how essential oils interact with it.

Skin Irritation

The majority of essential oils are perfectly safe when used on the skin in the dilutions used by most aromatherapists, i.e. 3% for most massage blends, and less for children and people with sensitive skin. When using oils that are known to be potentially somewhat irritant I use 1.5% or even as little as 1% in some instances.

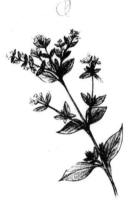

Some oils have such an ability to irritate that they must never be used on the skin, even in dilution, and not surprisingly a number of these are derived from 'hot' spice plants. Some of these, such as Horseradish and Mustard are classed as hazardous oils and never used, but one or two others, including Clove (Bud, Stem and Leaf) and Cinnamon (Bark and Leaf) may be listed because they have some important uses in inhalations and vaporisations.

Different parts of the same plant may be less or more irritant and there are also variations between different varieties of the same species. For example, Cinnamon Leaf is somewhat less irritant than Cinnamon Bud. Dwarf Pine is highly irritant and not to be used at all on the skin while Scotch Pine is among the least irritant oils. Most citrus oils are mildly irritant, but Lemon seems to be more aggressive than the others, and oils with a 'Lemon' scent, though not from the citrus group, such as Lemongrass, Lemon Verbena and Melissa also need to be used with caution.

Melissa

Obviously, as suggested in the first paragraph, different people will react differently to potential irritants, and people with ultra-sensitive skins (often very fair people or redheads) may experience irritation from oils that are not usually regarded as likely to do this. Commonsense and caution should go hand in hand when deciding on the choice of oils and strength of dilution. Irritation is more likely to arise from the use of oils in the bath than during massage, if the oils are used undiluted for bathing. For most oils, and for many people, 6 drops of undiluted oil in the bath is quite safe, but anybody with a sensitive skin should dilute all oils in a carrier before using them for bathing, and oils known to be mildly irritant should be restricted to not more than 3 drops in a bath, whoever is using them.

Occasionally, oils with a very mild irritant effect are used deliberately to produce reddening of the skin in a controlled and beneficial way. Such oils are described as rubefacient (i.e. reddening) and they produce a sensation of warmth, and increased local circulation which can be very comforting and healing in painful muscular conditions, rheumatism, etc. The most useful of the rubefacient oils are Black Pepper, Juniper, Marjoram and Rosemary.

A complete list of skin-irritant oils is included in Appendix A.

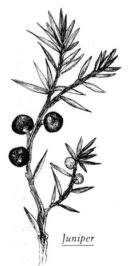

Juniper

Skin Sensitisation

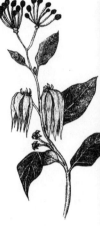

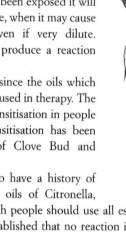

A very small number of oils have been found to cause sensitisation of the skin. This is not the same as irritation, since that is a simple reaction following contact with the irritant substance. In sensitisation, once the skin has been exposed it will be more sensitive to the same irritant in future, when it may cause a rash, blotches, itching or blistering even if very dilute. Occasionally other, similar substances will produce a reaction once the skin has been sensitised.

In practice this is not a major problem, since the oils which produce this effect most markedly are rarely used in therapy. The only oil in general use which will produce sensitisation in people with normal skin, is Cinnamon Bark. Sensitisation has been reported in a few instances with oils of Clove Bud and (surprisingly) Ylang-Ylang.

People with very sensitive skins, or who have a history of eczema or dermatitis, should avoid using oils of Citronella, Geranium, Ginger and Pine and indeed such people should use all essential oils with caution and well diluted until they have established that no reaction is caused by any particular oil.

Ylang-Ylang

see complete list of **HAZARDOUS OILS** *in* **APPENDIX A.**

Smell, Sense of

The sense of smell, or olfaction, is less well understood than any of the other senses: sight, hearing, touch and taste (although the latter is partially connected with the sense of smell). Research done in the past decade has increased our knowledge of the physiological processes by which our bodies experience odours, and of course such discoveries enrich our understanding of how essential oils can affect both body and mind so powerfully.

The olfactory nerves lie in the upper part of the nose. Unlike the nerves involved in touch, hearing, etc., they are directly connected to the brain. Indeed, they have been described as 'brain cells outside the brain'. Because of this, the sense of smell is the most immediate of our senses.

From the main body of each olfactory cell, several fine filaments called cilia extend into the layer of moisture (mucus) in the nose, and the tips of these filaments are equipped with receptors which detect the presence of any aromatic particles. Essential oils, and other odorous substances, are very volatile, i.e. they evaporate into vapour easily when exposed to the air. In this form they are breathed into the nose. The inside of the nose is always moist, and the particles of the aromatic vapour dissolve in this moisture. The olfactory nerves can only detect aromatic particles when they are in this liquid form.

Information about these particles passes along the cilia to the body of the cell. From here longer nerve fibres transmit this information to the brain, passing through the bony plate at the top of the nose. The brain identifies the particular smell, and we become conscious of perceiving it. All this happens almost instantaneously.

In recent years, the invention of electron microscopes with enormous powers of magnification, have revealed more about the way in which the cilia detect odorous particles. The receptors at the tips of the cilia are varied in shape. The molecules that make up anything that has a smell are also different shapes and sizes according to their origin, and when the smell-receptors come into contact with molecules that match their own shape, this triggers off the process that transmits information to the brain. The brain identifies the smell according to which type of receptor has picked it up. This does not mean that the information transmitted indicates 'rose' or 'tomcats'; such distinctions come from associated areas of the brain where memories of earlier smell experiences are stored. What the cilia can transmit is that the smell is sweet or acid, flowery, woody, heavy or light and so forth. Most odours are quite complicated, and made up of many different elements. The variety of shapes of the smell-receptors enables us to register all these complexities, and the total input is then interpreted by the brain as that particular odour.

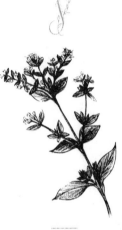

However, that is not the whole story, for the nose can detect far more different smells than the ears can detect sounds. Taste and sight are even simpler, as all taste and all vision is registered through only three or four different kinds of nerve cells. But the nose registers as many as ten thousand different types of smell sensation, and there do not appear to be ten thousand different kinds of receptors, so it seems likely that, as well as their shape and size, the rate of vibration of individual smell molecules plays a part in distinguishing between the myriad of smells that exist.

As well as being the most immediate of the senses, smell is also the most fleeting – perception of odours is sharpest when the odour is first smelt but decreases in intensity very quickly. This can be seen in two phenomena known as 'fading' and 'tiring'.

Fading takes place when we are exposed to one smell for a period of time, and can be illustrated by the example of a cook who does not smell the food he is cooking because he has been in the kitchen for some time. Somebody coming into the kitchen will notice the delicious aroma, and if the cook went out for a while and came back into the kitchen later, he would notice it, too, because he had been away from it for a while, so his nose would react as if it were a new stimulus.

Tiring takes place when we are exposed to a number of different smells within a fairly short time. We quickly lose the ability to distinguish clearly between one smell and another and they all begin to smell rather alike. You may have experienced this when trying out perfumes in a shop. If you try to sample more than three or four essential oils in succession the same phenomenon occurs.

In understanding the physical actions of essential oils on the body, it helps to know that the area of the brain in which smell is registered is linked by nerve-pathways to the hypothalamus, a structure at the base of the brain which is involved in regulating many important body activities. These include the endocrine system, which governs the secretion of hormones affecting growth, sex, metabolism and other functions; the autonomic nervous system which controls most of the unconscious activities that maintain life, such as digestion, rate of heartbeat and breathing and so forth; control of body temperature and hunger. Smelling good food makes us feel hungry; 'bad' smells, such as decaying meat can make us vomit, and certain odours may arouse sexual feelings. Maybe one day we will know why this is, but for the understanding of aromatherapy, it is enough to know that these reactions do happen. Why and how odours affect our emotions and memories is even less clear, though some ideas about this are discussed in the entry for **MIND**.

I am sometimes asked whether people who have no sense of smell can benefit from aromatherapy treatment. In fact they can, because essential oils are absorbed into the bloodstream, either through the skin or via the lungs when they are inhaled, so they can have a beneficial action on the body even if the recipient cannot smell them. It is doubtful, though, whether the same mental or emotional response to the oils could be experienced.

see also the entry for **MIND.**

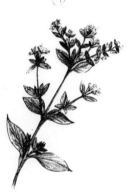

Sore Throat

A sore throat can be due to a variety of causes – bacterial infection, mechanical irritation from coughing, or a trickle of catarrh from the nose, for example.

In every case, steam inhalations will ease the discomfort. Oils of Benzoin, Lavender or Thyme are very helpful, and will help to deal with the infection causing the soreness.

For more detail read the entries for **INHALATIONS, LARYNGITIS, TONSILLITIS.**

Spasm

Thyme

In order to produce movement, a muscle has to contract (shorten). When the movement is completed, the muscle relaxes, and returns to its original length. All this takes very little time, though the contraction and relaxation may be constantly repeated, especially when we consider the muscles that form our internal organs (the smooth muscles).

In abnormal conditions a muscle may contract but fail to return to its relaxed condition afterwards. The muscle is then said to be in spasm. Spasm can affect both the smooth muscles and the voluntary muscles which move our limbs and body, and it is always painful. Spasm may follow injury or over-exertion and other possible causes include poor blood supply to the area, deficiency of sodium or other elements in the blood, fatigue, excessive exercise or injury, but quite often the cause of a spasm is not known. Stress frequently seems to be a factor.

Essential oils which relieve spasm in the smooth muscles include Bergamot, Camomile, Clary Sage, Fennel, Juniper, Lavender, Marjoram and Rosemary, and the most effective way to use them is in hot compresses over the affected organ. Gentle massage over the area is another good method.

Rosemary

Spasm in the external, voluntary muscles is best helped by massaging as deeply as possible around the painful area. Always 'warm up' the area with some more gentle, surface massage and friction before attempting any deeper pressure. Good oils to use include Black Pepper, Lavender, Marjoram and Rosemary. Both the action of the oils themselves and the physical effect of the massage will bring increased circulation to the area which is usually sufficient to release the spasm.

Spike Lavender
Lavandula spica or L. latifolia

Spike Lavender has a more penetrating, camphoraceous aroma. It is antibacterial, strongly antiviral, mucolytic and expectorant, which makes it an important oil for treating respiratory tract problems, especially bronchitis, sinusitis and throat infections. There are two chemotypes: Spanish Spike Lavender contains a much higher level of ketones than the French, which makes it a relatively toxic oil but most of the Spike Lavender available does come from Spain. As you can see, it does have some valuable properties, but use it with caution. It is probably best blended in small amounts with other oils.

Spikenard
Nardostachys jatamansi

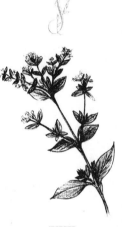

281

Spikenard, sometimes known as Nard, is native to northern India and has been prized for its healing properties and perfume since antiquity. It should NOT be confused with Spike Lavender (as it has been by some people who ought to know better!).

Spikenard is an aromatic herb, closely related to Valerian, with a most unusual root system: from a single root it develops two kinds of shoots, one of them an underground flower shoot or rhizome, in which most of the essential oil is found. The oil is extracted by steam distillation, and ranges from pale to deep amber in colour. The main constituents are bornyl acetate, isobornyl valerianate, borneol, patchouli, alcohol, terpineol and eugenol. The smell is very hard to define: Dioscorides said it smelt like goats! There is a rather 'animal' quality to the aroma, which is deep, peaty and earthy.

In its native India, Spikenard has always been valued as a perfume, medicinal herb and in skin care. It was highly prized in the Middle East and Mediterranean regions thousands of years ago, for it is mentioned in the Bible: in the Song of Solomon, and in the gospel of St. John where we find the story of Mary Magdalen anointing Christ's feet with 'ointment of Spikenard, very costly'. Dioscorides (when he wasn't being rude about the smell) described Spikenard as 'warming, drying and diuretic' and good for heavy periods, vaginal discharges, kidney and liver problems, inflammation of all kinds and for dispersing accumulated toxins.

Modern use suggests that Spikenard does have a balancing effect on the menstrual cycle. The white discharge to which Dioscorides referred is one symptom of vaginal thrush and Spikenard is an antifungal oil, so it could be useful to combat the candida albicans organisms.

The oil is helpful for allergic skin reactions and all kinds of rashes. Being a balancing oil, it can be used in facial massage and skin care preparations for all types of skin but is particularly valuable for mature skin. Victoria Edwards says, 'The oil redresses the skin's physiological balance and causes permanent regeneration.'

It might be worth trying Spikenard for the treatment of cellulite, as it is diuretic and detoxifying, but also because it is a deeply relaxing oil and cellulite is made worse by stress. It may help hormone imbalances, sometimes associated with cellulite.

It is certainly a wonderful oil for anybody tense and anxious, and has the ability, rather like Frankincense, to help people let go of old pain or emotional blocks that they are holding inside. Aromatherapists who work with chakra energy or auric massage would find this a very appropriate oil. Mary Magdalen's use of Spikenard to anoint Jesus on the night of the Last Supper suggests that it may also have significance for therapists working with the terminally ill. Jesus knew that his death was approaching, and the Magdalen knew this too: her anointing of his feet with Spikenard was a form of sacrament in preparation for that moment. Aromatherapists working in hospices might like to include Spikenard among the oils to help people nearing the end of their earthly lives.

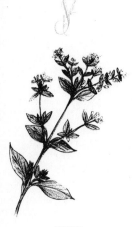

Sprains

The most effective treatment for a sprain is a cold compress, and firm but not too tight, strapping with a crepe bandage. A SPRAIN SHOULD NEVER BE MASSAGED.

The description sprain is used for a joint injury in which the ligament which supports the joint has been damaged. The joint will be swollen and often feel hot, and will usually be too painful to allow it to be used normally. Analgesic essential oils such as Lavender or Camomile are the most helpful, and will help to reduce inflammation and heat while easing the pain. The joint should be rested as much as possible, and strapping is important to provide support until the ligament has healed. The less the joint is moved, the sooner the ligament can mend. Cold compresses should be repeated as often as possible.

The ankle is the joint which is most often sprained. If a sprained ankle does not improve quickly or if any other joints appear to be sprained, treat very carefully and refer to a doctor, as the swelling may be due to a small fracture, synovitis or other cause.

see entry under **COMPRESSES** *for the method of making and applying them.*

Sprays

Essential oils can be used to great advantage in sprays, particularly to replace potentially dangerous aerosols. Depending on the choice of oil, the spray can be used to repel insects, to deodorise a room, to help prevent the spread of infection during epidemics or simply to create a pleasantly perfumed atmosphere.

Eucalyptus

A few drops of the chosen oil should be mixed with a little alcohol, and then added to water and shaken vigorously. If you intend to use the spray immediately, you can mix oils directly with water, provided that you shake the mixture well before using, and maybe once or twice during spraying. The oils will not, of course, mix with water, but will stay suspended in it for long enough to enable you to carry out the spraying. Proportions are not particularly important in sprays, but I usually use about 5% of oils to water or 10% during epidemics.

The best kind of spray to use is the ceramic kind sold for spraying indoor plants, but glass bottles which have originally held perfume or a deodorant can be recycled for holding small amounts of spray. The next best choice would be an ordinary plastic plant spray, but you should not leave an essential oil mixture standing in one of these as the essential oil may react with the plastic and become contaminated. Just make as much spray as you expect to use the same day and throw away any surplus.

Bergamot is one of the most deodorising oils, and is also a very good insect repellent, either alone or mixed with Lavender. Any of the Lemon-scented oils – Melissa, Lemon Verbena, Lemongrass or Citronella – will deter insects too.

Oil of Eucalyptus is recommended by Jean Valnet for spraying during epidemics and it can be used at frequent intervals in the room where a sick person is being cared for, to help minimise the spread of infection. Rosemary and Juniper are other oils which can be used in the same way. When there is an epidemic, spray each room several times a day.

As a room perfume, you can spray virtually any essential oil you enjoy.

A simple spray can be used to apply essential oils to the skin when it might be too painful to put them on directly. For example, a child suffering with chickenpox can be gently sprayed with a mixture of Camomile, Lavender and Eucalyptus, which will lower the child's temperature and soothe the spots. For this, the water should be very slightly warmed to avoid the shock of cold water on a feverish skin. You might adapt the same method to apply Lavender or Camomile or both to somebody with painful sunburn.

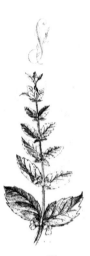

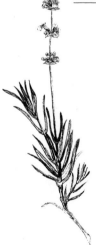

Melissa

283

St. John's Wort
Hypericum perforatum

The infused oil of St. John's Wort has exceptional healing and soothing properties. It has a very long history of use for the treatment of wounds, burns, bruises, and pain of various kinds: in the Middle Ages the Crusaders used it to treat battle wounds and many different uses of the plant are found in folk medicine all over Europe.

The oil is made by infusing the flowering tops in a bland oil and is a beautiful red colour. It is analgesic and anti-inflammatory and can be used in massage for fibrositis, neuralgia, muscular pain, sciatica, rheumatism, gout and arthritis. I have used it successfully in treating tendinitis. It is antiseptic and healing and good for minor burns, especially sunburn, and insect bites and stings, and is often incorporated in handcreams and skincare products. As always with infused oils, remember that they have their own chemistry and properties and add essential oils only in small amounts: between 1% and 2% of the total.

Sterility

Inability to conceive may stem from many and varied causes, and not all of them are likely to respond to aromatherapy treatment. However, there are several areas in which essential oils can be very helpful.

Quite often failure to conceive is linked to an irregular and scanty menstrual cycle, which makes the time of ovulation difficult to predict, or ovulation and periods may be completely absent. Rose is a oil which has a special affinity with the female reproductive system, and is a uterine tonic and cleanser. It is very effective in regulating the cycle, which suggests an action on the ovaries as well as the uterus. Geranium is another oil which has a balancing effect on hormonal secretion, and can also help in bringing about a regular and predictable pattern of ovulation and menstruation.

Rose has also been found to increase the sperm count in men where this was low, so it may be beneficial for both partners to use Rose in massage and baths when trying for a baby.

Trying unsuccessfully to have a baby can create many stresses and tensions, and these in turn set up a vicious circle where the tension becomes another obstacle to conception. Regular massage and bathing with relaxing oils can break this chain. I recommend Clary Sage, Jasmine, Neroli, Rose, Sandalwood, Rosewood and Vetivert in varying combinations or in alternation. Regular massage is the greatest help to a relaxed attitude, because the contact with the therapist can contribute as much as the mental/emotional/physical actions of the oils.

Very good nutrition is an important factor too.

It is certainly worth trying these gentle and health-promoting methods for several months before resorting to some of the more drastic methods used in orthodox medicine.

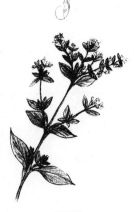

Rose

Stimulants

A stimulant is anything which has an enlivening effect on the body or mind. The use of essential oils as stimulants is safer than such things as caffeine, alcohol and stimulating drugs, but even so should not be abused. They can be very useful in the short-term, in a crisis, or when exceptional effort is needed, also in convalescence in small amounts, to help restore some vitality.

Stimulant oils include Basil, Black Pepper, Eucalyptus, Peppermint and Rosemary, and of these, I have found Rosemary to be the most effective.

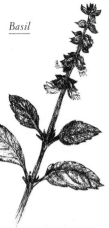
Basil

Massage with Rosemary oil, perhaps with a little Black Pepper added, is an almost magical reviver, but if nobody is available to give massage, baths are very effective too, or you can just sniff one of these oils from a hankie or tissue, or directly from the bottle. During long writing sessions, I put a drop of Rosemary oil on each wrist, so that I can smell it as my hands move over the typewriter. Basil, Peppermint and Eucalyptus are less useful as bath oils, as all can produce an unpleasant tingling of the skin, but a single drop added to some other oil or blend is enlivening. All are useful in burners or sprays. Peppermint tea is a good adjunct to using the oils.

These oils are not a substitute for proper sleep, nutrition and relaxation and should be seen as short-term aids when some special need arises, and not as long-term 'crutches'.

Stomach

The lining of the stomach can easily be damaged by essential oils, which is why I, in common with a growing number of aromatherapists, do not advocate taking essential oils by mouth, even in dilution. Undiluted essential oils used in this way can give rise to chronic ulceration, which has been found to be very difficult to treat, and some danger is associated even with diluted oils.

This is also the least efficient way to use essential oils, as they pass out of the body faster through the digestive tract than when they are inhaled or absorbed through the skin.

Some stomach problems, indigestion, nausea, etc., can be successfully treated by massaging or applying cold compresses over the stomach externally.

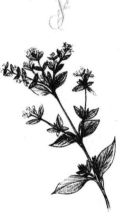

285

Stress

Stress, and stress related illness, are among the most prevalent health problems of 'civilisation' and certainly figure prominently on any aromatherapist's case-list.

Stress can be described as anything which disturbs the normal balance of mental and physical health and stress factors may be mental, physical or environmental in origin. For example, an accident or injury is a source of physical stress; bad lighting, noise, polluted air or ugly, dehumanised surroundings are sources of environmental stress. However, in discussing stress we tend to think more of the mental/emotional aspects, such as worries about work, finance, relationships or even the end of civilisation as we know it. Stress from any source makes us less able to withstand stress from any other source: for example, when we are worried, we may have minor or major accidents and we are more prone to 'catch' infectious illnesses when we are emotionally drained.

External sources of stress are not, in themselves, the problem, but the way in which we react to them. This has been described by Dr. Hans Selye as the General Adaptation Syndrome. After an initial reaction to some external threat or stress, the body adapts to the situation and can continue to function reasonably well, even though the source of stress is still present, for some time. This adaptation phase puts a certain degree of strain on the body, especially the adrenal glands, and if the level of stress increases, or if a fresh source of stress materialises, the ability to adapt to it may break down, and all kinds of symptoms, from allergy to heart attacks can follow.

One of the most useful things that anybody can do about stress is to recognise that they are threatened in this way, and take active steps to reduce the levels of stress suffered by the body. Along with such techniques as yoga, meditation, exercise, and creative activities, aromatherapy has an important function as a de-stressing technique. Some people consulting an aromatherapist are well aware that they are stressed, and have chosen this therapy for the deep relaxation that massage with essential oils can bring. Many others consult about the physical symptoms provoked by stress, and may need to be helped to understand that reducing the stress will help their overt problem.

A huge array of essential oils are at our disposal in coping with stress: all the sedative and antidepressant oils initially to induce relaxation. These include Bergamot, Camomile, Clary Sage, Jasmine, Lavender, Marjoram, Neroli, Rose, Rosewood and Vetivert.

Oils which strengthen the action of the adrenals may help in the short-term, but they should not be over-used. The most useful of these are Geranium and Rosemary. Rosemary is also a general stimulant, along with Black Pepper, Peppermint, Thyme, etc., and these can be used for short periods when stress has led to exhaustion.

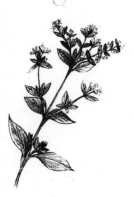

These oils are by no means the only ones that might be used, and represent only those I have found most effective. The therapist may also choose suitable oils based on the stress-related symptoms that emerge during the initial consultation.

Anybody who knows that they are under some stress, be it long-term or of a passing nature, can do a great deal to help themselves by using aromatic baths as an aid to relaxation. It helps to make bath time almost a ritual; setting aside a time when there will be no interruptions, taking the phone off the hook if necessary, choosing a favourite essential oil or blend to add to the bath and perhaps making a cup of relaxing herbal tea to take into the bathroom.

Obviously, it makes sense to do whatever possible to remove the source of stress. Talk to a trusted friend or a professional counsellor about work, financial or relationship problems, remove additive-laden foods from your diet, choose household products free from synthetic chemicals to reduce the number of physical stressors affecting your body. Joining an environmental pressure group and campaigning about water, air or agricultural pollution is far less stressful than doing nothing but worrying about the possible effect on your self or your family.

Rosemary

During a period of stress, the body is less able to absorb nutrients, so some supplementation especially of the B group of vitamins, and vitamin C is helpful. Ginseng, described as an 'adaptogen' helps the body to cope with the effects of stress, and many people find herbal iron preparations helpful.

But my best advice is: get massaged, and as often as you possibly can.

Stretchmarks

๛

The best time to treat stretchmarks is before they happen – this is definitely a situation where prevention is better than cure. They are a form of scarring, due to the stretching of the skin during pregnancy. Once stretchmarks have formed, they are very difficult to eradicate, though dedicated daily massage can reduce them.

From the fourth or fifth month of pregnancy, expectant mothers should massage their tummy and hips daily to increase the elasticity of the skin. Just massaging with an oil such as almond, or with a rich cream, is helpful, but Mandarin and Neroli oils make it more effective. A very good blend is 1% Mandarin, 2% Neroli in a base of Rosehip seed oil (Rosa rubiginosa). Rosehip oil contains between 30% and 40% of gamma linoleic acid which is very beneficial to the skin. If you wish, you could include up to 10% of Hazelnut oil, which is rich in Vitamin E.

Some women find creams easier to handle than oils, in which case you could use the Cocoa Butter cream formula in Appendix C with 10 drops of Mandarin and 15 drops of Neroli.

Sunburn

๛

Sunlight is important to health, particularly because the skin manufactures Vitamin D when exposed to sunlight. This doesn't mean that we need to bake ourselves for hours on end to be healthy! As little as ten minutes in the open air each day, even in winter, is all that is needed.

Over-exposure to the sun, and especially allowing the skin to burn, increases the risk of skin cancers and the thinning of the ozone layer has made this risk greater, even in temperate climates. Avoiding sunburn is the best strategy, but if burning does occur it should be treated like any other burn. Even mild sunburn needs to be considered seriously, because it often covers a large area of the body.

Camomile oil will soothe and cool burning skin. The fastest and most effective way to relieve a large area of redness and stinging is to take a lukewarm bath with 5 or 6 drops of Camomile oil added to the water. This can safely be repeated at intervals of a few hours until the burning sensation subsides. If it is a child who is burnt, dilute 3 or 4 drops of Camomile oil in a little almond oil before adding it to the bath.

More severe sunburn is best treated with Lavender oil, which is the first choice oil for burns of any kind. Make a solution of Lavender oil in boiled and cooled water (12 drops to each tablespoonful of water) and dab this on the burnt area if there is no blistering and the skin is not broken. If the skin is blistered, you can apply Lavender oil neat to the blisters.

Essential oil of Bergamot, most other citrus oils, Angelica Root and some others make the skin more sensitive to the sun's rays, so it burns more easily. This effect is known as photosensitisation. Don't use Bergamot oil in your bath, as a skin treatment, massage oil or perfume before going out in strong sunlight, or you may end up with quite

Camomile

serious burns. The photosensitising effect may last for 24 hours or more, but does not seem to operate if the Bergamot or other photosensitising oil is diluted to less than 2%. The same warning applies to perfumes and toilet waters of which Bergamot is an ingredient: for example, eau de cologne, Hungary water and citrussy toilet waters and aftershave lotions.

The best advice I can give on sunburn is that prevention is the best cure. Remember that essential oils do not prevent burning, and use a commercial preparation with a protection factor appropriate to your own skin and to the climate and conditions in which you will be sunbathing.

---

see also **BERGAMOT** *and* **PHOTOSENSITISATION.**

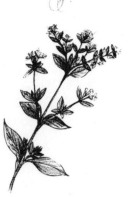

Synthetic Oils

A synthetic substance is one which has been put together from various materials in order to imitate another substance. The manufacture of synthetic essential oils is widespread and growing, because demand outstrips supply. The expanding perfume industry requires ever-increasing supplies of essential oils, in many cases more than the annual world-wide production of genuine oil. In almost every instance, it is cheaper to manufacture a synthetic oil than to grow, harvest and distil the genuine product.

The main raw material for these oils are natural terpenes, which are broken down and re-combined to make a huge variety of aromatic molecules. Pine trees are the main source of these terpenes, and trees are being felled in increasing numbers to provide them. The largest and most profitable raw material for synthetics, though, is benzene, a by-product of the petrochemical industry which is one of the world's worst polluters.

Synthetic oils have no therapeutic properties at all and may produce allergic reactions. They have no place in aromatherapy, and can only add to the pollution of our 'inner environment' as well as that of the planet.

288

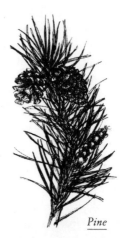

Pine

Tachycardia

Over-rapid heartbeat, often experienced at times of stress, anxiety, shock, etc.

The essential oil which is most often of use in slowing the beat is Ylang-Ylang. This can be given to smell on a tissue, or straight from the bottle in an emergency, but it is good to use it also in massages and aromatic baths as soon as possible after a crisis, and to continue to use this and other oils fairly regularly to prevent recurrence, if the person is susceptible to attacks. Other helpful oils include Camomile, Lavender, Neroli and Rose.

see also **PALPITATIONS.**

Tagetes
Tagetes minuta

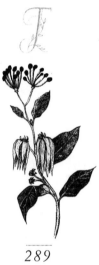

Tagetes, also known as Tagette, Taget, French Marigold, African Marigold or simply Marigold is a hazardous oil which, because of ambiguity about its name, is sometimes confused with the English Marigold or Calendula *(Calendula officinalis)*. Calendula does not exist in the form of an essential oil: very small amounts of an absolute are sometimes made, but it is mostly to be found as an infused oil which is very safe and valuable for skin problems.

Tagetes, on the other hand, is a toxic oil, containing a very high proportion of ketones (mainly tagetone, its principal constituent). It also contains some furocoumarins, which are photosensitising agents.

Tagetes is occasionally used in the treatment of corns, verrucas, etc., but there are perfectly safe oils which have the same effect.

When buying any oil labelled 'Marigold' be certain that you know the botanical origin, to avoid a potentially dangerous confusion.

Tangerine

see **MANDARIN.**

Tarragon
Artemisi dranunculus

Tarragon is sometimes described as being a digestive aid. This is true of the herb in its natural form, but in the concentration produced by distilling an essential oil it becomes hazardous. Like many of the Artemisia family, it can cause miscarriage if used during pregnancy, and it is a suspected carcinogen.

My advice is not to use this oil at all.

Teething

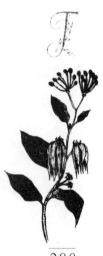

It is usually obvious when a tooth is about to erupt, as the baby will often have one red cheek on the side where the tooth is pushing through, and may be fractious, crying a lot and sleeping badly. Very often, the baby's general resistance is lowered while a tooth is erupting. Colds, coughs, earache and colic are often more frequent at this time, and nappy-rash may get worse, or may only be a problem during teething and not at other times.

The discomfort and various side effects can be helped with essential oils, remembering to observe the safety precautions listed in the entry for **CHILDREN**. The main method to use is simple massage on the affected side of the baby's face with diluted Camomile oil (1% to 1.5%). (Older babies, when cutting back teeth, may have two coming through at once, so massage both sides of the face.) German Camomile oil seems to be the most effective for this use, so put one or two drops, never more, into a 5 mls measuring spoon of carrier oil, and use this to very gently massage the check. Quite often a teething baby will rub or pull at one ear, either because the pain from the erupting tooth is referred to the ear, or because there is an actual ear infection at the same time. In this case, extend the massage to include the area all round the ear. Let the oil become warm in your hand before using it, or in very cold weather warm it a little over hot water before you put the oil on your hand to use.

A teething baby will often be very sleepless, so a drop of Lavender or Camomile in the bath (diluted before adding), or on the cot sheet or the baby's nightie, will help. If using Camomile to massage the face. I would be inclined to use Lavender to help sleep, but you can experiment and see which works best for your baby.

see also entries for **BABIES, CHILDREN, EARACHE, CAMOMILE** *and* **LAVENDER**.

Temperature

The normal temperature of the human body is around 98.4°F (37°C) though this fluctuates quite normally from slightly lower in the morning to higher in the evening. This level is controlled by a centre in the brain, which co-ordinates the various ways in which the body can regulate its own heat, such as sweating to lower temperature, or shivering to produce some heat from the muscles.

A number or essential oils have the effect of helping to raise, lower or normalise the body temperature. Bergamot, Eucalyptus, Lavender, Melissa and Peppermint oils will all help to reduce body temperature, and oils which promote sweating, such as Cypress and Rosemary will do so indirectly. They can be used in baths, or mixed with plenty of cool water and sponged over the body.

Brisk massage, even without the addition of essential oils, will help to raise the body temperature quite effectively, but if you add a warming oil such as Marjoram or Thyme it will be even better. Any of the oils described as rubefacient will increase the local circulation and help to induce a feeling of warmth, especially in cold extremities. These include Black Pepper, Juniper and Rosemary.

The temperature control mechanism is less efficient in babies and elderly people, so variations in their temperature need to be watched carefully.

see also **FEVER.**

Tenosynovitis

Inflammation of the tendons of the wrist (or less often, the ankle) and their surrounding sheath. The cause is nearly always over-use of the tendon due to repetitive movements though the inflammation is sometimes caused by rheumatism or a bacterial infection.

The condition is very painful and very slow to improve. Analgesic and anti-inflammatory oils will help, but rest is the most important part of the treatment. Treatment is discussed in detail in the entry for **REPETITIVE STRAIN INJURY.**

Terpenes

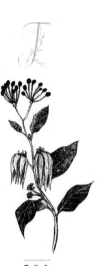

Terpenes are the most common category of organic molecules found in essential oils. Some terpenes are skin irritants, and you may come across essential oils, described as de-terpenated, which have had the terpene component removed to avoid this risk.

Terpenes can be sub-divided into Monoterpenes and Sesquiterpenes, and you will find the two groups described in their separate entries.

291

Thread Veins

The condition usually known as thread veins is due to stretching of the tiniest veins (capillaries) in the face.

Capillaries beneath the facial skin are easy to see, especially in fair-skinned people. If they become more noticeable than usual, they are usually described as 'broken', though 'stretched capillaries' might be a better description. The capillary walls are normally very elastic, and they dilate (enlarge) when the skin is hot, or as a response to spicy foods, alcohol, very hot drinks and other stimuli. When this happens, the person looks flushed, but as soon as the external stimulus wears off, the capillaries return to their original size.

If the capillary walls lose some of their elasticity, perhaps due to bad diet, excessive alcohol or stimulants such as coffee and strong tea, very severe climates or circulatory disorders, they may not shrink as much as they should, and then the face, and especially the cheeks, looks red all the time.

Gentle facial massage with essential oils that help to restore the natural elasticity of the blood vessels can eventually get rid of the redness, but it needs to be carried out faithfully every day, and it really does take many months to be effective. A slight improvement may be seen after a few weeks, but it may be six months or more before any significant change is noticeable.

Camomile, Parsley and Rose are the oils which I use for this treatment, usually in a lotion which can be gently massaged into the face twice a day. Infused oil of Arnica strengthens the tiny vessels, so it could be used as a base oil with a small amount of essential oil added. However, treatment is useless unless the diet is improved, alcohol, coffee and tea cut out or reduced to a minimum, and extremes of hot and cold avoided as much as possible. It is not good to wash the face in very hot water, and facial steaming, saunas and so forth must be avoided.

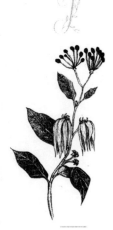

Throat

ॐ

---

see entries for **LARYNGITIS, SORE THROAT, TONSILLITIS, COLDS** *and* **COUGHS.**

Thrush

ॐ

Thrush is the common name for infection of a mucous membrane by the fungus candida albicans. It sometimes affects the mouth, particularly in young babies, but is most often a vaginal infection. Oral thrush is one of a complex of symptoms that often affect people who are H.I.V. positive.

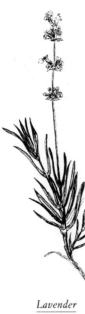

Thrush often follows a course of antibiotics, because these kill many of the helpful bacteria in the intestines. Everybody has the candida organisms present in the body, but in normal conditions the intestinal flora keep the candida from proliferating to a level where they cause trouble.

Aromatherapy treatment consists of baths, massage and local applications of Ti-tree, Lavender, Myrrh or a blend of any of these three, which are all anti-fungal. Ti-tree is also an immunostimulant, so it helps the body fight the infection. For oral thrush, you can make up a mouthwash, or use tincture of Myrrh.

At the same time, yoghurt tablets, or lacto-bacillus capsules should be taken to help re-establish the intestinal flora, and plenty of live yoghurt eaten. People who have prolonged or repeated bouts of thrush may need to follow a special anti-candida diet which restricts all sugars severely, as the fungus thrives on all kinds of sugars and starches, especially the refined kinds. Yeast, yeast derivatives and fermented foods, such as miso, soy sauce, vinegar, etc. must also be excluded.

Treatment with essential oils and diet must be continued for a considerable time, even though symptoms may disappear quite quickly. Three months, and possibly six months may be needed to bring the candida invasion of the body under control, and discontinuing treatment

Lavender

too soon will lead to a reappearance of symptoms quite soon. As with any prolonged aromatherapy treatment, vary the choice of oils from time to time.

Thrush and cystitis often alternate with each other in a painful and depressing cycle, because the antibiotics' given for the cystitis suppress the body's natural way of controlling candida organisms. Using essential oils to treat the cystitis, either alone or in conjunction with antibiotics if necessary, and using yoghurt or lacto-bacillus to counter the side-effects of the drugs, can break this cycle.

Thuja
Thuja occidentalis

ௐ

Thuja is a highly toxic essential oil, and an abortifacient due to the high proportion (60%) of thujone it contains. It should not be used at all in aromatherapy.

Thyme
Thymus vulgaris

ௐ

Thyme is yet another of the Labiatae family, and another native of the Mediterranean. It was known as a medicinal plant to all the early civilisations of the Mediterranean basin, and both Hippocrates and Dioscorides described its uses. There are several varieties of Thyme, but the common Thyme is the one most used in aromatherapy. Its familiar and pervasive scent is the origin of its name, which derives from the Greek 'thymos' – to perfume. The oil is distilled twice, to remove irritant substances present in the plant. The active constituents of a typical Thyme oil include thymol and carvacrol, together making up about 60% of the volume, with terpinene, cymene, borneol and linalol, but Thyme shows more chemical variation than almost any other plant (a point I will return to later). Carvacrol and thymol are frequently isolated and used in pharmacy.

The herb has always been used in cooking, and like many of the essential oils derived from culinary herbs, that of Thyme delays the putrefaction of meat. When we consider the conditions in which food was cooked and kept before refrigeration, especially in warm climates, the wisdom of adding this herb to so many dishes is obvious, and as happens so often with the culinary herbs, this wisdom has been substantiated in relatively recent times by laboratory tests, using bacilli cultured in meat broth. Essential oil of Thyme slowed down the proliferation of bacteria and prevented the broth from going bad for three days. It is also a digestive stimulant, useful for people with a sluggish digestive system, or in convalescence when the whole body is less efficient than usual. It is an intestinal antiseptic, valuable in gastric infections.

Another traditional use of Thyme has been in treating colds, coughs and sore throats, and here again the 'old wives' knew what they were about, for Thyme is an excellent pulmonary disinfectant, useful for all respiratory infections, as well as being very effective against mouth

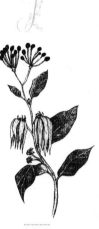

293

Thyme

and throat infections. It can be used as an inhalation for nose, throat and chest infections, or as a mouthwash or gargle. Even as little as 0.1% of essential oil of Thyme in a toothpaste is effective against bacteria which cause mouth and gum infections.

It is also a urinary tract antiseptic, useful for all infections of the bladder or urinary tract, and as it is a diuretic as well, this doubles its effectiveness.

Perhaps one of the most important actions of Thyme in all forms of infection, is that it stimulates the production of white corpuscles, so strengthening the body's resistance to invading organisms. It stimulates the circulation generally, and raises low blood pressure. It is particularly good for people who are fatigued, depressed or lethargic, making it very useful in convalescence, and it stimulates the appetite which is so often poor after an illness. Thyme helps to revive and strengthen both body and mind and it is reputed, like Rosemary, to stimulate the brain and improve memory.

Thyme is used in baths to help insomnia, and this is not as paradoxical as it may seem in the light of its stimulating properties, for we find once again, as with so many oils, a balancing effect. Thyme will enliven when you need to be wakeful, but help you sleep when you need to.

It is sometimes used for hair rinses, aromatic waters for the skin and in compresses for sores and wounds. It has been used in soapy solutions for disinfecting the hands before surgery, being a much stronger antiseptic than many of those commonly used in hospitals. Thyme is sometimes used in hot compresses to relieve rheumatic pain, and the fresh herb, crushed, is a good first-aid for insect bites and stings. Don't try using the neat essential oil for this, as it will sting the skin itself. It also stings in the bath, unless previously dissolved.

However, there are several variants of Thyme oil which are less irritant. These are all extracted from *Thymus vulgaris,* but although the plants are botanically identical, those found in different locations sometimes show a marked and consistent difference in the composition of their essential oil (see the entry on **CHEMOTYPES**). Three valuable chemotypes of Thyme oil are those containing a preponderance of Thymol (known as Thymus c/t Thymol), another with mainly Linalol, which is very gentle, non-irritant and suitable for treating even quite young children, and another known as Thymus c/t Thuyanol IV which is a very powerful antiviral oil. One or two specialist suppliers import these chemotypes which have definite advantages over the basic Thyme oil.

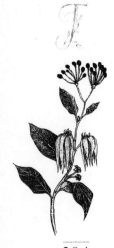

Tisanes

෨

see **HERB TEAS.**

Ti-Tree (or Tea-Tree)
Melaleuca alternifolia

෨

I prefer to use the traditional spelling Ti-tree for this oil, rather than the newer form, Tea-tree, in order to avoid confusion with the tea that is drunk *(Camellia thea).* Ti-tree has no connection at all with the cup that cheers and belongs to a quite different botanical family. Along with Cajeput and Niaouli, it belongs to a sub-species of the Myrtaceae family, which also includes Clove, Eucalyptus and Myrtle. An outstanding property common to all essential oils from the Myrtaceae group is their anti-infectious action, and in Ti-tree this is particularly powerful.

The active principles of Ti-tree oil include large amounts of terpineol with cineol, pinene, terpinenes and various alcohols. The oil may be pale yellow or almost colourless and has a powerful medicinal odour, a little like Eucalyptus. Because there are many varieties and sub-species of Melaleuca, confusion and substitution can arise but, fortunately, there are plenty of well-authenticated sources of genuine Ti-tree.

Although this is by far the most important of the Melaleuca oils used in aromatherapy, it has not been in use in Europe as long as Cajeput or Niaouli (though it is probable that some oils sold in the past with those names were, in fact, Ti-tree). Our knowledge of the properties and uses of this oil derived originally from a very long history of use by the aboriginal people of Australia, where the tree grows, and have been confirmed and extended by its ever-increasing use in aromatherapy.

Ti-tree oil has a very wide range of applications, but they all depend on two important inter-related facts:

1. This oil is unusual in that it is active against all three categories of infectious organisms: bacteria, fungi and viruses.
2. It is a very powerful immunostimulant, so when the body is threatened by any of these organisms, Ti-tree increases its ability to respond.

The immunostimulant action of Ti-tree is perhaps its most important property, and is especially useful in debilitating illnesses such as glandular fever, and for people who repeatedly succumb to infections or who are very slow to recover from any illness. I would certainly include Ti-tree in any treatment for M.E. and because of its action on the immune system, it is one of the most important oils we have at our disposal for helping people who are H.I.V. positive.

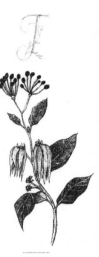

It is valuable for colds, influenza and the infectious illnesses of childhood. If used in the bath at the first signs of a cold or 'flu, one of the effects of Ti-tree is to stimulate profuse sweating, which has long been recognised in naturopathy and other forms of natural healing as a valuable response to infection. Quite often this is enough to stop a cold or 'flu developing and, if not, will reduce its severity and help to prevent secondary infections. This is not suppressing the infection but efficiently fighting it.

In general, Ti-tree is not a skin irritant and can, in fact, be used undiluted on the skin. However, I have known a very few people become sensitive to this oil so those with sensitive skins should use Ti-tree cautiously at first, though even as little as 3 drops in a full bath for an adult has been shown to have the anti-infectious action described above.

Neat Ti-tree oil is an effective treatment for cold sores. Dab it on at the first burning sensation that precedes the blisters. Some people find it more effective if mixed in a little alcohol first (vodka does this well). The blisters of shingles and chickenpox can be treated in the same way.

Verrucae and warts can be eradicated by placing a single drop of neat Ti-tree oil on the centre every day and covering with a plaster. It may take several weeks to see any result, but is effective in the long run.

I use Ti-tree in skin-washes for acne, alternating it with the oils more traditionally used, such as Lavender and Bergamot. The decidedly 'medicinal' smell is welcomed especially by teenage boys who might be wary of sweeter-smelling lotions. It is also good for the large, inflamed and often painful spots which some women tend to get around the nose and chin in the days preceding menstruation. A single drop of Ti-tree dabbed on each spot rapidly reduces the heat and pain and clears the spot up quite quickly.

There are, of course, a good number of essential oils which are active against bacteria and viruses, but anti-fungal oils are relatively few, and Ti-tree is a welcome addition to their number. It is an effective treatment for fungal infections like ringworm and athlete's foot, but a more important application is in controlling Candida albicans. This yeast-like organism normally lives harmlessly in the gut but can get out of control and proliferate, giving rise to a variety of symptoms. (See entries for **CANDIDA** and **THRUSH** for more detailed discussion.) Ti-tree helps to control the Candida organisms by reducing the rate at which they reproduce and strengthening the body's ability to resist them.

As a preventative measure, Ti-tree has been used to build up the strength of patients before surgery. By using the oil in baths and massages for some weeks prior to an operation, and continuing with massage (avoiding the immediate area of the operation wound or scar) afterwards, post-operative shock can be reduced.

These uses for Ti-tree are far from exhaustive. Try it in inhalations for catarrh and sinusitis, in burners and vaporisers during epidemics, mixed in a protective cream for nappy rash, and also in the rinsing water for nappies as a preventative measure. There is a wide range of commercial products based on Ti-tree: lozenges, toothpastes, lotions, creams, etc. and, provided they contain enough of the essential oil, these offer a safe and convenient format for home use.

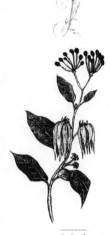

Tonic

An essential oil, herbal preparation, etc., which strengthens and restores vitality to the body, especially during convalescence, or any time when the organism as a whole is debilitated, or under stress.

Tonic oils include Angelica, Basil, Black Pepper, Cinnamon, Clove, Geranium, Ginger, Lavender, Lemon, Marjoram, Myrrh, Nutmeg, Rosemary and Thyme. Most of these are gently stimulating, and indeed you will see that there is an overlap with the group of stimulant oils. It is sensible to use these oils in conjunction with good nutrition, multivitamin and mineral supplements and adequate rest, alternated with gentle exercise.

Basil, Geranium, Lavender, Marjoram, Myrrh, Rosemary and Thyme are all good bath and massage oils. If at all possible, massage is the best way of restoring tone to a run-down person, but baths are a good second-best and a good back-up treatment to use between massages. The other oils mentioned can be used in baths or massage oils in very low percentages, with the exception of Cinnamon. Use these in burners or vaporisers, inhale them directly from the bottle or on a hankie or tissue, and try to include the corresponding herb or spice in cooking.

Angelica

see also **STIMULANTS** *and* **CONVALESCENCE.**

Tonsillitis

The tonsils are formed of lymphoid tissue, and lie in the upper part of the throat (pharynx). In common with the spleen, thymus and lymphatic system they form part of our defence against infection. Like the thymus, they are larger in childhood, and dwindle in adulthood, possibly because antibodies to a great number of illnesses are formed during childhood as the child progressively comes into contact with the various bacteria and viruses responsible for infection.

Tonsillitis, or inflammation of the tonsils, is due to infection of these organs themselves, often by streptococci. Steam inhalations at frequent intervals will both relieve the pain and help to combat the infection. Thyme is one of the best oils to use, as it is not only a very powerful antiseptic, but also has a mild local anaesthetic effect which reduces the discomfort. (See entry for **INHALATIONS** for the method to use.) Lavender and Benzoin are other good oils.

Repeated attacks of tonsillitis indicate a low state of resistance, and steps need to be taken to improve this. An improvement in diet, garlic tablets or capsules taken every night, massage with Ti-tree and other oils and large amounts of Vitamin C are all indicated.

The practice of removing the tonsils, particularly during childhood, is now fortunately far less common than it was 20 or 30 years ago, and if natural treatment with essential oils, plus nutritional measures are followed, it should only very rarely be necessary.

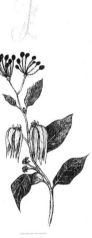

Toothache

There are one or two aromatherapy first-aid methods which will relieve the pain of toothache until the sufferer can get to a dentist. The classic method is familiar to many people who otherwise know nothing of aromatherapy – to put a little oil of Cloves into the cavity of the painful tooth. Clove acts as a local anaesthetic, and is also a very powerful disinfectant which can help to prevent infection of the root until proper dental treatment is possible. Put a drop of Clove on a cotton-bud and apply to the tooth. If there is a large cavity, for example if a filling has fallen out, or the tooth is broken, put one or two drops of Clove oil on a small twist of cottonwool and press into the cavity. When the anaesthetic effects wear off, the Clove oil can be re-applied.

Another method, perhaps more helpful for a dull ache than an acute pain, is to make a hot compress with oil of Camomile and place this over the cheek. The compress should be renewed as it cools. This is the best method to use if an abscess is forming, or you suspect that it might. The heat and the action of the Camomile oil will help to draw infection to the surface so that the abscess will clear faster, and the tooth can then be treated.

see under **ABSCESSES**, *also* **COMPRESSES** *for method of making and applying.*

Toxicity

The great majority of essential oils are non-toxic and perfectly safe when handled sensibly; that is to say, in the small quantities and low dilutions described in this book, and used by responsible therapists. There are, though, some which are highly toxic, even in small amounts, and others which may give rise to toxicity if used over a long period of time. There are also several groups of people who are far more vulnerable to possible damage from the use of essential oils than most of us. They are: babies and young children, pregnant women, people suffering from epilepsy, and the elderly; and special caution should be taken when using essential oils for anybody in one of these categories. This is more fully discussed in the entries for each of these groups of people.

The most toxic essential oils have never been commonly used in therapy, and are difficult to obtain. However, there is a group of oils which could be considered as 'borderline', in that they present certain risks, but are quite easy to get hold of, and it is perhaps here that the greatest care is needed. Some of these are described in books, particularly those originating in France, without any cautions regarding their use, but we need to bear in mind that in France the majority of aromatherapists are doctors, who have undertaken a training in the use of essential oils after their general medical training. They may, on occasion, use with great caution and with a complete understanding of their possible effects on the body, some oils which could be lethal if misused. In much the same way, both homoeopaths and allopathic doctors use minute amounts of toxic plants to produce a cure, but this does not mean that the lay person, or an aromatherapist without a medical background (and in Great Britain that means almost all of us) should attempt to do the same.

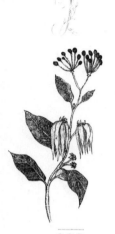

There are also some oils whose possible toxic effects have not been fully understood until recently, through new research and through clinical observation, and these too may be described as though they are completely safe in a number of older reference works.

298

Among the oils which are potentially dangerous, but which you may be able to buy without difficulty, are Camphor, Mugwort (often sold under its French name of Armoise), Pennyroyal, Sassafras, Thuja, Wintergreen and Wormwood. All these oils present risk of poisoning, and it is best to leave them strictly alone.

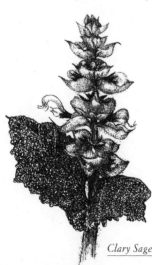

Sage is an oil which has been commonly held to be quite safe, but my personal observation suggests otherwise, and other therapists are now producing evidence which confirms this. I would suggest using Clary Sage as a safer alternative in almost every situation. Some varieties of Thyme are potentially hazardous and I would certainly use this oil in very low concentrations only, and avoid Thyme, or use the gentle Thyme chemotype with linalol, if treating children.

The essential oil from Bitter Almonds is very dangerous indeed, as it contains cyanide. (The almond oil used as a carrier for massage is obtained from the sweet almond and is perfectly safe.) Almond essence sold for food flavouring has either had the cyanide removed by a chemical process, or is more commonly a synthetic product.

Aniseed, again often given its French name, Anise, has serious effects if used over a long period of time. It can damage the nervous system and the circulation and can be addictive in the same way as

Clary Sage

narcotic drugs. It is wise, in any case, to avoid using any essential oil repeatedly over a long period of time, as residues may build up in the body and give rise to toxic effects. Even with the safest essential oils, the body simply stops responding to them if they are used continually, so it is more sensible to vary the oils used, or take a little 'holiday' from your favourite oils from time to time.

The most toxic oils frequently have the effect of damaging the kidneys and/or the liver, and prolonged use of the dubious oils can do the same. This is because these organs have the job within our bodies of filtering out many dangerous substances, so high concentrations of poisons eventually accumulate in them.

I would like to emphasise that in speaking of toxicity – or, in plain terms, poisoning – I am not only referring to taking essential oils by mouth. This is by far the most dangerous method of use, and you will realise from many other entries in this book that I neither use nor recommend the use of essential oils in this way. The majority of responsible aromatherapists share this view and most of the professional organisations require their members to give an undertaking not to recommend internal use.

However, essential oils are very effectively absorbed into the body, whether we inhale them or apply them to the skin, and they find their way into the bloodstream. It is this very fact which makes aromatherapy the effective system which it is, but it also means that toxic oils can be taken into the body by the same routes.

A complete list of toxic essential oils is given at the end of this book.

see also entries under **SKIN IRRITATION, EPILEPSY, ELDERLY. PREGNANCY, BABIES,** *etc.*

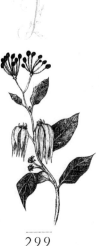

Tranquillisers

Tranquillisers are a class of drugs used to reduce symptoms of anxiety, most of which are benzodiazepines. These include Valium, Librium, Ativan and many other brand-names. A smaller group of other drugs including propranolol are used to reduce sweating, palpitations, etc., caused by anxiety.

Thousands of people have become addicted to these legally-prescribed drugs, and taking them for only a few months can produce dependency. Headaches, abnormal fatigue, depression, digestive, menstrual and sexual disturbances are known side-effects, as well as possible skin rashes, nausea and other problems.

Aromatherapy offers a safe and effective alternative to the use of tranquillisers in stressful situations, and has also proved effective in helping people to abandon the use of these drugs, even after taking them for years.

If it is possible to help a stressed and anxious person before they resort to tranquillisers, there is fortunately a wide range of essential oils which can help to reduce stress, especially when allied to massage given by a sensitive therapist. Lavender, Neroli and Ylang-Ylang are perhaps the first oils that spring to mind, though Benzoin, Bergamot, Camomile, Clary Sage, Helichrysum, Melissa, Rose and Sandalwood would all be excellent choices. As always, the client's preference for one or more of these should be your guide to the final choice, and as treatment is likely to continue for a period of time, this should be varied quite often. Aromatic baths are a good adjunct to regular massage, and an oil or blend that is really liked can be used as a perfume.

Sometimes people who are already taking tranquillisers will consult an aroma-therapist for help in discontinuing them. The most important point to remember is that the amount of the drug being taken should be reduced gradually. Sudden withdrawal can be extremely unpleasant and possibly dangerous. A general rule is to reduce the daily dosage by one-quarter at first, and if the client feels able to cope, to reduce the remaining dose by a further one-quarter, and so on. Each stage of this process may take as little as a week or as long as several months. The longer the tranquillisers have been used, the longer it is likely to take to get off them. It is important that the prescribing doctor is informed before this process begins, and consulted at intervals throughout it. Most doctors are very pleased to help patients get off tranquillisers, and will support their efforts by prescribing the drug in a lower-dosage formulation that makes gradual reduction easier.

I suggest several aromatherapy treatments – i.e., massage with any of the oils previously mentioned, before any reduction of the drug is attempted. Aromatic baths are an important part of the treatment, not least because the client is in control of them, and this reduces any feeling of dependence on the therapist. The oils used should be changed frequently, to avoid the risk of any one oil being regarded as a 'crutch' in place of the tranquillisers. Physical addiction to essential oils is almost impossible, but a kind of emotional addiction can arise: also the oils simply become less effective if used too continuously. The client may need support and treatment for some time after the last dose of tranquillisers has been taken.

Supplementation with vitamins, especially C and the B complex, will reinforce the aromatherapy treatment, as deficiencies have been observed in many people suffering from anxiety. Some people may benefit from counselling or psychotherapy.

see also **ADDICTION.**

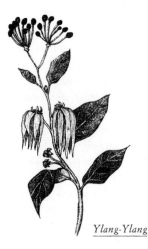

Ylang-Ylang

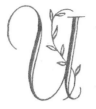

Ulcers, Mouth

❧

see **MOUTH ULCERS.**

Urethritis

❧

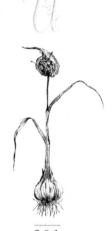

Inflammation of the urethra – the tube carrying urine from the bladder to the outside. Urination is frequent and painful, with a sensation of heat and stinging. Inflammation may travel upwards in to the bladder, especially in women, leading to cystitis.

Most urethritis is caused by infection with the bacteria *E. coli,* normally present in the gut where it is harmless, but becomes a threat when it migrates to other parts of the body. However, urethritis can also be a symptom of gonorrhoea, so it should always be investigated.

At the first sign of irritation, repeated local swabbing can sometimes prevent the infection developing. Bergamot is really the best oil to use. Dilute 3 or 4 drops first in a little vodka, and add this to half a litre of boiled and cooled water. Swab after every urination. Add 6 drops of Bergamot to a full bath and soak for 20 minutes, twice a day if possible. If no relief is obtained, do not delay in consulting a doctor.

see also entries for **CYSTITIS** and **URINARY TRACT.**

Uric Acid

❧

Uric acid is a by-product of the digestion of proteins, which is normally filtered out of the blood by the kidneys and excreted in the urine. However, some people produce more uric acid than the kidneys can easily get rid of, or the kidneys themselves do not dispose of the acid efficiently. When this happens, deposits of uric acid build up in the body, giving rise to disease, especially arthritis and gout. Essential oil of Lemon has a very specific action in counteracting the excess acidity of the system, as does fresh lemon juice. Use a little Lemon oil in massage blends for arthritis, etc., and encourage the client to drink fresh Lemon juice regularly. Although the fruit is itself acid, it has an alkaline reaction in the body. Other essential oils which can be helpful in such toxic accumulations are detoxifying oils such as Fennel and Juniper.

Urinary Tract

By the urinary tract we mean the tubes which carry urine from the kidneys where it is made (the ureters), the bladder, and the single tube carrying urine from the bladder to the outside (the urethra). In women the urethra is about 1.5 ins (4 cm) in length, while in men it is considerably longer as it has to pass through the penis. Because of this, women are generally more susceptible to bladder infections, chiefly cystitis, caused by bacterial infection from the outside. Many attacks of cystitis originate as urethritis, and the infection passes quite quickly up the urethra into the bladder. Very prompt treatment at the beginning of an attack can sometimes prevent the infection being transmitted in this way.

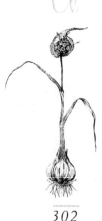

Eucalyptus

(See the entry for **CYSTITIS** for method.) No bladder infection should ever be neglected because of the risk of infection spreading via the ureters to the kidneys. While continuing with aromatherapy treatment, do not hesitate to consult a doctor if symptoms have not gone within two days, or if they are severe with fever, blood or pus in the urine.

Quite a number of essential oils are urinary tract antiseptics, the most valuable being Bergamot, Camomile, Eucalyptus, Juniper, Sandalwood and Ti-tree. They should be applied in repeated hot compresses over the lower abdomen. At the same time, copious drinks of spring water and Camomile tea should be taken. Fresh garlic or capsules will reinforce the treatment.

Hot compresses are also used to relieve the discomfort of prostatitis in men. The prostate gland becomes enlarged – a problem usually arising in middle age or later, and because this gland surrounds the outlet of the urethra from the bladder, it obstructs the flow of urine. If the problem is neglected until it becomes acute, or when the onset is sudden, the retention of urine may be total, placing great strain upon the kidneys. Hot compresses of Camomile, Juniper or Pine, placed immediately over the bladder area, will often produce a flow of urine, but medical help must also be urgently obtained. Compresses over the lower back (kidney area) may also help.

see also entries for **CYSTITIS** *and* **URETHRITIS.**

Urticaria

Urticaria is an allergic skin reaction that takes its name from the fact that the symptoms are similar to nettle stings.

Stings release histamine in the body, which causes the tiny blood vessels beneath the skin to leak fluids into the tissues around them, and creates burning and itching sensations. Allergic reactions to other substances starts a very similar chain of events. The substance that starts this off (an allergen) may be a food, or an external irritant such as dust, detergent, etc. Red itchy blotches appear on the skin and they may take the form of raised lumps. Quite often they disappear fairly quickly, only to break out again on a different part of the body. In severe cases they may appear as large, red weals, particularly on areas that are rubbed by clothes.

Many people suffer attacks of urticaria during periods of stress, but not at times when they are calm and relaxed, and this is a feature common to all allergic reactions. The body under stress is unable to cope with irritants that are harmless in more favourable conditions.

Camomile and Melissa are traditionally used to treat allergies, and will quickly relieve most attacks of urticaria. An important factor is that both these oils work on the mental/emotional level as well as the physical, having a calming and de-stressing action, so they work on the underlying cause of the allergy as well as the immediate effect.

Some people respond better to one oil and some to the other, or you may wish to combine them to be sure of giving some immediate relief. If the rash covers a large area of the body the simplest and most soothing treatment is to immerse the patient in a lukewarm bath with 4 drops of Camomile and 2 of Melissa. Do not exceed the number of drops mentioned or the bath may make the skin even more irritated instead of soothing it.

If the rash is localised, it might be easier to apply diluted Camomile and/or Melissa directly to a small area. Dilute to 1% in boiled and cooled water and sponge onto the itchy area, or soak a gauze in the solution and wrap it around the area. Carrier oils and oil-based creams make the condition worse, but if you have an unperfumed, non-oily lotion available, you could add a few drops of Camomile to that. Any of these treatments can be repeated every few hours until the rash and itching have cleared.

If you think that stress is a major factor, it would be wise to continue treatment with massage, baths, etc. after the actual skin eruption has healed.

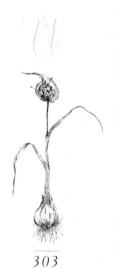

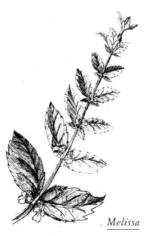

Melissa

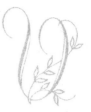

Vaginitis

Inflammation of the vagina, usually caused by organisms such as Candida albicans and Trichomonas. See the entry for **THRUSH** for suggested treatment.

Vaporisers

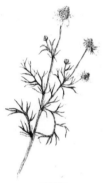

SEE AEROSOLS AND BURNERS.

Varicose Veins

The abnormal swelling of veins in the legs is a symptom of a generally poor circulatory system, with a loss of elasticity in the walls of the veins and particularly in their valves. When they are functioning normally, these valves prevent blood from flowing back (away from the heart), but if their efficiency decreases some blood may stagnate in the vein, which then becomes swollen and twisted, causing aching and abnormal fatigue of the legs. The tendency for the valves to fail in this way is sometimes inherited, but the main causes are prolonged standing, poor nutrition and obesity – often a combination of two or more of these factors. Pregnancy may also cause the onset of varicose veins due to the increased weight, and pressure, in the pelvic area.

Aromatherapy treatment needs to be aimed chiefly at improving the general tone of the veins, and should be combined with dietary and other advice. One of the most important oils for strengthening the veins is Cypress, which should be used as a bath oil, and applied, very gently, over the area of the affected veins. Massage can be used above the affected area of the vein (i.e. on that part of the leg which is nearer the heart), but must NEVER be used below the varicosity, as this will only increase the pressure in the vein. Cypress oil can either be blended in a carrier oil at 3% or made up in a cream. A cream is probably the most convenient form in which to give the oil to a client to take home for daily use.

Garlic capsules are a good way to strengthen the circulatory systems, and you can recommend 3 capsules a day, as well as fresh garlic in the diet. Vitamins E and C should be taken as supplements initially, but in the long-term it is necessary to make sure that they are supplied in sufficient amounts in foods.

Resting with the legs higher than the head for at least 20 minutes every day is very helpful and will also decrease the immediate discomfort. The inverted postures of yoga are an excellent way of doing this, or you could suggest using a slant-board, or lying on the floor with the legs and feet supported by a chair.

Gentle exercise is helpful – again yoga would be my first choice, with swimming second. Walking, and gentle stretching exercises are suitable, but jogging, skipping, aerobics and other exercises which involve repeated impact can do more harm than good. However, such exercise would be so uncomfortable for anybody with varicose veins that they would be unlikely to try it for more than a very short time.

It may take many months to produce any improvement in the varicose veins, and as in any situation where prolonged treatment is needed, it is important to vary the essential oils used from time to time. I sometimes use Lavender, Juniper or Rosemary as alternatives to Cypress, but whichever oils are chosen, perseverance with daily application will be needed.

Verbena
Lippia citriodora

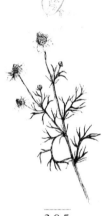

Verbena (or Lemon Verbena) is a native of Chile and Peru, which was introduced to Europe in the 18th century, but a good deal of confusion exists around the naming of this oil. Certain authors give the Latin name as *Andropogon citratus,* which is in fact Lemongrass, or give Lemongrass as an alternative name to Verbena, although they are totally different plants. This is probably due to the fact that there is some similarity in the lemony smell, and the cheaper oil of Lemongrass is sometimes used to adulterate Verbena oil, which is more costly to produce. Further confusion arises between this and Vervain, or *Verbena officinalis,* particularly as Verbena oil is often sold under its French name of Verveine. Because of this confusion, descriptions of Verbena oil sometimes include properties which should be more rightly attributed to *Verbena officinalis,* an odourless, bitter plant used in herbal medicine.

True Verbena oil is obtained by steam distillation from the flowering stalks of the plant, and is a lovely greeny-yellow colour. The yield is quite small, which accounts for the high cost of real Verbena oil. The main constituent is citral (between 30% and 45%) with limonene, myrcene, linalol, geraniol and others.

Palau y Verdera, one of the first writers to describe Verbena, about twenty years after its introduction into Europe, described it as an excellent digestive stimulant, stomachic and antispasmodic, useful in all kinds of digestive upsets and for congestion of the liver; a tonic and stabiliser for the nervous system, useful for vertigo, palpitations and hysteria.

We can recognise all of these properties in Verbena oil, and it is particularly indicated for digestive problems that are the result of anxiety or stress. Regular massage with Verbena can help to reduce stress levels, and the leaves can also be made into a delicious tea, with digestive properties. Combining both methods is probably the most effective course of treatment. Commercially, Verbena is used in several liqueurs with digestive properties. It is regarded by some as a hangover cure!

The 'tea' or infusion also makes a delicious and cooling summertime drink, which can be used as a gentle febrifuge in feverish conditions. It is mildly sedative and may help insomnia, though Arab civilisations have traditionally regarded it as an aphrodisiac! I can neither confirm nor disprove this.

Massage with Verbena oil will also help insomnia, anxiety and stress. If using it in

CAUTION
Verbena may cause
skin sensitisation and
photosensitisation. No
reliable safety data is
available, but it would
be wise to treat
Verbena as suspect
until proved otherwise.

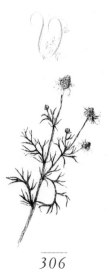

night-time baths for this purpose, be extremely careful, for more than two or three drops in an average bath will cause stinging and blistering of the skin. Just two drops in a bath, with perhaps three or four drops of Lavender, is an excellent sedative bath which will help with many sleep problems.

Verrucas

Verrucas (or more correctly, verrucae) are a form of wart occurring on the soles of the feet, and are also known as plantar warts. Like all warts they are caused by a virus, and will disappear of their own accord when the body develops its resistance to the viral infection. However, because of the pressure exerted on the sole of the foot, they are exceedingly painful and usually need to be treated without waiting for them to go away spontaneously. A simple and effective treatment with essential oil can be found under the entry for LEMON (q.v.). Ti-tree is a very good alternative.

The virus is highly contagious, and verrucas are almost always the result of contact in places where people congregate in bare feet, such as swimming pools and changing rooms in gymnasia and sports centres.

Local treatment is effective if there is a single verruca, or maybe two or three, but if there are a lot of verrucae present, or if new ones keep appearing, massage to increase the body's immune response to the virus will make treatment more effective. Long strokes up the leg, from the ankle towards the thigh, are used with oils of Rosemary, Geranium, Grapefruit or Juniper, or a blend of any two of these. It may also be a good idea to look at other factors, such as poor diet or stress, which may be lowering immunity.

see also entries for WARTS, LEMON and TI-TREE.

Veterinary Uses

Essential oils have a number of applications to the care and treatment of animals. One of the most useful is the prevention and control of fleas, tics and other parasites in the coats of domestic animals. Bergamot, Eucalyptus, Geranium, Lavender and other essential oils are effective insect repellents, and it is possible to avoid completely the use of synthetic chemicals for flea control on cats and dogs by rubbing one or more of these oils in their coats. Dogs generally take more kindly to this kind of grooming than cats, and can be sponged with a mixture of the above oils in tepid water which is then brushed or combed through the coat. For cats, I use Lavender oil, or Manuka, which has an even gentler aroma, putting a few drops on the palms of my hands and stroking it over the fur. Some cats will tolerate this and others will not. If you have a long-haired cat, put the oil on its brush when carrying out the normal grooming. You can use the same method for dogs if you do not want to wet the coat.

Lavender and Ti-tree are valuable for treating minor wounds: add a few drops of the oil to boiled and slightly cooled water for bathing bites, scratches and other battle wounds. Wounds inflicted by claws or teeth often become badly infected, with much heat, pain and pus because the tiny puncture in the skin closes over before the deeper tissues have healed. Hot compresses of Ti-tree, frequently repeated, will draw out the pus and disinfect the wound so it can heal properly.

Cypress is effective against canker in the ears. Wipe inside the ear flap twice a day with a drop of the oil on cotton wool or a cotton-bud.

Horse-owners use a variety of essential oils to treat stiff and painful joints suffered by their mounts. Hot compressing is the most effective method, and any oil that would be used for a similar condition in a human patient is suitable.

I have known people keeping sheep on a small scale (half a dozen sheep kept for their wool) to use a strong solution of Lavender oil instead of a commercial sheep dip, though this would probably not be viable on a larger scale.

NOTE: Unless you are a qualified veterinary surgeon, it is illegal to treat an animal owned by anybody but yourself, but you may wish to use the above suggestions to help your own household pets.

Vetivert
Vetiveria zizanoides

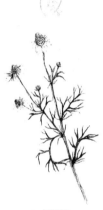

Vetivert is a scented grass native to India and Sri Lanka but now cultivated in the Caribbean and elsewhere. It is botanically related to Lemongrass, Citronella and several other scented grasses.

The essential oil is distilled from the roots and is dark brown and thick in consistency. It requires a very long, slow distillation period and the whole process is very labour intensive, involving digging of the roots and washing them before they can be distilled. The main constituents are vetiverone, vetiverol, vetivines and cadinene. The smell is subtle and not easy to define: it has a depth and smokiness somewhat reminiscent of both Myrrh and Patchouli, but when diluted lemony overtones become more apparent. The perfume is perhaps more pleasing in dilution and adds a subtle note to many blends. It 'marries' very well with Sandalwood, Jasmine, Cedarwood, and – perhaps surprisingly – Lavender. In very small amounts it could be considered as an alternative base note in virtually any blend.

Vetivert roots have been used for their perfume in India for thousands of years, and the oil is used in modern perfumery as a base note and fixative. The oil has many uses in skin care, especially for oily skin and acne. As it has such a 'dark' aroma, it might appeal more to young men with problem skins than some of the lighter, more flowery oils. It is used in commercial cosmetics both for its fragrance and the benefit to the skin.

Less well-known is the fact that Vetivert is an immunostimulant, and increases our ability to withstand stress without becoming ill. It has a mild rubefacient effect, so some therapists use it for arthritis, rheumatism and muscular pain.

However, perhaps the most important actions of Vetivert are on the psyche. Its Indian name, meaning 'Oil of Tranquillity' expresses its character beautifully.

Vetivert is deeply relaxing, so valuable in massage and baths for anybody experiencing stress, anxiety, insomnia or depression. To soak in a Vetivert bath is one of the most de-stressing experiences I know. Because of its earthy quality, being extracted from the roots, it is a very grounding, stabilising oil, useful for people who 'live in the clouds' a bit too much, for those who focus excessively on intellectual activity to the exclusion of the physical and anybody who at times feels a bit insecure. It would be a good oil to use after a shock or during a traumatic period in life, such as divorce, separation or bereavement.

Violet Leaf
Viola odorata

☙

An absolute can be obtained from the leaves of Violets which is mainly used in high class perfumery. Small amounts are occasionally available to aromatherapists, though at extremely high prices. All parts of the Violet plant (petals, leaves, rhizome) contain an alkaloid named violine from which the plant derives is properties, with parmone, salicylic acid, glucosides etc. The absolute has a fresh, dry aroma resembling hay.

It is antiseptic, and has healing properties which are especially valuable in treating skin problems, especially acne, oily skin and large pores. It may have some effect on thread veins. Violet leaves have been used in the treatment of rheumatism, headaches, catarrh and harsh coughs with difficult breathing. It is reported to have pain-killing properties, which one would expect from the presence of salicylic acid but there is no shortage of analgesic oils, and it is unlikely you would choose Violet for this use due to its cost.

Mrs Grieve mentions that Violet leaves have been used in the treatment of cancer in various preparations, including infusions, compresses and a poultice made from the fresh leaves, and she cites some cures, so it might be worth investigating the possibility of using Violet Leaf absolute alongside other therapies, either orthodox or not, in helping cancer patients. A colleague who has been working with people with A.I.D.S. has found this a valuable oil, too. These are possible uses where the high cost would be justified.

Viral Infections

☙

Viruses are the invading agent responsible for most epidemic illnesses, including colds and influenza, chicken pox, smallpox, poliomyelitis and measles. In addition, a great many vague undiagnosed fevers and many instances of diarrhoea are due to viral infection. Some forms of pneumonia originate with viral infection while others are bacterial. Most of these are discussed under their individual headings.

A few essential oils are powerfully antiviral, the most important being Bergamot, Eucalyptus, Manuka, Ravensara and Ti-tree. Of these, Manuka, Ravensara and Ti-tree are probably the most powerful. They also stimulate and strengthen the body's immune response to the infection.

Baths and vaporisation (and where the respiratory tract is involved, steam inhalations) are the best form of treatment, because there is nearly always fever, and during fever massage is contra-indicated. Vaporisations, whether by means of a burner, electric fragrancer, an aerosol diffuser or such simple means as a few drops on a light bulb or on a wet cloth hung over a radiator, not only help the patient, but are one of the best ways of decreasing the risk of the infection being transmitted to other people in the household.

see entries for **COLDS, INFLUENZA, CHICKENPOX, MEASLES,** *etc.*

Vodka

☙

Vodka can be used to dissolve essential oils for use as gargles, mouthwashes, aftershaves, skin tonics, and for adding to the bath.

It is not a totally effective dilutant (only 100% alcohol or bland oils are), but as it is not possible to buy 100% alcohol in the British Isles without a licence, vodka can be substituted for many home-use applications. The higher the degree proof, the more effectively the vodka will dissolve the essential oil. As the dilution is not total, always shake any such mixture thoroughly before use.

Volatility

This is the term to describe the ease and speed with which any substance disperses on contact with the air. It refers particularly to the time taken for a liquid to evaporate, and can be scientifically measured. Essential oils, and in fact all aromatic substances, are highly volatile, i.e. they evaporate very quickly, and this is an intrinsic part of their aromatic nature, for our noses can only detect odours in the form of a vapour or gas.

Essential oils, though all highly volatile, do not all evaporate at the same speed, and this difference in the time taken to evaporate directly affects the length of time the smell of the oil will linger, and the time it will take to be absorbed into the body when applied to the skin. Those oils which take longer to evaporate (i.e., the least volatile) will continue to perfume the skin, or any substance to which they are applied, for many hours and in some cases even days, while those which are the most volatile will disappear quickly.

In any blend of oils, the oil which is most volatile is the one which will be most easily detected when first smelling the blend, while the slowest, or least volatile, is the smell which will last after the others have faded. In perfumery, these differences are classed on a scale analogous to a musical scale, the most volatile substances being described as Top Notes, the least volatile and most long-lasting as Base Notes, with a graduated scale of Middle Notes between. Some aromatherapists refer to such scales when making blends, and may even see different therapeutic properties attaching to the Top, Middle and Base notes. However, a major disadvantage of this approach is that it is somewhat subjective. Neither aromatherapists nor perfumiers agree as to where to place various oils on such a scale, and this is hardly surprising when we consider how much an oil can vary from season to season, according to the weather; or from place to place due to variations in soil and climate.

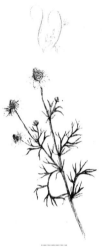

Vomiting

Vomiting can often be relieved by either massaging very gently over the stomach area, or applying a warm compress to that area. Appropriate oils are Camomile, Lavender, Lemon and Peppermint.

If the vomiting is associated with cold, a warming oil such as Black Pepper or Marjoram may be more effective. Camomile and Lavender are probably the best choices if sickness is related to emotional upset.

Camomile, Fennel or Peppermint herbal infusions should be sipped and the Bach Rescue Remedy will often give dramatic relief.

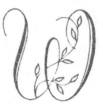

Warts

✑

Small round tumours of the skin, caused by a virus infection. The Latin name verruca is applied to those which appear on the soles of the feet.

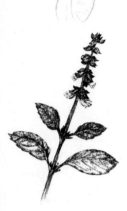

Any wart will disappear of its own accord in time, as the body develops immunity to the virus, but if it is unsightly or uncomfortable, a very simple and effective local treatment is to use Ti-tree oil neat, directly on the wart. Take a single drop of Ti-tree on the end of a toothpick or orange stick, and drop it on to the centre of the wart. Put a dry plaster over the wart and keep it covered. This treatment should be repeated every day until the wart shrivels and drops off. Some warts will disappear in less than a week, and others may take up to a month to do so. Once the wart has gone, massage a little wheatgerm oil, which is rich in vitamin E, into the area until any scarring or soreness has healed. Lavender and/or Marigold oil can be added to the wheatgerm to speed healing. Lemon is an alternative to Ti-tree, and can be used in alternation with it. Some people suffer from the appearance of large numbers of warts in a relatively short space of time, suggesting a low level of resistance to the virus. Garlic capsules (between 3 and 6 a day) will help to strengthen the immune response, as will lymphatic massage with essential oils of Rosemary, Geranium, Juniper or a blend of these. Sometimes such 'plagues' of warts may appear following a trauma, such as a road accident, bereavement, etc. and treatment appropriate to such a situation will also be needed.

A good level of nutrition will also help the body in dealing with the virus, particularly appropriate levels of all vitamins and minerals, especially Vitamin E.

see also **VERRUCAS.**

Whitlow

✑

A whitlow is an infection of the finger-tip, at the side of the nail, which may creep under the nail itself. Pus collects, and particularly if it is trapped under the nail, can be very painful. Sometimes the nail has to be removed.

Hot compresses of Bergamot, Camomile, Lavender or Ti-tree should be applied round the finger repeatedly, a fresh one being applied as soon as the previous one has cooled. This will draw out pus and promote faster healing. Once the whitlow has broken and pus has been released, neat Lavender oil can be applied and covered with a gauze dressing, held in place with a strip of adhesive plaster. Do not use a plaster that covers the area and excludes air, or the finger will get very damp and healing will be delayed.

A high level of Vitamin C supplementation is a valuable adjunct to the treatment with essential oils, and it may also be useful to take a general look at the diet of the person involved, as whitlows often affect those with a generally poor standard of nutrition.

Whooping Cough

෨

In common with the other infectious illnesses of childhood, the severity of whooping cough can be modified by using essential oils.

The use of steam kettles in the sickroom has long been known to give some relief from the exhausting coughing fits, and adding essential oils to any source of steam will be doubly valuable. Good oils to use are Ti-tree or Niaouli (closely related to each other), Rosemary, Lavender, Cypress, Thyme and various blends of these. Steam vaporisations are valuable whatever the age of the child – though of course the kettle or other appliance should be placed well out of reach of a young child.

Older children can have chest rubs with a blend of 5 drops Niaouli, 10 drops Cypress and 10 drops Lavender in 50 mls of almond, sunflower or other bland oil. Rub the child's chest and back, three or four times a day with this blend to reduce the coughing spasms.

In every case, call a doctor, as whooping cough can be a long, drawn-out and very debilitating illness, and the child becoming weakened risks succumbing to complications such as pneumonia.

However, using essential oils as suggested will reduce this risk and help to shorten the illness.

Wounds

෨

Virtually all essential oils are antiseptic and therefore helpful in cleansing and treating wounds, but some are more notably so. Several of them also help to promote healing and kill pain, so obviously a combination of these properties makes a good oil for treating wounds. A further requirement is that the oil will not damage or irritate the exposed flesh (some of the most powerfully antiseptic oils are more suitable for washing surfaces, vaporising in sickrooms, etc., than for applying directly to broken skin).

The combination of properties reduces our choice to a small handful of oils, but as each of these is a really powerful healer, this is no disadvantage. Lavender has been used for this purpose for thousands of years (indeed, its name is derived from the Latin 'lavare', to wash, since it was used to wash out wounds). Myrrh was similarly used by the ancient Greeks, and Ti-tree, although a relatively recent introduction to Europe, has a long history of use by the Aboriginal people of Australia.

The essential oil can be used neat on minor wounds – it will sting for a moment but this will quickly pass. The safest method, which avoids touching the wound is to put a few drops of the oil on a plaster and then put this over the cut. For larger injuries, put the essential oil on a piece of gauze, and cover the wound with this, but be sensible about the extent to which you should attempt to treat without medical help. If in any doubt, especially if the edges of a wound may need to be held together with one or more stitches, use the essential oil as first aid and take the injured person to a doctor or casualty department as soon as possible.

Many other essential oils are suitable for treating wounds, including Benzoin, Bergamot, Camomile, Eucalyptus, Juniper and Rosemary, but I regard Lavender and Ti-tree as the most important and useful, with Myrrh in reserve for any wound that is slow to heal, especially if it is weepy.

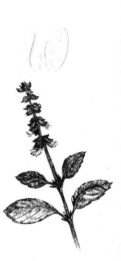

Wrinkles

Wrinkles occur as the skin gets older, because the connective tissue which forms a great part of the inner layers (or Dermis) of the skin, loses its elasticity. Imagine an elastic band. When it is new it will spring back into place after it has been stretched, but when the rubber gets old it will stay stretched instead of returning to its original size. Similarly, skin which is repeatedly stretched, such as in smiling, frowning or screwing up the eyes, quickly goes back to its original state when young, but not as the connective tissue ages.

Regular massage with essential oils can do a certain amount to reduce wrinkling, although the best time to apply such treatment would be, ideally, before any wrinkles have formed! Massage stimulates the local circulation, and this ensures good supplies of oxygen to the minute blood vessels in the inner layers of skin. The cells in the inner skin need oxygen for health and growth, as does every cell in the body. Massage directly onto the face needs to be ultra-gentle, since any pulling of the skin would only make the problem worse, but it is very helpful to give vigorous massage to the scalp, which stimulates the circulation to the whole head. This is something which can easily be done every day as a self-help measure: rub the head as if shampooing, and tap with the fingertips all over the scalp. Massage, and the input of plenty of oxygen, also helps to tone the muscles underlying the skin and this can give a more youthful appearance.

Two of the most useful essential oils are Frankincense and Neroli, both of which have been used in skin care for thousands of years. The Egyptians used Frankincense for cosmetic purposes as well as for embalming and religious ceremonies and it does seem to have a preservative action on the skin. In some instances it may even reduce existing wrinkling, but it does certainly help to prevent further wrinkles forming. Neroli is particularly valuable in that it stimulates the body to produce healthy new cells, and this can help to keep the skin looking smooth by delaying the ageing process in the layers of connective tissue.

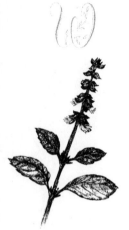

The carrier oil used for the massage is important too, and richer oils such as avocado or jojoba are the most helpful, with the addition of 25% wheatgerm oil.

Anything which is good for the general health and vitality of the body is helpful, too, especially exercise of all kinds, which, like massage, increases circulation and improves muscle tone.

Good nutrition is important, especially foods which provide good amounts of Vitamins B, C and E, and a vitamin and mineral supplement might help. Smoking, alcohol and excessive amounts of tea and coffee lower the vitality of the skin, and increase the tendency to wrinkle.

You will notice that I have referred to the inner layers of the skin. The outer layer of skin, or Epidermis, is composed of cells which are already dead, just as our hair and nails are, so any treatment which is aimed at improving the appearance of the skin must always take into account the living layers of skin where new cells are constantly being formed.

Rosemary

Xeroderma

⨖

An abnormal dryness of the skin, such as is found in Icthyosis. The skin has fewer sebaceous glands than usual, so it lacks natural lubrication. It may appear scaly (hence the name Icthyosis from the Greek word for a fish). It is quite different from ordinary dryness of the skin, in which the normal number of sebaceous glands are present, but are secreting less than they should, and it is not easy to treat.

Rich creams can be helpful, with essential oils that benefit dry skin in general, such as Camomile, Geranium, Lavender and Neroli, but these need to be applied frequently, and nothing that can truly be considered a cure is known. Treatments described for Psoriasis can sometimes help.

see **CREAMS** *for suitable formulae, also* **PSORIASIS.**

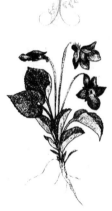

X-rays

⨖

X-rays, also known as Roentgen rays, are a form of electro-magnetic radiation. They resemble light rays, except that they have a very much shorter wave length. Whereas they were previously used very widely as a form of treatment, as well as for diagnosis, this has now been superseded by less dangerous methods for almost all conditions except certain skin cancers and other superficial growths where it remains a valuable therapy outweighing the possible dangers.

Diagnostic use of X-rays is also restricted to those circumstances where there is no safer alternative method, since the dangerous side-effects have become increasing well understood. Diagnostic X-rays are less damaging than X-rays used in therapy, but they still carry some risk.

Lavender oil is very valuable as a treatment for skin which has been damaged by X-ray therapy. Though healing may take a long time, therapists in Norway have had very good results with cancer patients who had skin burns as a result of their treatment.

Anybody who has received X-ray therapy, or who is worried about exposure .to X-rays used in diagnosis, could try the special bath formula described under **RADIATION**.

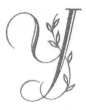

Yin/Yang

The concept of Yin and Yang is part of the Taoist philosophy underlying the practice of traditional acupuncture and shiatsu, but extends to aromatherapy in that some writers have attempted to classify essential oils in this way.

Yin and Yang are descriptions given to opposite and complementary energies, or qualities, which are present in everybody and everything. Yin is seen as feminine, dark, moist, cool, contracting and Yang as masculine, light, dry, hot and expanding. However, nothing is wholly Yin or wholly Yang, and there is always a little Yin in a predominantly Yang organism, and vice versa. Also the balance of Yin and Yang is not static but constantly changing.

In the human body, a proper balance of Yin and Yang is seen as being necessary to complete health. If one or the other predominates, mental or physical problems will arise, and the therapist's task is to try to re-establish the balance, so that health is restored.

The classification of essential oils into Yin and Yang groups is somewhat controversial, and not every therapist agrees on which oils should be put into which category. Some oils which are very clearly 'feminine', cooling, and so forth, such as Rose or Camomile can easily be seen as Yin, and others which are of an obviously strong or fiery nature, such as Black Pepper, Ginger, Jasmine and so forth can be described as Yang. However, many oils are difficult to fit into either category, and may even seem Yin at one time and Yang at another, according to the soil, climate and growing season, and for these reasons I would not attempt to classify oils in this way.

However, the concept can still be a useful guide when choosing essential oils for any particular person, and can be added to all the other ways we have of describing the therapeutic and other properties of the oils in order to deepen our understanding of them.

see also the entry for **ACUPUNCTURE**.

Ylang-Ylang
Cananga odorata

A small tropical tree which grows in the Philippines, Java, Sumatra and Madagascar, gives us the essential oil known as Ylang-Ylang. The name Ylang-Ylang means 'flower of flowers' in the local dialect, and is sometimes given to the tree *Anona odorantissima*, though there is some doubt as to whether these are in fact two different trees, or simply the same one exhibiting some differences when grown in different soil and climate.

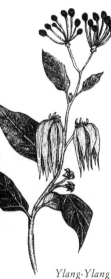

There are pink, mauve and yellow-flowered varieties, and the finest essential oil comes from the yellow-flowered trees. The first part of the oil which is drawn off during the steam distillation process is of the highest quality, and is sold under the name of Ylang-Ylang, while that which comes from the latter part of the process – known as the 'tail' of the distillate – is of a poorer grade and is usually sold under the name of Cananga. In either case, the therapeutic properties are the same, but the perfume of Cananga is less refined. The best oil of all is obtained from flowers picked in early summer, and early in the morning.

Both oils contain methyl benzoate, methyl salicilate, eugenol, geraniol, linalol, safrol, ylangol, terpenes, pinene, benzyl acetate, and a combination of acetic, benzoic, formic, salicylic and valeric acids. The oil varies from almost colourless to a pale yellow, and the aroma is extremely heavy and sweet. Some people find it sickly, and it is often best used in blends with oils such as Lemon or Bergamot which will somewhat offset the sweetness.

Ylang-Ylang

Perhaps the most important physical property of Ylang-Ylang is its ability to slow down over-rapid breathing (hyperpnoea) and over-rapid heartbeat (tachycardia). These symptoms may appear when somebody is shocked, frightened or anxious, and, sometimes when they are extremely angry, and immediate use of Ylang-Ylang can be very helpful in such circumstances. However, anybody who has such symptoms in the longer term clearly should be receiving advice and care from a doctor, homoeopath or acupuncturist though the oil can be used as a back-up treatment with great benefit.

Ylang-Ylang is one of the oils which will help to reduce high blood pressure, often found in association with hyperpnoea or tachycardia.

It is used widely in perfumery and cosmetics, and is suitable for both dry and oily skins, having a balancing action on the secretion of sebum. The sweet perfume makes it popular for these uses commercially, for it is quite a lot less costly than the other 'heady' floral oils, such as Rose and Jasmine. It has been described as resembling Hyacinth, though I can find little resemblance between the two scents. It is thought to have a tonic effect on the scalp, and in the 19th century was used as an ingredient in a hair preparation known as Macassar oil, which was so widely used that Victorian housewives needed to protect their chair-backs against the oily stains – hence 'antimacassars'. If you wanted to try it as a hair preparation, an alcoholic solution would be less likely to damage the furniture.

Like Jasmine, Rose and Sandalwood oils, Ylang-Ylang is antidepressant, aphrodisiac and sedative, and can be used to help people who have sexual difficulties, for these are so often the result of stress and anxiety. The calming and relaxing effect of Ylang-Ylang may be responsible for its designation as an aphrodisiac, as it can be used, wisely, to break the vicious circle of anxiety about sexual inadequacy, anxiety actually creating such inadequacy, which leads to further anxiety.

The oil often seems to be best when used in combination with others, not only for the purpose of lightening the perfume.

Take care when using Ylang-Ylang, for too high a concentration or using it for too long a time, can give rise to nausea and/or headache.

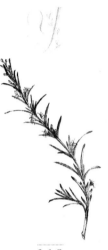

315

Yoga

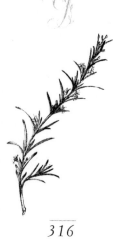

In a number of entries in this book you will find references to yoga as a valuable aid to relaxation and the reduction of stress. Many people who consult an aromatherapist do so because they are under stress, or because they are suffering physical symptoms which are the result of stress and anxiety.

While the aromatherapist can do a great deal to induce relaxation and reduce stress in the short-term with massage, suitable choice of oils and advice on aromatic baths and other uses, this is passive stress-reduction, and in the long term there is a real need for the stressed person to learn some active methods of helping him or herself. Yoga is one of the most effective of these, along with meditation (q.v.). I have found repeatedly that when yoga is combined with regular aromatherapy massage, the person needing help will benefit much more than if either of these methods is used on its own.

One reason why yoga appears to combine so well with aromatherapy is that, like aromatherapy, it works on many levels. It can be viewed simply as a system of physical exercise, or as a profound philosophy, and yoga teachers vary in the amount of emphasis they place on the different aspects. All yoga teachers give some instruction on how to ally the breathing to the physical movements, but some will spend more time than others on breathing exercises. Again, many yoga teachers include some form of simple meditation in their lessons, and some of them will spend time discussing yoga philosophy, or give out leaflets, or recommend books on the subject to students who are interested in this aspect. You may prefer one teacher's approach to another's, and perhaps you will need to try several yoga classes before you discover the one that feels most appropriate to your own needs and outlook. There are classes in almost every town in the British Isles, often as part of the local authority's adult education provision. To find a teacher who has had a thorough, two-year training, contact the British Wheel of Yoga.

Yoga is non-competitive, and suitable for people of all ages, whether they have health problems or not. No yoga teacher will force you, or even encourage you, to attempt anything which is beyond your physical capacity, or which you feel worried about doing. Always tell your teacher on first joining the class if you have any specific problem, such as high blood pressure, or long-term back trouble, and also remember to mention any short-term trouble, such as headache or catarrh, a pulled muscle or backache, so that your teacher can advise you on which asanas to avoid and which will benefit you.

When you first join a yoga class, you may find that you are not able to do all the asanas perfectly: this is of no importance, as it is not the final pose, but the correct effort made to reach it which will benefit you, and your teacher will make sure that you are trying to attain the posture in a safe and effective way. Never compare your ability with that of other people in the class, or even with your own ability at some other time.

Disabled people can benefit from yoga too, and it has been found especially helpful in certain specific ailments, notably asthma and multiple sclerosis. Some teachers specialise in working with people with disabilities.

Conversely, aromatherapy and particularly massage, can help to improve your yoga. If you have certain areas of the body which are stiffer than others, some specific massage will often help to loosen the muscles so that you can reach yoga postures which will further benefit those muscles. If you are unable to visit a therapist, or wish to reinforce the value of the massage, aromatic baths, particularly using Lavender, Rosemary or

Marjoram and taken shortly before you go to your lesson, will also have the effect of making you more supple.

Of course, you will derive more benefit from yoga if you practice for a short time each day, in addition to your lesson, which will usually be weekly. There are many books and tapes to help with home practice, but it is very important to remember that they are only meant to act as a back-up to regular lessons with a teacher. Never attempt to teach yourself yoga without supervision by a properly trained and qualified teacher, as you may do yourself more harm than good.

Yoghurt

Quite apart from its important nutritional properties, yoghurt is used by many aromatherapists in facial and other skin treatments. Used as a face-pack, either alone, or mixed with a little honey, yoghurt has a rejuvenating and softening effect on the skin. It is particularly useful for treating the skin of the neck which can become discoloured, especially at the end of winter, after months of central heating or wrapping up in scarves, high collars, etc. Yoghurt has a mild bleaching action, and will restore a healthier colour to the neck.

It is possible to mix essential oils into full-cream yoghurt, as the fat content is sufficient to dissolve the oil. However, the majority of yoghurts on sale are made from skimmed milk, and it is not advisable to try to mix essential oils with them, as the oil will not completely dissolve.

When treating intestinal problems, yoghurt is an extremely valuable adjunct to aromatherapy, because it provides a suitable environment for the 'friendly' bacteria of the colon. This is particularly important when a patient has previously been treated with antibiotics, or if they are taking such drugs concurrently with aromatherapy treatment, as antibiotics will kill the helpful bacteria along with the dangerous invading organisms against which they have been prescribed.

It is important to use only natural, live yoghurt.

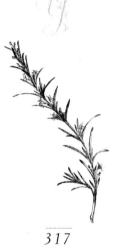

317

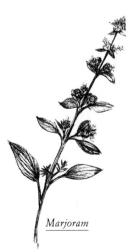

Marjoram

Zdravetz

Geranium macrorrhizum, or *Robertium macrorrhizum*

◈

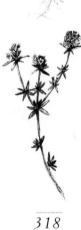

The name Zadravetz is derived from a Bulgarian word 'zdrave', meaning 'health' and the plant has been used as a medicinal herb for as long as anybody can recall. In Bulgaria, which is the main area of production, it is greatly valued as an aphrodisiac. It is a small perennial, native to the Balkan region, though it is also found wild in Northern Italy and has become naturalized in other parts of south-eastern Europe. The plant is very hardy and grows best on rocky soil at high altitudes, up to about 2,400 metres.

The essential oil is distilled in Bulgaria, and for that reason is sometimes described as 'Bulgarian Geranium oil' – a confusing label as it implies Geranium oil grown in Bulgaria, while Zdravetz in no way resembles the more usual Geranium, in either its aroma or its uses.

It is greenish-yellow and slightly viscous at room temperature. It solidifies into a crystalline mass at temperatures only slightly below that, and is sometimes, mistakenly, described as a concrete. The major constituents are germacrol (about 50% of the whole), elemone and elemol, with tiny traces of a wide range of other constituents, which would account for its complex aroma. This is quite elusive, not easy to describe but very pleasing, predominantly woody but with herbal and floral notes. I find it slightly reminiscent of Clary Sage. The first impression is not powerful, but it is very long-lasting. In this respect, the oil can be compared to Sandalwood, and in fact santalene is one of the minor constituents.

The main use of Zdravetz oil has traditionally been in perfumery, where it is a very good fixative. In Bulgaria it is sometimes used to adulterate Rose oil, though I cannot imagine why as, to my nose at least, it bears no resemblance to Rose!

Not surprisingly, for an oil that has been mainly used in the perfume industry, it blends very well with a wide variety of other oils. It makes an intriguing blend with Bergamot, Petitgrain and in fact all the citrus oils, acting very much as a base note, also with Jasmine, Geranium and Lavender. Very small proportions of Zdravetz, maybe 1% of the total essential oil content (not counting any carrier or dilutant), are best – more than that tends to 'swamp' the other components.

Zdravetz oil is a relative newcomer to aromatherapy, so we do not have a long history of therapeutic use to draw on. However, the resemblance to Clary Sage and Sandalwood would certainly seem to confirm its traditional use as an aphrodisiac and it would be well-worth exploring its potential as an alternative to the established aphrodisiac oils. Its use in perfumery is another pointer in this direction, since the major aim of perfume has always been to enhance sexual attraction.

With time, we may well find other uses for Zdravetz, but for now it can be regarded as a valuable addition to our repertoire for helping clients with sexual problems.

Zinc

Our bodies need a certain amount of the mineral zinc (usually 10–15 mgs daily) for healthy bone growth, reproduction, healing of wounds and the health of the skin and nervous tissues. It is associated with the good functioning of the senses of taste and smell – so vital in aromatherapy. Zinc deficiency can lead to partial or complete loss of the sense of smell, which will return with adequate supplementation if this is the cause.

Many environmental and other factors in modern life destroy zinc, or impair our ability to utilise it in the body. These include car exhaust fumes, food refining, the contraceptive pill and other drugs, so many people have far less than the optimum level of zinc in their bodies. Good food sources are fish and shellfish, eggs, wholegrains, peas and yeast, but supplementation is probably necessary if there are symptoms of deficiency, such as loss of the sense of smell or taste, brittle nails or white spots or lines under the nails.

People with certain skin diseases often respond well to an increase in the amount of zinc in their diet. Psoriasis, which is a notoriously difficult condition to treat, is often helped by upwards of 15 mg of zinc a day, so you should bear this in mind when treating a psoriasis sufferer with aromatherapy.

Zinc is involved in the production of viable sperm, and deficiency has been connected with infertility in men.

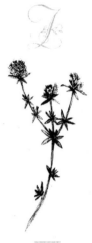

Zona

Zona, a Greek word meaning 'belt' or 'sash' is the more correct name of the painful and distressing condition usually referred to as shingles, and derives from the fact that the accompanying rash often appears in a band around the torso.

The condition is caused by the same virus as chickenpox, Herpes zoster, which can lie dormant in the body after an attack of chickenpox, and flare up many years later, usually in adult life, and most often when the person is stressed or physically run down.

The virus affects sensory nerves before they enter the spinal cord, and causes clusters of blisters on the area of skin served by the affected nerves. These can be very painful indeed, and the pain is usually felt before the blisters appear. It may be accompanied by fever for a few days, but this is not always so. After the blisters have disappeared, pain may persist, sometimes for many weeks or months with fatigue and general debility.

The essential oils of Bergamot, Eucalyptus and Ti-tree are very helpful in easing the pain and drying the blisters. These oils are analgesic, and have an antiviral action, and they seem to work better in combination than either of them alone. It is interesting to note that Bergamot is one of the finest antidepressant oils in the whole repertoire of the aromatherapist, and people who develop shingles are often tense, anxious or depressed before the attack. The pain of an attack is, in itself, cause of further depression, so this oil would be valuable if that were its only action. But the fact that it is also active against the herpes virus makes it doubly so.

If the area of blisters and pain is small, a 50/50 blend of Bergamot and Ti-tree can be applied neat. The best method and that which causes least pain, is to use a soft paintbrush to apply the oil. If a larger area is affected, you might either make a solution of the oils in alcohol, or use them to add to baths. A combination of painting the blistered and painful area several times a day, and an aromatic bath at night is probably the most effective.

Although the accepted orthodox view is that nothing can be done for shingles except to ease the symptoms, and that the attack cannot be shortened, my own experience is otherwise. I have treated or observed a number of cases where the use of Bergamot and Eucalyptus has reduced the length of time that the blisters persisted, and the amount and duration of pain, to considerably less than what is normally experienced or expected.

Where pain persists long after the blisters have disappeared, Lavender and Camomile oils can be alternated with, or substituted for Bergamot, Eucalyptus or Ti-tree, or a blend, such as Bergamot/Lavender can be used.

Zone Therapy

Zone Therapy is another name for Reflexology. It refers to the fact that different areas, or 'zones' on the feet correspond to different organs or areas of the body. For a fuller description, see **REFLEXOLOGY**.

APPENDIX A
Hazardous Essential Oils

OILS THAT SHOULD NOT BE
USED AT ALL IN AROMATHERAPY

These oils are generally considered too dangerous to be used in aromatherapy. They are all either narcotic, toxic, capable of causing a miscarriage, likely to provoke epileptic-type fits or can seriously damage the skin. Some of them present more than one of these hazards.

ALMOND, BITTER	*Prunus amygdalis, var. amara*
ANISEED	*Pimpinella anisum ·*
ARNICA	*Arnica montana*
BOLDO LEAF	*Peumus boldus*
CALAMUS	*Acorus calamus*
CAMPHOR	*Cinnamomum camphora*
CASSIA	*Cinnamomum cassia*
CINNAMON BARK	*Cinnamomum zeylanicum*
COSTUS	*Saussurea lappa*
ELECAMPANE	*Inula helenium*
FENNEL (BITTER)	*Foeniculum vulgare*
HORSERADISH	*Cochlearia armorica*
JABORANDI LEAF	*Pilocarpus jaborandi*
MUGWORT (ARMOISE)	*Artemisia vulgaris*
MUSTARD	*Brassica nigra*
ORIGANUM	*Origanum vulgare*
ORIGANUM (SPANISH)	*Thymus capitatus*
PENNYROYAL (EUROPEAN)	*Mentha pulegium*
PENNYROYAL (N. AMERICAN)	*Hedeoma pulegioides*
PINE (DWARF)	*Pinus pumilio*
RUE	*Ruta graveolens*
SAGE	*Salvia officinalis*
SASSAFRAS	*Sassafras albidum*
SASSAFRAS (BRAZILIAN)	*Ocotea cymbarum*
SAVIN	*Juniperus sabina*
SAVORY (SUMMER)	*Satureia hortensis*
SAVORY (WINTER)	*Satureia montana*
SOUTHERNWOOD	*Artemisia abrotanum*
TANSY	*Tanacetum vulgare*
THUJA (CEDARLEAF)	*Thuja occidentalis*
THUJA PLICATA	*Thuja plicata*
WINTERGREEN	*Gaultheria procumbens*
WORMSEED	*Chenopodium anthelminticum*
WORMWOOD	*Artemisia absinthium*

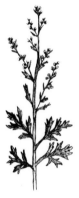

OILS THAT SHOULD ONLY BE
USED WITH CAUTION IN AROMATHERAPY

In addition to the above, there are a number of oils with valuable therapeutic properties, but which need to be carefully used with an understanding of possible undesirable effects. With the exception of Bergamot, which is safe as long as exposure to sunlight is avoided, it may be wiser for the general reader to avoid these oils, leaving them to the trained therapist.

OILS THAT SHOULD NOT
BE USED BY PEOPLE WITH EPILEPSY

FENNEL (SWEET)	*Foeniculum vulgare*
HYSSOP	*Hyssopus officinalis*
ROSEMARY	*Rosmarinus officinalis*

(Plus Sage and Wormwood which are on the 'not to be used at all' list.)

OILS THAT SHOULD NOT
BE USED DURING PREGNANCY

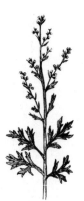

BASIL	*Ocimum basilicum*
BIRCH	*Betula alba, B. lenta, B.alleghaniensis*
CEDARWOOD	*Cedrus atlantica*
CLARY SAGE	*Salvia sclarea*
CYPRESS	*Cupressus sempervirens*
GERANIUM	*Pelargonium asperum*
HYSSOP	*Hyssopus officinalis*
JASMINE	*Jasminium officinale*
JUNIPER	*Juniperis communis*
MARJORAM	*Origanum majorana*
MYRRH	*Commiphora myrrha*
NUTMEG	*Myristica fragrans*
PEPPERMINT	*Mentha piperata*
ROSEMARY	*Rosmarinus officinalis*
TARRAGON	*Artemisia dranunculus*
THYME	*Thymus vulgaris*

OILS TO AVOID DURING THE
FIRST THREE MONTHS OF PREGNANCY

These oils should be avoided during the first three months of pregnancy, and used cautiously during the remaining months. Use in small amounts and well diluted (1% to 2% for massage: 3 to 4 drops added to a carrier oil for baths). If there is any previous history of miscarriage, do not use at all.

CAMOMILE	*Anthemis nobilis, et al.*
GERANIUM	*Pelargonium asperum*
LAVENDER	*Lavandula vera*
ROSE	*Rosa centifolia v damascena*

OILS WITH A RISK OF TOXICITY
OR CHRONIC TOXICITY

Use these oils with caution, and do not continue use for more than a few days at any one time.

BASIL	*Ocimum basilicum*
CEDARWOOD	*Cedrus atlantica*
CINNAMON LEAF	*Cinnamomum zeylanicum*
EUCALYPTUS	*Eucalyptus globulus*
FENNEL (SWEET)	*Foeniculum vulgare*
HYSSOP	*Hyssopus officinalis*
LEMON	*Citrus limonum*
ORANGE	*Citrus aurantium*
NUTMEG	*Myristica fragrans*
THYME	*Thymus vulgaris*

SKIN IRRITANTS AND SKIN SENSITISERS

Always dilute these oils to 1% before use.

ANGELICA	*Angelica archangelica*
BLACK PEPPER	*Piper nigrum*
CINNAMON LEAF	*Cinnamomum zeylanicum*
CITRONELLA	*Cymbopogon nardus*
CLOVE (ALL PARTS)	*Eugenia caryophyllus*
GINGER	*Zingiber officinalis*
LEMON	*Citrus limonum*
LEMONGRASS	*Cymbopogon citratus*
LEMON VERBENA	*Lippia citriodora*
ORANGE	*Citrus aurantium*
NUTMEG	*Myristica fragrans*
PEPPERMINT	*Mentha piperata*

PHOTOSENSITISING OILS

Do not use on the skin before exposure to the sun.

ANGELICA	*Angelica archangelica*
BERGAMOT	*Citrus bergamia*
LEMON	*Citrus limonum*
ORANGE	*Citrus aurantium*

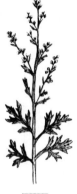

323

APPENDIX B
The Major Properties of Essential Oils

This list is by no means exhaustive. I have aimed to show the most important essential oils in general use for the properties listed.

ANALGESIC reduces pain: *Bergamot, Camomile, Lavender, Marjoram, Rosemary*

ANAPHRODISIAC reduces sexual response: *Marjoram*

ANTIBIOTIC combats infection within the body: *Cajeput, Garlic, Manuka, Niaouli, Ravensara, Ti-tree*

ANTIDEPRESSANT helps to lift the mood: *Bergamot, Clary Sage, Geranium, Grapefruit, Jasmine, Lavender, Mandarin, Melissa, Mimosa, Neroli, Orange, Petitgrain, Rose, Sandalwood, Ylang-Ylang*

ANTI-INFLAMMATORY reduces inflammation: *Bergamot, Camomile, Lavender, Myrrh*

ANTISEPTIC prevents or combats bacterial infection locally: *Bergamot, Eucalyptus, Juniper, Lavender, Manuka, Ravensara, Rosemary, Ti-tree* All essential oils are antiseptic to a greater or lesser degree.

ANTISPASMODIC prevents or relieves spasms (especially of the intestines and uterus): *Camomile, Cardamon, Clary Sage, Ginger, Marjoram, Orange*

ANTIVIRAL kills or inhibits the growth of viruses: *Bergamot, Eucalyptus, Garlic, Lavender, Manuka, Ravensara, Ti-tree*

APHRODISIAC increases sexual response: *Clary Sage, Jasmine, Neroli, Patchouli, Rose, Sandalwood, Vetivert*

ASTRINGENT tightens the tissues, reduces fluid loss: *Cedarwood, Cypress, Frankincense, Juniper, Myrrh, Rose, Sandalwood*

BACTERICIDE kills bacteria: *Bergamot, Cajeput, Eucalyptus, Juniper, Lavender, Manuka, Niaouli, Rosemary*

BECHIC eases coughing: *Lavender, Sandalwood, Thyme*

CEPHALIC clears the mind, stimulates mental activity: *Basil, Grapefruit, Rosemary, Thyme*

CHOLAGOGUE stimulates the flow of bile: *Camomile, Lavender, Peppermint, Rosemary*

CYTOPHYLACTIC a cell regenerator: *All essential oils, especially Lavender, Neroli and Ti-tree*

DEODORANT reduces odour: *Bergamot, Clary Sage, Cypress, Eucalyptus, Lavender, Litsea Cubeba, Neroli, Petitgrain*

DETOXIFYING helps cleanse the body of impurities: *Birch, Fennel, Garlic, Juniper, Rose*

DIURETIC increases production of urine: *Birch, Camomile, Cedarwood, Fennel, Geranium, Juniper*

EMMENAGOGUE encourages menstruation: *Basil, Camomile, Clary Sage, Fennel, Hyssop, Juniper, Marjoram, Myrrh, Peppermint, Rose, Rosemary, Sage*

EXPECTORANT helps expel phlegm: *Benzoin, Bergamot, Eucalyptus, Marjoram, Myrrh, Sandalwood*

FEBRIFUGE reduces fever: *Bergamot, Camomile, Eucalyptus, Melissa, Peppermint, Ravensara, Ti-tree*

FUNGICIDAL kills or inhibits growth of yeasts, moulds, etc.: *Lavender, Myrrh, Ti-Tree*

HEPATIC strengthens the liver: *Camomile, Cypress, Lemon, Peppermint, Rosemary, Thyme*

HYPERTENSIVE raises blood pressure: *Clary Sage, Hyssop, Rosemary*

HYPOTENSIVE lowers blood pressure: *Lavender, Marjoram, Melissa, Ylang-Ylang*

IMMUNO strengthens the body's defensive stimulant reaction to infection: *Garlic, Lavender, Manuka, Ravensara, Rosewood, Ti-tree*

MUCOLYTIC breaks down catarrh: *Myrrh, Ravensara*

NERVINE strengthens the nervous system: *Camomile, Lavender, Marjoram, Melissa, Rosemary*

RUBEFACIENT produces local warmth and redness when applied to the skin: *Birch, Black Pepper, Eucalyptus, Juniper, Marjoram, Pimento, Rosemary*

SEDATIVE calms the nervous system: *Benzoin, Bergamot, Camomile, Clary Sage, Frankincense, Lavender, Marjoram, Melissa, Neroli, Rose, Ylang-Ylang*

STIMULANT increases activity of the body generally, or of a specific organ: *Basil, Black Pepper, Eucalyptus, Geranium, Peppermint, Rosemary*

SUDORIFIC promotes sweating: *Basil, Camomile, Juniper, Manuka, Peppermint, Ravensara, Ti-tree*

TONIC strengthens the body generally or a specific organ: *Basil, Birch, Black Pepper, Frankincense, Geranium, Juniper, Lavender, Marjoram, Myrrh, Neroli, Rose, Ti-tree*

UTERINE has a tonic action on the womb: *Clary Sage, Jasmine, Rose*

VASOCONSTRICTOR causes small blood vessels to contract: *Camomile, Cypress, Rose*

VASODILATOR causes small blood vessels to expand: *Marjoram*

VULNERARY helps wounds to heal: *Benzoin, Bergamot, Camomile, Lavender, Myrrh, Ti-tree*

325

APPENDIX C
Recipes and Formulae

1. BATHS

A REFRESHING MORNING BATH

ROSEMARY	4 drops
PETITGRAIN	2 drops

or

ROSEMARY	3 drops
GRAPEFRUIT	3 drops

(Either of these would also be good in the early evening, after a day's work, as a 'reviver' before the evening's activities.)

A morning bath to counteract excessive fatigue:

ROSEMARY	3 drops
PINE	2 drops
THYME	1 drop

or

ROSEMARY	2 drops
THYME	2 drops
GRAPEFRUIT	2 drops

A BATH TO RELIEVE OVERWORKED MUSCLES

LAVENDER	3 drops
MARJORAM	2 drops
JUNIPER	1 drops

(for evening use)

or

ROSEMARY	3 drops
MARJORAM	2 drops
PINE	1 drop

(for morning use)

BATHS TO AID RELAXATION AND PROMOTE SLEEP

LAVENDER	4 drops
PETITGRAIN	2 drops

or

LAVENDER	3 drops
MARJORAM	3 drops

or

NEROLI	3 drops
PETITGRAIN	3 drops

or

CAMOMILE	4 drops
LAVENDER	2 drops

or

LAVENDER	3 drops
FRANKINCENSE	3 drops

or

LAVENDER	3 drops
CLARY SAGE	3 drops

(All these are also recommended to relieve anxiety and stress generally.)

BATHS TO HELP WITH SYMPTOMS OF COLDS, 'FLU AND OTHER VIRAL INFECTIONS

LAVENDER	3 drops
MANUKA	2 drops
RAVENSARA	1 drop

(for evening use)

or

RAVENSARA	2 drops
ROSEMARY	2 drops
TI-TREE	2 drops

(for morning use)

USE THESE BATHS PARTICULARLY AT THE ONSET OF A COLD, ETC.

LAVENDER	3 drops
THYME	2 drops
TI-TREE	1 drop
(if the throat is sore)	

or

LAVENDER	2 drops
FRANKINCENSE	2 drops
SANDALWOOD	2 drops
(if there is a cough)	

DETOXIFYING BATHS

JUNIPER	3 drops
GRAPEFRUIT	2 drops
LAVENDER	1 drop
(for evening use)	

or

GERANIUM	3 drops
ROSEMARY	2 drops
JUNIPER	1 drop
(for morning use)	

APHRODISIAC BATHS

SANDALWOOD	5 drops
BLACK PEPPER	1 drop

or

JASMINE	5 drops
PIMENTO	1 drop

or

ROSE	4 drops
NEROLI	2 drops

or

YLANG-YLANG	3 drops
NEROLI	2 drops
VETIVERT	1 drop

All these blends and quantities are intended for a full bath for an adult.

The essential oils can be used neat or mixed in a carrier before adding to the water.

For children between about 5 and 12 years, use 3 to 4 drops of essential oil and always mix in a carrier before adding to the bath.

Any of the above blends could also be used as a massage oil, by adding the 6 drops to 10 mls of carrier oil.

BABIES' BATHS

CAMOMILE	1 drop
LAVENDER	1 drop
dissolved in 5 mls soya oil	
(a soothing bath)	

or

MANDARIN	1 drop
HELICHRYSUM	1 drop
dissolved in 5 mls soya oil	
(refreshing and good for baby's skin)	

Always mix the essential oils in the carrier before adding to the bath.

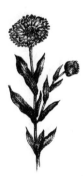

327

2. SOME SIMPLE CREAMS

GALEN'S COLD CREAM

40 grams almond oil
10 grams beeswax
40 grams rosewater
10 drops Rose absolute

This makes a firm cream which liquefies almost immediately on contact
with the skin. It can be used as a cleansing cream, handcream or as an
alternative to oil for certain types of massage. You could substitute
orange-flower water or any appropriate hydrolat for the rosewater, and
any essential oils suitable for your purpose instead of the Rose.

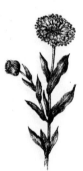

COCONUT OIL CREAM

50 grams coconut oil
20 grams almond oil
25 grams rosewater (or orange-flower water, etc.)
20 drops essential oil(s) of your choice

This is a richer cream. Valuable for dry skin and after sunbathing.

COCOA BUTTER CREAM

50 grams infused Calendula oil
35 grams cocoa butter
10 grams beeswax
45 grams flower hydrolat
10 drops Lavender oil
10 drops Myrrh
5 drops Lemon (or a total of 25 drops of any oils you choose)

This is the richest of the three creams. It is very good for dry, cracked or
chapped skin, as a handcream for people who work outdoors or in any
job that is damaging to their hands, for cracks in the heels, etc.

Method

The method is the same for all three creams.

Weigh all ingredients accurately. (Shred beeswax with a very sharp knife before weighing.) Put the almond and/or other oils in a bowl which should be either stainless steel or Pyrex, and add the beeswax, if used. Put the flower-water in another bowl and stand both bowls in a large shallow pan of water over a gentle heat. Stir the bowl containing the oil(s) and beeswax until all the ingredients are melted, then remove from heat.

Start adding the flower-water to the oil mixture, a drop or two at a time while beating with a rotary whisk. Continue to add the flower-water very gradually, beating all the time, as if making a mayonnaise.

When all the flower-water has been absorbed into the oil/wax mixture, stop beating at once. If using an electric mixer, set it on the lowest speed, as over-beating can make the cream separate.

Finally, stir in the essential oil and put into a jar or jars. Leave in a cool place or fridge until set. Alternatively, divide the cream into several small jars before adding the essential oil, in which case you can use a variety of different oils in different jars.

These amounts make a relatively small amount of cream. Once you have mastered the technique, you can double or treble the quantities to make larger batches. The creams will keep for quite a long time, as the essential oils act as natural preservatives, but if making large batches, keep in the fridge until needed and then dispense small amounts into individual jars.

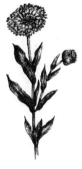

329

3. TONERS and AFTERSHAVES

FOR OILY SKIN

250 mls orange-flower water   *or*   200 mls orange-flower water
15 mls vodka   100 mls witch hazel
3 drops Grapefruit   3 drops Grapefruit
3 drops Lavender   3 drops Geranium
     2 drops Manuka
(this one is best for very oily
skins and for acne)

FOR SENSITIVE OR ALLERGIC SKIN

250 mls distilled water
10 mls vodka
4 drops German Camomile

FOR DRY SKIN

250 mls rosewater
10 mls vodka
4 drops Rose absolute
2 drops Frankincense

FOR NORMAL SKIN

250 mls rosewater
15 mls vodka
3 drops Palmarosa
3 drops Rose

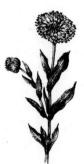

AFTERSHAVE

250 mls orange-flower water
25 mls vodka
6 drops Sandalwood, or other essential oil

This is a good aftershave for men with sensitive skins, including teenage boys who have only recently begun to shave. Sandalwood is a bactericide and helps to control and prevent barber's rash. Experiment with other essential oils such as Cedarwood, Cypress, Grapefruit and Vetivert.

Method

Put the vodka into a clean, dry bottle, add the essential oils and shake until dissolved. If using witch hazel, add this next, and shake again. Add the floral water or hydrolat last and shake well. Shake well before using each time. Use the highest proof vodka you can obtain.

4. MOUTHWASHES

250 mls cheap brandy	*or*	250 mls cheap brandy
30 drops Peppermint		50 drops Ti-tree
20 drops Thyme		30 drops Grapefruit
10 drops Myrrh		(for use if there are mouth
10 drops Fennel		ulcers or gum infection)

Method

Put the brandy in a clean, dry bottle, add all the essential oils and shake well. To use, shake well and add 2 or 3 teaspoons to half a tumbler of warm water.

APPENDIX D
Useful Addresses

PROFESSIONAL ORGANISATIONS

All these organsations can supply details of qualified therapists. Some make a small charge for this. Most will also be able to provide details of training courses for would-be therapists. Please send a large s.a.e. with all enquiries.

International Federation of Aromatherapists
61–63 Churchfield Road
London, W3 6AY
Telephone: 020 8992 9605
www.ifaroma.org

Aromatherapy Consortium
P.O. Box 6522
Desborough
Kettering
Northants, NN14 2YX
Telephone: 0870 774 3477

American Aromatherapy Association
P.O. Box 3679
South Pasadena, CA 91031
Telephone: (818) 457 1742

National Association for Holistic Aromatherapy
3327 W. Indian Trail Road PMB 144
Spokane, WA 99208
Telephone: (509) 325 3419
www.naha.org

British Herbal Medicine Association
1 Wickham Road
Boscombe
Bournemouth
Dorset, BH7 6JX
Telephone: 01202 433691
www.bhma.info

National Institute of Medical Herbalists
Elm House
54 Mary Arches Street
Exeter, EX4 3BA
Telephone: 01392 426022
www.nimh.org.uk

British College of Naturopathy and Osteopathy
Lief House
3 Sumpter Close
120–122 Finchley Road
London, NW3 5HR
Telephone: 020 7435 6464

British Chiropractic Association
59 Castle Street
Reading
Berkshire, RG1 7SN
Telephone: 0118 950 5950
www.chiropractic-uk.co.uk

British Homeopathic Association
Hahnemann House
29 Park Street West
Luton, LU1 3BE
Telephone: 0870 444 3950
www.trusthomeopathy.org

National Federation of Spiritual Healers
Old Manor Farm, Studio
Church Street
Sunbury on Thames
Middlesex, TW16 6RG
Telephone: 01932 783164
www.nfsh.org.uk

British Reflexology Association
Monks Orchard
Whitbourne
Worcester, WR6 5RB
Telephone: 01886 821207
www.britreflex.co.uk

GENERAL ORGANISATIONS

British Holistic Medical Association
PO Box 371
Bridgwater
Somerset, TA6 9BG
Telephone: 01278 722000
www.bhma.org

Has medical, non-medical and lay members. Conferences, lectures, etc.

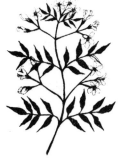

331

Institute for Complementary Medicine

P.O. Box 194
London, SE16 7QZ
Telephone: 020 7237 5165
www.i-c-m.org.uk

Information on all branches of
alternative medicine.

SPECIALIST ORGANISATIONS

Association for New Approaches to Cancer (ANAC)

PO Box 194
Chertsey
Surrey, KT16 0WJ
Telephone: 01372 471 017
www.newapproaches.co.uk

Penny Brohn Cancer Care

Chapel Pill Lane
Pill
Bristol, BS20 0HH
Telephone: 01275 370 100
www.pennybrohncancercare.org

Institute of Optiumum Nutrition

Aralon House
72 Lower Mortlake Road
Surrey, TW9 2JY
Telephone: 020 8614 7800
www.ion.ac.uk

S.A.D. Association

PO Box 989
Steyning
W. Sussex, BN44 3HG
Telephone: 01903 814942
www.sada.org.uk

Women's Nutritional Advisory Service

PO Box 268
Lewes
E. Sussex, BN7 2QN
Telephone: 01273 487366
www.naturalhealthas.com

Some of the above are voluntary
organisations and others are professional
services charging fees. Please send s.a.e.
with all enquiries.

TUITION

London School of Aromatherapy (L.S.A. North)

P.O. Box 11850,
Turriff
Aberdeen, AB53 8YA
Freephone: 0800 716 847

Aromatherapy courses designed by the
author. Send s.a.e. for details of training
in London, other areas of the UK and
overseas.

Clare Maxwell-Hudson

Lower Ground Floor
20 Enford Street
London, W1H 1DG
Telephone: 020 7724 7198
(Massage tuition)
www.cmhmassage.co.uk

California School of Herbal Studies

PO Box 39
Forestville
CA 95436, USA
Telephone: (707) 887-7457
www.cshs.com

SUPPLIERS OF MATERIALS AND EQUIPMENT

Fragrant Earth

Orchard Court
Magdalen Street
Glastonbury
Somerset, BA6 9EW
Telephone: 01458 831216
Fax: 01458 831361
www.fragrant-earth.co.uk

High quality organic essential oils,
hydrolats, vegetable oils, etc., and
aromatherapy charts and posters
designed by Patricia Davis.

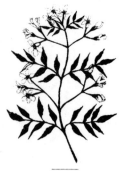

Norman and Germaine Rich
2 Coval Gardens
London, SW14 7DG
Telephone: 020 8878 2976

High quality essential oils, some organic,
carrier oils, etc.

Absolute Essentials
P.O. Box 82
Hereford, HR4 0ZE
Telephone: 0800 716847
E-mail: absolutessential@aol.com

Organic and wild-grown essential oils.
Mail-order to UK and most countries.

Aroma Vera, Inc.
5310 Beethoven Street
Los Angeles
CA 90016, USA
Telephone: (1 800) 669-9514
www.aromavera.com

Leydet Aromatics
PO Box 2354
Fair Oaks
CA 95628, USA
Telephone: (916) 965-7546
www.leydet.com

Marshcouch
14 Robinsfield
Hemel Hempstead
Herts, HP1 1RW
Telephone: 01442 263199
www.marshcouch.com

Folding massage tables, multi-height
tables and accessories.

SPECIALIST
PUBLICATIONS

International Journal of Aromatherapy
Elsevier Limited
Linacre House
Jordan Hill
Oxford, OX2 8DP
Telephone: 01865 474000

In Essence
IFPA
82 Ashby Road
Hinckley
Leics, LE10 1SN
Telephone: 01455 637987
www.ifparoma.org

The Aromatic Thymes
18–4 East Dundee Road
Suite 200
Barrington, IL 60010
USA
Telephone: (847) 304 0975

NAHA Aromatherapy Journal
National Association for Holistic
Aromatherapy
3327 W. Indian Trail Road PMB 144
Spokane, WA 99208
Telephone: (509) 325 3419
www.naha.org

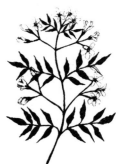

APPENDIX E
Further Reading

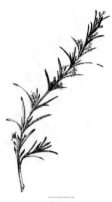

BOOKS ABOUT AROMATHERAPY

THE ART OF AROMATHERAPY *Robert Tisserand* C.W. Daniel Co. Ltd.

THE PRACTICE OF AROMATHERAPY *Jean Valnet* C.W. Daniel Co. Ltd.

MARGUERITE MAURY'S GUIDE TO AROMATHERAPY *Marguerite Maury* C.W. Daniel Co. Ltd.

GATTEFOSSÉ'S AROMATHERAPY *R.M. Gattefossé* C.W. Daniel Co. Ltd.

AROMATHERAPY FOR WOMEN AND CHILDREN *Jane Dye* C.W. Daniel Co. Ltd.

SUBTLE AROMATHERAPY *Patricia Davis* C.W. Daniel Co. Ltd.

THE ENCYCLOPAEDIA OF ESSENTIAL OILS *Julia Lawless* Element

AROMANTICS *Valerie Worwood* Pan Books

BOOKS ABOUT HERBAL MEDICINE

KITTY CAMPION'S BOOK OF HERBAL HEALTH *Kitty Campion* Sphere Books Ltd.

THE LIVING HERBALIST *Jill Davies* Elm Tree Books

THE NEW HOLISTIC HERBAL *David Hoffman* Element

THE COMPLETE BOOK OF HERBS *Lesley Bremness* Dorling-Kindersley

There are many other excellent books on plant medicine, but these four are written with the home user, rather than the professional herbalist, in mind.

BOOKS ABOUT MASSAGE

MASSAGE FOR HEALING AND RELAXATION *Carola Beresford Cooke* Arlington Books

THE MASSAGE BOOK *George Downing* Penguin

THE COMPLETE BOOK OF MASSAGE *Clare Maxwell Hudson* Dorling-Kindersley

These books give excellent and clear instructions for a simple massage, though personal tuition is strongly advised.

GENERAL

GREEN PHARMACY *Barbara Griggs* Jill Norman & Hobhouse

YOUR HEALTH AND BEAUTY BOOK *Clare Maxwell Hudson* Macdonald

HOLISTIC LIVING *Patrick Pietroni* J.M. Dent & Sons

BIBLIOGRAPHY

Bardeaux, Fabrice La Medicine Aromatique 1976

La Pharmacie du Bon Dieu 1973

Bernadet, Marcel La Phyto-Aromathérapie Pratique 1983

Culpeper, Nicolas The English Physician 1652

Edwards, Victoria Common Scents, Vol 1,No.2 1989

Gerard, John The Historie of Plants 1597

Grieve, Mrs. M. A Modern Herbal 1931

Griggs, Barbara Green Pharmacy 1981

Hoffman, David The Holistic Herbal 1983

Kenton, Lesley Ageless Aging 1984

Lawless, Julia The Encyclopaedia of Essential Oils 1992

Masson, Robert Folies et Sagesses de la Medicine Naturelle 1972

Maury, Marguerite Le Capital Jeunesse 1961

Sibe, Dominique 70 Huiles Essentielles 1982

Tisserand, Robert The Art of Aromatherapy 1977

The Essential Oil Safety Data Manual 1985

Valnet, Jean Aromathérapie 1964

Phytothérapie 1972

Worwood, Valerie Aromantics 1987

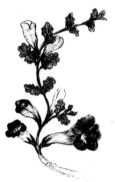

335